The Healing Power of Foods

Nutrition Secrets for Vibrant Health and Long Life

Michael T. Murray, **N.D.**

Prima Publishing
P.O. Box 1260BK
Rocklin, CA 95677
(916) 632-4400

Library of Congress Cataloging-in-Publication Data

Murray, Michael T.
The healing power of foods: nutrition secrets for vibrant health and long life / Michael T. Murray.
p. cm.
Includes bibliographical references and index.
ISBN 1-55958-317-7 :
1. Nutrition. I. Title.
RA784.M844 1993
613.2—dc20 93–16251
CIP

96 97 98 99 AA 10 9 8 7 6 5 4

Printed in the United States of America

How to Order:
Quantity discounts are available from Prima Publishing, P.O. Box 1260BK, Rocklin, CA 95677; telephone: (916) 632-4400. On your letterhead include information concerning the intended use of the books and the number of books you wish to purchase.

To Terry Lemerond, president of Enzymatic Therapy, for his tremendous commitment to integrity and quality. The positive impact that Terry has made on my life and on the lives of so many other people he has touched is immeasurable. Thank you, Terry.

Contents

Preface

"Let your food be your medicine and let your medicine be your food."
—Hippocrates

There is an ever growing appreciation of the role of diet in determining our level of health. It is now well established that certain dietary practices cause—and certain others prevent—a wide range of diseases. In addition, more and more research indicates that certain diets and foods offer immediate therapeutic benefit.

As people learn more about the value of proper nutrition, they often become confused. There seem to be many different opinions on nutrition. The purpose of this book is to provide answers to some fairly simple questions:

What is a healthy diet?
How do I know what to eat and in what quantities?
How much protein, fiber, and other food factors do I need in my diet?
What properties do individual foods possess?
If foods are medicines, what foods offer the greatest benefit for specific health problems?

My desire over the past 15 years to answer these questions for myself has led me to incredible discoveries. My goal in writing this book was two-fold. First, I wanted to provide the latest information on what is known about the role of food and health. Second, and more important, I wanted this information to inspire readers to make more healthful food choices. I believe that such choices will result in a healthier and happier existence.

The quality of one's life is directly related to the quality of the foods one routinely ingests. The human body is the most remarkable machine in the world, but most Americans are not feeding their body the high-quality fuel it deserves. If a machine does not receive proper fuel or maintenance, how long can it be expected to run in an efficient manner? If your body is not fed the full range of nutrients it needs, how can it be expected to remain in a state of good health?

Your body, the vessel of your soul, is something to cherish. Treat it as your most prized possession. Ralph Waldo Emerson said, "The first wealth is health." I agree with this and I urge you to make health a habit. Make a commitment to leading a healthy life and eating a healthful diet. "But what is a healthful diet?" you ask. That, my friend, is what I hope to describe to you in *The Healing Power of Foods*.

Live, in Good Health, with Passion and Joy!

Michael T. Murray, N.D.

Acknowledgments

Since this book represents a great deal of what is currently known about the role of diet in determining health, numerous people need to be acknowledged. Foremost, perhaps, are the researchers, physicians, and scientists who over the years have strived to understand human nutrition better. While my work has simply consisted of compiling information, their role has been to create it. The evolution in understanding about human nutrition and medicine is largely a result of long, hard hours of study and research by individuals who never experience the public spotlight. Without their work, this book would not exist.

I would also like to thank everyone at Prima, especially Ben Dominitz and Jennifer Basye; everyone at Trillium Health Products, especially Steve, Rick, Bob, and the staff nutritionists (Brenda, Barbara, Kristin, and Daniella); Melanie Field at Bookman Productions; and Steven Gray for his excellent copyediting.

This book was truly a team effort, and my most important teammate was my wife, Gina. Her love, support, and patience are the major blessings in my life. I have also been blessed with truly wonderful parents (Cliff and Patty Murray), parents-in-law (Robert and Kathy Bunton), and friends. Special friends whom I would like to acknowledge for their support over the years are Terry Lemerond, Dr. Joseph Pizzorno, John Weeks, and Greg Ris.

And finally, I would like to thank you, the reader, for granting me the opportunity to share with you—*The Healing Power of Foods.*

PART I

The Healing Power of Foods

1

The Healthful Diet

In order to know what a healthful diet is, we must first take a look at what our body is designed for. Is the human body designed to eat plant foods, animal foods, or both? Respectively, are we herbivores, carnivores, or omnivores? Based on detailed anatomical and historical evidence, researchers believe that humans evolved as "hunter-gatherers"; that is, humans appear to be omnivores capable of surviving on both gathered (plant) and hunted (animal) foods.[1]

But, while the human gastrointestinal tract is capable of digesting both animal and plant foods, certain physiological features indicate that the human body can accommodate plant foods much more easily than the harder-to-digest animal foods.[2] Specifically, our teeth consist of 20 premolars and molars that are perfect for crushing and grinding plant foods, and eight front incisors that are well-suited for biting into fruits and vegetables. Only our front four canine teeth are designed exclusively for meat eating. Our jaws swing both vertically to tear and laterally to crush, while carnivores' jaws only swing vertically. Additional evidence to support the body's preference for plant foods is the long length of the human intestinal tract. Carnivores typically have a short bowel while herbivores have a bowel length comparable to that of humans. Thus, the human bowel length favors plant foods.

For further insight into what humans should eat, many researchers look to other primates, such as chimpanzees, monkeys, and gorillas. Nonhuman primates are also omnivores (or as often described, herbivores and opportunistic carnivores). They eat mainly fruits and vegetables but may also eat small animals, lizards, and eggs if given the opportunity. In a study of 21 primates, researchers found that, in general, the percentage of animal food consumption is inversely proportional to body weight. The smaller primates eat more animal foods, as a percentage of overall caloric intake, while the larger primates eat far less animal foods. The gorilla and the orangutan eat only 1 percent and 2 percent, respectively, animal foods as a percentage of total calories. The remainder of their diet comes from plant foods. Since average human weight falls between the weights of the gorilla and of the orangutan, it has been suggested that humans should eat around 1.5 percent of their calories from animal foods.[3] Most Americans derive well over 50 percent of their calories from animal foods.

The meat that our ancestors consumed differed considerably from the meat we find in the supermarkets today. Domesticated animals have always had higher fat levels than their wild counterparts, but people's desire for tender meat has led to the breeding of cattle whose meat has a fat content of 25 to 30 percent (or higher), compared to a fat content of less than 4 percent for free-ranging animals or wild game. In addition, the type of fat is considerably different. Domestic beef consists primarily of saturated fats, with virtually undetectable amounts of omega-3 fatty acids. In contrast, the fat of wild animals contains over five times more polyunsaturated fat per gram and has significant amounts of beneficial omega-3 fatty acids (approximately 4 percent).[4]

What does all this mean? Basically it means that humans are physiologically best suited to a diet composed primarily of plant foods. This contention is supported not only by the preceding information but by the tremendous volume of evidence showing that deviating from a predominantly plant-based diet is a major factor in the high Western incidence of heart disease, cancer, stroke, arthritis, and many other chronic degenerative diseases. Many health and medical organizations now recommend that the human diet should focus primarily on plant-based foods—vegetables, fruits, grains, legumes, nuts, seeds, and so on. Such a diet is thought to offer significant protection against the development of chronic degenerative disease.[5]

The Role of Diet in Chronic Degenerative Disease

The evidence supporting diet's role in chronic degenerative diseases is substantial. Two basic facts support this link:

1. A diet rich in plant foods (whole grains, legumes, fruits, and vegetables) protects against many diseases that are extremely common in Western society.
2. A diet that provides a low intake of plant foods contributes to the development of these diseases and provides conditions under which other causative factors become more active.[6]

Much of the link between diet and chronic disease was first established in the work of two medical pioneers, Denis Burkitt, M.D., and Hugh Trowell, M.D., authors of *Western Diseases: Their Emergence and Prevention,* which was first published in 1981. The work of Burkitt and Trowell actually represents a continuation of the landmark work of Weston A. Price, a dentist and author of *Nutrition and Physical Degeneration.*[7] In the early 1900s, Dr. Price traveled the world, observing changes in teeth and palate (orthodontic) structure as various cultures discarded traditional dietary practices in favor of a more "civilized" diet. Price was able to follow individuals as well as cultures over periods of 20 to 40 years, and he carefully documented the onset of degenerative diseases as their diets changed. Based on extensive studies examining the rate of diseases in various populations (epidemiological data) and his own observations of "primitive" cultures, Burkitt formulated the following sequence of events:

- FIRST STAGE: The primal diet of plant eaters contains large amounts of unprocessed starch staples; there are few examples of such chronic degenerative diseases as osteoarthritis, heart disease, diabetes, and cancer.
- SECOND STAGE: Commencing Westernization of diet, obesity and diabetes commonly appear in privileged groups.
- THIRD STAGE: With moderate Westernization of the diet, constipation, hemorrhoids, varicose veins, and appendicitis become common complaints.
- FOURTH STAGE: Finally, with full Westernization of the diet, chronic degenerative diseases such as osteoarthritis, rheumatoid arthritis, gout, heart disease, and cancer become extremely common.

Population studies, as well as clinical and experimental data, have linked the so-called "Western diet" to a number of now common diseases. In 1984, the National Research Council's Food and Nutrition Board established the Committee on Diet and Health to undertake a comprehensive analysis of diet and major chronic diseases.[8] The Food and Nutrition Board develops the Recommended Dietary Allowance guidelines, which specify the desirable amounts of essential nutrients in the diet. Their findings, as well as those of the U.S. Surgeon General and other highly respected medical groups, have underscored the need for Americans to change their eating habits to reduce their risk for chronic disease. Table 1.1 lists diseases that have been linked convincingly with a diet low in plant foods. Many of these now common diseases were extremely rare before the twentieth century.

Table 1.1 Diseases Highly Associated with a Diet Low in Plant Foods

Disease Category	*Specific Ailment*
Metabolic	obesity, gout, diabetes, kidney stones, gall stones
Cardiovascular	heart disease, high blood pressure, strokes, varicose veins, deep-vein thrombosis, pulmonary embolism
Colonic	constipation, appendicitis, diverticulitis, diverticulosis, hemorrhoids, colon cancer, irritable bowel syndrome, ulcerative colitis, Crohn's disease
Other	dental caries, autoimmune disorders, pernicious anemia, multiple sclerosis, thyrotoxicosis, various skin conditions

Trends in U.S. Food Consumption

During this century, food consumption patterns have changed dramatically. Figure 1.1 compares the percentage of calories in the average American diet from protein, carbohydrate, and fat during the period from 1909 to 1985. Total dietary fat intake has increased from 32 percent of all calories

Figure 1.1 Changes in fat, protein, and carbohydrate consumption from 1909 to 1985.

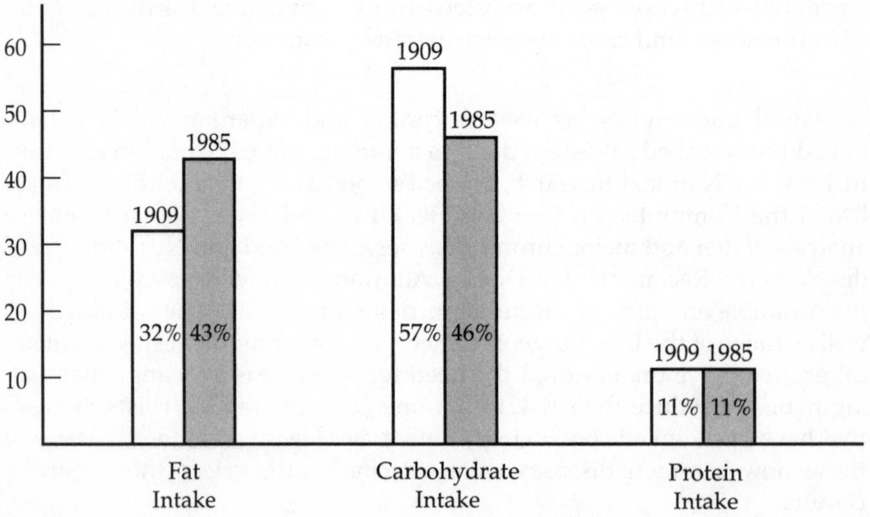

in 1909 to 43 percent in 1985. Meanwhile, overall carbohydrate intake has dropped from 57 percent to 46 percent. Protein intake has remained fairly stable at about 11 percent.[9]

Compounding these detrimental changes are the individual food choices that account for them (see Table 1.2). Dramatic increases in the consumption of meat, fats and oils, and sugars and sweeteners have occurred in conjunction with markedly decreased consumption of noncitrus fruits, vegetables, potatoes, and grain products. As a result, the percentage of dietary calories from starches or complex carbohydrates, as found naturally occurring in grains and vegetables, has dropped from 68 percent in 1909 to 47 percent in 1980. Currently, more than half of all carbohydrates the average American consumes are in the form of sugars (sucrose, corn syrup, and the like) added to foods as sweetening agents. High consumption of refined sugars has been linked to many chronic diseases, including obesity, diabetes, heart disease, and cancer.

The Government and Nutrition Education

Throughout the years, various governmental organizations have published dietary guidelines, but the recommendations of the United States Department of Agriculture (USDA) have become the most widely known. In 1956, the USDA published "Food for Fitness—A Daily Food Guide." This became popularly known as the Basic Four Food Groups. The Basic Four categorized foods as follows:

1. The Milk Group—milk, cheese, ice cream, and other milk-based foods
2. The Meat Group—meat, fish, poultry, and eggs, with dried legumes and nuts as alternatives
3. The Fruit and Vegetable Group
4. The Bread and Cereal Group

One major problem with the Basic Four Food Groups model is that it graphically suggests that the food groups are equal in health value. The result has been overconsumption of animal products, dietary fat, and refined carbohydrates, and insufficient consumption of fiber-rich foods such as fruits, vegetables, and legumes. This in turn has caused diet to be responsible for many premature deaths, chronic diseases, and increased health-care costs. According to the U.S. Surgeon General's 1988 Report on

Table 1.2 Trends in Quantities of Foods Consumed per Capita

	Lb/Year		
Foods	*1909–1913*	*1967–1969*	*1985*
Meat, poultry, and fish			
Beef	54	81	79
Pork	62	61	62
Poultry	18	46	70
Fish	12	15	19
Total	171	221	224
Eggs	37	40	32
Dairy products			
Whole milk	223	232	122
Low-fat milk	64	44	112
Cheese	5	15	26
Other	28	100	86
Total	339	440	450
Fats and oils			
Butter	18	6	5
Margarine	1	10	11
Shortening	8	16	23
Lard and beef tallow	12	5	4
Salad and cooking oil	2	16	25
Total	41	54	67
Fruits			
Citrus	17	60	72
Noncitrus			
Fresh	154	73	87
Processed	8	35	34
Total	179	168	193

SOURCE: National Research Council, *Diet and Health: Implications for Reducing Chronic Disease Risk* (Washington, D.C.: National Academy Press, 1989).

Nutrition and Health, diet-related diseases account for 68 percent of all deaths in this country (see Table 1.3).

As the Basic Four Food Groups became outdated, various other governmental and medical organizations developed guidelines of their own designed either to reduce the incidence of chronic degenerative disease (like cancer or heart disease) or to reduce the public's risk for all chronic diseases. The recommendations of the U.S. Surgeon General, the U.S. Senate, the U.S. Department of Health and Human Services, the American Heart Association, the National Cancer Institute, the American Diabetes

Foods	*Lb/Year* 1909–1913	1967–1969	1985
Vegetables			
Tomatoes	46	36	38
Dark green and yellow	34	25	31
Other			
Fresh	136	87	96
Processed	11	35	29
Total	227	183	194
Potatoes, white			
Fresh	182	67	55
Processed	0	15	28
Total	182	82	83
Dry beans, peas, nuts, and soybeans	16	16	18
Grain products			
Wheat products	216	116	122
Corn products	56	15	7
Other grains	19	13	26
Total	291	144	155
Sugar and sweeteners			
Refined sugar	77	100	63
Syrups and other sweeteners	14	22	90
Total	91	122	153
Miscellaneous	10	17	14

Association, and the National Research Council's Committee on Diet and Health are remarkably similar. Tables 1.4 on page 12 and 1.5 on page 14 identify the most prominent common features. We may summarize these as follows:

1. Reduce total fat intake to 30 percent or less of total calories; reduce saturated fatty acid intake to less than 10 percent of total calories; and reduce cholesterol intake to less than 300 mg daily.
2. Eat five or more servings of a combination of vegetables and fruits, especially green and yellow vegetables and citrus fruits.

Table 1.3 Top Ten Causes of Death in the United States in 1987

Rank	*Cause of Death*	*Number*	*% of Total Deaths*
1	**Heart diseases**	**759,400**	**35.7**
2	**Cancers**	**476,700**	**22.4**
3	**Strokes**	**148,700**	**7.0**
4	Unintentional injuries	92,500	4.4
5	Chronic obstructive lung disease	78,000	3.7
6	Pneumonia & influenza	68,600	3.2
7	**Diabetes mellitus**	**37,800**	**1.8**
8	Suicide	29,600	1.4
9	Chronic liver disease & cirrhosis	26,000	1.2
10	**Atherosclerosis**	**23,1000**	**1.1**
	All Causes	2,125,100	100.0

Causes of death in which diet plays a part are in bold.

SOURCE: From the Surgeon General's Report on Nutrition and Health, National Center for Health Statistics, *Monthly Vital Statistics Report*, vol. 37, no. 1 (April 25, 1988).

3. Increase intake of fiber and complex carbohydrates by eating six or more servings per day of a combination of breads, cereals, and legumes.
4. Maintain protein intake at moderate levels.
5. Balance food intake and physical activity to maintain appropriate body weight.
6. Limit intake of alcohol, refined carbohydrates (sugar), and salt (sodium chloride).

The USDA's Eating Right Pyramid

In an attempt to create a new model for nutrition education, the USDA developed the "Eating Right Pyramid." On April 24, 1991, after 3 years of development, the completed pyramid was submitted to USDA Secretary Edward R. Madigan for publication. The very next day, Madigan appeared to succumb to pressure from the meat and dairy industries and from food manufacturers when he delayed the chart's publication. One year and $1 million later, the USDA finally approved the pyramid (see Figure 1.2).

The pyramid has not changed the Basic Four's categories of food groups per se; instead it visually stresses the importance of making fresh

Figure 1.2 The Eating Right Pyramid of Foods.

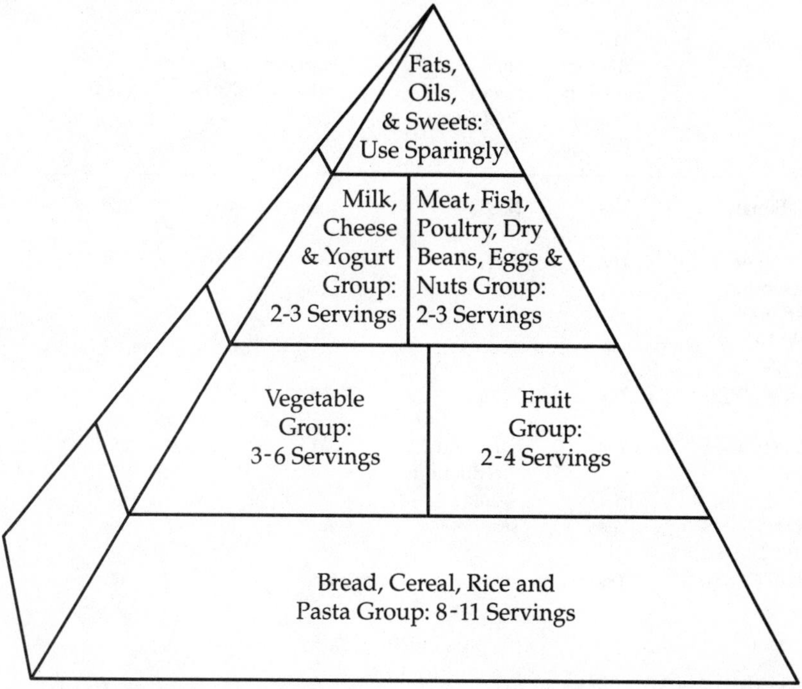

fruits, vegetables, and whole grains the foundation of a healthy diet. This focus on plant foods is what the meat and dairy industries objected to.

Is it appropriate to have the USDA make these recommendations? The USDA serves two somewhat conflicting roles: 1. It regulates and represents food industries. 2. It educates consumers about nutrition. How impartial can the USDA be, given the influence of the meat and dairy industries on it? Throughout the USDA's existence, evidence suggests, it has yielded to pressure from the meat and dairy industries.

A Rational Alternative

Many medical experts feel the USDA's Eating Right Pyramid simply does not make a strong enough statement. On April 8, 1991, the Physician's Committee for Responsible Medicine (PCRM), a nonprofit organization based in Washington, D.C., proposed an alternative to both the Basic Four Food Groups and the Eating Right Pyramid.[10] PCRM's proposal was that the old Basic Four be replaced by the New Four Food Groups: fruits,

Table 1.4 General Dietary Health Recommendations to the U.S. Public, 1977 to 1990

	Maintain Appropriate Body Weight, Exercise	*Limit or Reduce Total Fat (% kcal)*	*Reduce Saturated Fatty Acids (% kcal)*	*Increase Polyunsaturated Fatty Acids (% kcal)*	*Limit Cholesterol (mg/day)*	*Limit Simple Sugars*
U.S. Senate (1977)	Yes	27–33	Yes	Yes	250–350	Yes
Council on Scientific Affairs (AMA) (1979)	Yes	No	No	No	No	Yes
DHEW (1979)	Yes	Yes	Yes	NS	Yes	Yes
NRC (1980)	Yes	For weight reduction only	No	No	No	For weigh reductic only
USDA/DHHS (1980, 1985)	Yes	Yes	Yes	No	Yes	Yes
DHHS (1988)	Yes	Yes	Yes	No	Yes	Yes
USDA/DHHS (1990)	Yes	Yes	Yes	No	Yes	Yes

Note: NC = No coment; NS = Not specified. AMA = American Medical Association; DHEW = Department of Health, Education, and Welfare; NRC = National Research Council; USDA = U.S. Department of Agriculture; DHHS = U.S. Department of Health and Human Services.

Source: National Research Council. 1989. *Diet and Health: Implications for Reducing Chronic Disease Risk* National Academy Press, Washington, D.C.

vegetables, grains, and legumes. Foods obviously missing from this proposal are meats and dairy products; PCRM suggested that these foods be considered optional under the new plan.

Although PCRM's New Four Food Groups proposal is unlikely ever to be adopted by the USDA, it offers the best guidelines from a health-promotion standpoint. A diet based primarily on plant foods makes sense

ncrease Complex arbohydrates % kcal from total arbohydrates)	Increase Fiber	Restrict Sodium Chloride (g)	Moderate Alcohol Intake	Other Recommendations
'es	Yes	8	Yes	Reduce additives and processed foods
JC	NC	12	Yes	Consider high-risk groups
es	NS	Yes	Yes	More fish, poultry, legumes; less red meat
'o	No	3–8	For weight reduction only	Variety in diet; consider high-risk groups
at adequate starch and fiber		Yes	Yes	Variety in diet; consider high-risks groups
es	Yes	Yes	Yes	Fluoridation of water; adolescent girls and women increase intake of calcium-rich foods; children, adolescents, and women of childbearing age increase intake of iron-rich foods
hoose diet with plenty of vegetables, fruits, and grain products		Yes	Yes	Variety in diet

for good health and for environmental responsibility. In *Diet for a New America,* John Robbins paints a graphic portrait of the consequences of typical American eating habits on individual health, on the environment, on our natural resources, and on our planet as a whole.[11] This book is essential reading for anyone concerned about the environment, personal health, and the earth (see Table 1.6).

Table 1.5 Recommendations to Reduce Risk of Specific Chronic Diseases

	Maintain Appropriate Body Weight, Exercise	*Limit or Reduce Total Fat (% kcal)*	*Reduce Saturated Fatty Acids (% kcal)*	*Increase Polyunsaturated Fatty Acids (% kcal)*	*Limit Cholesterol (mg/day)*	*Limit Simple Sugars*
Osteoporosis						
NIH (1984)	Exercise	NC	NC	NC	NC	NC
Diabetes						
ADA (1987)	Yes	<30	Yes	No	<300	Yes
Heart Disease						
Inter-Society Commission for Heart Disease Resources (1984)	Yes	<30	8	10	<250	NC
NIH (1985)	Yes	<30	<10	Up to 10	250–300	*
AHA (1988)	Yes	<30	<10	Up to 10	<300	NS
Cancer						
NRC (1982)	NC	~30	Yes	No	NC	NC
ACS (1984)	Yes	~30	Yes	No	NC	NC
NCI (1987)	Yes	Yes	Yes	No	NC	NC

*Endorsed recommendations of AHA (1982) and Inter-Society Commission for Heart Disease Resources (1984).

NOTE: NC = No comment; NS = Not specified. ADA = American Diabetes Association; NIH = National Institutes of Health; AHA = American Heart Association; NRC = National Research Council; ACS = American Cancer Society; NCI = National Cancer Institute.

Increase Complex Carbohydrates (% kcal from total *carbohydrates)*	*Increase Fiber*	*Restrict Sodium Chloride (g)*	*Moderate Alcohol Intake*	*Other Recommendations*
NC	NC	NC	NC	Raise calcium to 1,000 mg/day (premenopausal), 1,500 mg/day (postmenopausal); use calcium supplements if needed; use vitamin D for calcium absorption
55–60	Yes	Yes	Yes	Nonnutritive sweeteners permitted but not recommended; limit protein to RDA level; avoid supplements except in special cases
Increase to make up caloric deficit	NC	5 g/day	NC	NS
*	*	NC	NC	Specific recommendations for high-risk groups; also physicians, public, and food industry
≥50	NS	≤3g/day of sodium	1–2 oz ethanol/day	Protein to make up remainder of calories; wide variety of foods
Through whole grains, fruits, and vegetables	NS	By limiting intake of salt-cured, pickled, and smoked foods	Yes	Emphasize fruits and vegetables; avoid high doses of supplements; pay attention to cooking methods
Same as NRC (1982)	Yes	Same as NRC (1982)	Yes	Same as NRC (1982)
Yes, more whole grains, fruits, and vegetables	To 20–35 g/day	NC	Yes	Variety in diet; avoid fiber supplements

SOURCE: National Research Council, *Diet and Health: Implications for Reducing Chronic Disease Risk* (Washington, D.C.: National Academy Press, 1989).

Table 1.6 *Diet for a New America* Facts

- The risk of breast cancer among women who eat meat daily is 3.8 times higher than that among women who eat meat less than once a week.
- The water pollution attributable to U.S. agriculture, including runoff of soil, pesticides, and manure, is greater than that attributable to all municipal and industrial sources combined.
- More than half of all water consumed for all purposes in the United States is consumed for livestock production.

Features of a Healthful Diet

Quite simply, a healthful diet provides optimum levels of all known nutrients and low levels of food components that are detrimental to health such as sugar, saturated fats, cholesterol, salt, and food additives. A healthy diet is rich in whole, "natural," and unprocessed foods. It is especially high in plant foods—fruits, vegetables, grains, beans, seeds, and nuts—because these foods contain valuable nutrients and additional compounds that have remarkable health-promoting properties.

2

Safe Eating

Many consumers are extremely concerned about the safety of the food they eat and the water they drink. Specifically, they are concerned about the effects that food additives, pesticides, and pollutants have on their bodies. Are these concerns founded? Yes. Much evidence supports the negative effects of these substances on our health and on the environment. Before we discuss the negative effects of pesticides and food additives, however, we should note that even whole, "natural" foods contain compounds that have been linked to cancer in animal studies. What is the difference between these naturally occurring substances and synthetic food additives? In general, the difference is that the whole food also provides a wide range of compounds that protect the body from harm, while food additives are typically added to nutritionally poor foods (junk foods). For example, many common vegetables (including celery, radishes, and beets) are rich sources of nitrates. The concern about nitrates is that they can be converted into nitrites and then into cancer-causing compounds known as nitrosamines by bacteria in the gut. However, other compounds in the vegetables, like vitamin C, prevent the harmful conversions from taking place. In contrast, the nitrites added to cured meats are easily converted into cancer-causing nitrosamines. Cured meats are also high in saturated fats, salt, and other food additives. This chapter will discuss the health risks of food additives, pesticides, and the water supply.

Food Additives

Food additives are used to prevent spoiling or to enhance flavor. They include such substances as preservatives, artificial colors, artificial flavorings, and acidifiers. Although the government has banned many synthetic food additives, not all additives currently used in our food supply are demonstrably safe. Indeed, many synthetic food additives still in use have been linked to such diseases and chronic conditions as depression, asthma or other allergy, hyperactivity or learning disabilities in children, and migraine headaches.

The FDA has approved the use of over 2,800 different food additives. In 1985 the per capita daily consumption of these food additives was approximately 13 to 15 g.[1] This astounding figure leads to many questions. Which food additives are safe? Which should be avoided? An extremist might argue that no food additive is safe. However, many food additives do fulfill important functions in our modern food supply. Many compounds approved as additives are natural in origin and possess health-promoting properties; others are synthetic compounds with known cancer-causing effects. Obviously, the most sensible approach is to focus on whole, natural foods and to avoid foods that are highly processed.

The Feingold Hypothesis

The hypothesis that food additives can cause hyperactivity in children stemmed from the research of Benjamin Feingold, M.D., and is commonly referred to as the "Feingold hypothesis." According to Feingold, many hyperactive children—perhaps 40 to 50 percent—are sensitive to artificial food colors, flavors, and preservatives, as well as to naturally occurring salicylates and phenolic compounds.[2]

Feingold's claims were based on his experience with over 1,200 cases in which food additives were linked to learning and behavior disorders. Since Feingold's presentation to the American Medical Association in 1973, the role of food additives in causing hyperactivity has been hotly debated in the scientific literature. Thus far, however, researchers have focused on only 10 food dyes versus the 3,000 food additives with which Feingold was concerned.

At first glance, the majority of the double-blind studies designed to test the hypothesis appear to have shown essentially negative results.[3] Closer examination of these studies and further investigation into the literature, however, indicate that food additives do play a major role in hyperactivity.[4] This is somewhat contrary to the conclusions expressed in the final report filed by the National Advisory Committee on Hyperkinesis and Food Additives to the USA Nutrition Foundation in 1980. On the other hand, the U.S. National Institutes of Health, Consensus Conference on Defined Diets and Childhood Hyperactivity, have agreed to reconsider the Feingold diet in the treatment of childhood hyperactivity.[5]

This reconsideration is largely due to the overwhelming evidence produced in several studies[6] and the fact that, despite major inadequacies in the negative studies, about 50 percent of those who tried the Feingold diet in these studies displayed a decrease in symptoms of hyperactivity.[7]

It is interesting to note that, while U.S. studies have been largely negative, the reports from Australia and Canada have been more supportive.[8] Feingold had contended that there was a conflict of interest on the part of the Nutrition Foundation, an organization supported by the major food manufacturers—Coca Cola, Nabisco, General Foods, and so on. Significantly the Nutrition Foundation has financed most of the negative studies.[9] Feingold contended that the conflict of interest arose because these companies would suffer economically if food additives were found to be harmful. Other countries have significantly restricted the use of artificial food additives because of their possible harmful effects.[10] The effects of specific food additives will be discussed next.

Colors

The total annual consumption of food colors in the United States is approximately 100 million pounds for the entire population.[11] Food color additives are officially designated as either certified or exempt from certification.[12] Food color additives that are exempt from certification are primarily natural in origin. This reflects the popular belief that natural compounds are safer, and the belief appears to hold up under scientific scrutiny. Table 2.1 lists the current status of food color additives.

One of the most widely used food colors is FD&C yellow dye #5, or tartrazine. Tartrazine is added to almost every packaged food, as well as to many drugs, including some antihistamines, antibiotics, steroids, and sedatives.[13] In the United States, the average daily per capita consumption of certified dyes is 15 mg, of which 85 percent is tartrazine.[14] Among children, consumption is usually much higher.

Although the overall rate of allergic reactions to tartrazine is quite low in the general population, allergic reactions due to tartrazine are extremely common (20 to 50 percent) in individuals sensitive to aspirin and in other allergic individuals.[15] Like aspirin, tartrazine is a known inducer of asthma, hives, and other allergic conditions, particularly in children.[16] In addition, tartrazine (like benzoate and aspirin) increases production of a compound that increases the number of mast cells in the body.[17] Mast cells are involved in producing histamine and other allergic compounds. A person whose body contains more mast cells typically is more prone to allergies. For example, examinations of patients with hives have shown that more than 95 percent exhibit an increase in mast cells.[18]

In studies using provocation tests to determine sensitivity to tartrazine and other food additives in patients with hives, positive reactions have been found in 5 to 46 percent of patients.[19] Diets that eliminate tartrazine as well as other food additives in sensitive individuals have frequently proved to be of great benefit in patients with hives and other allergic conditions such

Table 2.1 Current Status of Food Additives

Exempt from Certification	*Certified Colors Currently in Use*	*Certified Colors Prohibited from Further Use*
Annatto extract	FD&C red no. 3	FD&C red no. 1
Beet powder	FD&C yellow no. 5	FD&C red no. 2
Beta-apo-8-carotenol	FD&C yellow no. 6	FD&C red no. 4
Beta-carotene	FD&C blue no. 2	FD&C green no. 2
Canthaxathin		FD&C violet no. 1
Caramel		FD&C yellow no. 2
Carrot oil		FD&C yellow no. 3
Cochineal extract		FD&C orange no. 1
Corn endosperm oil		
Dried algae meal		
Ferrous fluconate grapeskin extract		
Fruit juice		
Paprika		
Riboflavin		
Saffron		
Synthetic iron oxide		
Thetes meal and extract		
Titanium dioxide		
Toasted cottonseed flour		
Turmeric		

as asthma and eczema.[20] Obviously, people suffering from allergic conditions should eliminate artificial food colors from their diets.

Sweeteners

The two primary artificial sweeteners currently in use are saccharin and aspartame (sold under the trade names NutraSweet and Equal). They are both among the most controversial of food additives. Advocates argue that the benefits they supposedly provide outweigh the potential adverse health effects. The perception is that consuming these sweeteners will lead to a reduction in the total number of calories consumed, which in turn will lead to weight loss or weight stabilization. Unfortunately, this is not the case. Detailed studies have not shown that these sweeteners reduce the total number of calories consumed or indeed have any significant effect on body weight.[21] Studies suggest that aspartame may actually increase appetite.[22]

On the negative side, what are the risks associated with these sweeteners? Saccharin is a known cancer-causing compound in rats.[23] And while these effects have not been noted in humans, saccharin has been shown to cause cancer in rats only if it is administered over two generations.[24] Therefore, future generations might have to pay for the current one's consumption of saccharin. Such an effect on future generations would perhaps finally provide the firm evidence the Council of Scientific Affairs requires. This council has concluded that "Until there is firm evidence of its [saccharin's] carcinogenicity in humans, saccharin should continue to be available as a food additive."[25] But, if saccharin offers no benefit to health, as studies have shown,[26] and a cloud of doubt hangs over the question of its safeness, why should it be used?

Aspartame is composed of aspartic acid, phenylalanine, and methanol. Aspartame was approved for food use by the FDA in 1981, despite the final recommendation of the FDA advisory panel on aspartame that no approval be granted until safety issues could be resolved.[27] Richard Wurtman, a pioneer in the study of nutrition and the brain, cautioned the FDA that, based on his extensive research, he believed that aspartame could significantly affect mood and behavior.[28] Wurtman and other researchers have demonstrated that administering aspartame to animals at levels comparable to those of high human consumption can alter brain chemistry.[29] Furthermore, other researchers have suggested that the methanol portion of the sweetener could also have adverse effects.[30] Methanol is quite toxic; the amount of methanol in 1 g of aspartame is approximately 100 mg. A child consuming 700 mg of aspartame would exceed by almost 10 times the Environmental Protection Agency's recommended daily maximum consumption of methanol.[31] The effect of long-term ingestion of subtoxic doses of methanol from aspartame has yet to be determined.

While the long-term effects of aspartame are largely unknown, some people are quite sensitive to aspartame and report immediate reactions.[32] Problems associated with aspartame ingestion include seizures, migraine headaches, hives, and disturbances in nerve function. Aspartame is particularly problematic for some individuals who suffer from migraine headaches.[33] Again, one has to ask, do the supposed benefits outweigh the risks? Since there is some risk associated with aspartame and no proven benefit, its use cannot be recommended.

Antioxidants

Without antioxidants, many foods would spoil quite rapidly. The two most widely used are butylated hydroxyanisole (BHA) and butylated hydroxytoluene (BHT). Like saccharin, these food additives have caused cancers in rats. However, other studies suggest that these antioxidants do actually protect against the development of cancers. In fact, many "experts" in life extension have recommended that these substances be taken as a food supplement at very high doses (up to 2 g per day). In light of extensive research, this recommendation is extremely unwise. Such a dose is 100 times greater than the estimated acceptable intake of BHA, BHT, or the sum of both, as set by the Joint Food and Agriculture Organization of the United Nations/World Health Organization Expert Committee on Food Additives.[34] It also supplies more than 100 times the acceptable intake's estimated inhibitory activity and may actually promote cancer. While BHA and BHT may be safe at low levels in foods, in the future they will most likely be replaced by naturally occurring antioxidants.

Preservatives

Preservatives like sodium benzoate, nitrates, nitrites, and sulfites retard spoilage by checking the growth of microorganisms. All of these preservatives have come under attack recently. As discussed earlier, nitrates and nitrites are known carcinogens.[35] Sulfites and benzoates, on the other hand, can produce allergic reactions. Clearly, preservatives should be avoided, especially by people prone to allergies. The best way to do this is to consume fresh, whole foods.

Benzoic acid and benzoates are the most commonly used food preservatives.[36] Although for the general population the rate of allergic response is thought to be less than 1 percent, the frequency of positive challenges in patients with chronic hives or asthma varies from 4 to 44 percent.[37] Even more of a problem are sulfites. Sulfites were once widely used on produce at restaurant salad bars. Because most people were not aware that sulfites were being added, and because most people who had a sensitivity to sulfites were unaware that they did, many unsuspecting people experienced severe allergic or asthmatic reactions. For years the FDA refused even to consider a ban on sulfites, despite admitting that these agents provoked attacks in an unknown number of people and in 5 to 10 percent of asthma victims. Not until 1985, when sulfite sensitivity was linked to 15 deaths between 1983 and 1985, did the FDA agree to review the matter. In 1986, the FDA finally banned sulfite use on produce and required labeling of other foods, such as wine, beer, and dried fruit, that have had sulfites added. The average person consumes an average of 2 to 3 mg of sulfites per day, while wine and beer drinkers typically consume up to 10 mg per day.[38]

Pesticides

In the United States each year, over 1.2 billion pounds of pesticides and herbicides are sprayed or added to crops. That amounts to roughly 10 pounds of pesticides for each man, woman, and child. Although the pesticides are designed to combat insects and other organisms, experts estimate that only 2 percent of the pesticide actually serves its purpose, while over 98 percent of the pesticide is absorbed into the air, water, soil, or food supply. Most pesticides in use are synthetic chemicals of questionable safety. Major long-term health risks of these include increased likelihood of cancer and birth defects; major health risks of acute intoxication include vomiting, diarrhea, blurred vision, tremors, convulsions, and nerve damage.[39]

To get a glimpse at the scope of the problem, let's examine the case of the farmer. A farmer's lifestyle is generally healthful: a farmer eats fresh food, breathes clean air, works hard, and tends to avoid such unhealthy habits as cigarette smoking and alcohol use. Despite this lifestyle, several studies have found that farmers are at greater risk for certain cancers, including lymphomas, leukemias, and cancers of the stomach, prostate, brain, and skin.[40]

Are pesticides, herbicides, and other synthetic chemicals responsible for this increased cancer risk? The studies say yes. Large studies of farmers in Canada, Australia, Europe, New Zealand, and the United States have demonstrated that the greater the exposure to these chemicals, the greater the risk for non-Hodgkin's lymphoma.[41]

What is the government's position? Because the evidence documenting the cancer-causing capabilities of pesticides in animals is inadequate, the formal opinion of many "experts" is that they pose no significant risk to the public or to the farmer. This opinion reflects a major dilemma faced by scientists. What is more valid—studies in laboratory animals or population studies in humans? More and more human evidence of increased cancer and birth defect rates after pesticide exposure is accumulating, indicating that pesticides are not as safe as the "experts" claim they are.

The history of pesticide use in this country is riddled with the names of pesticides that were once widely used and then later banned due to health risks. Perhaps the best-known example is DDT. Widely used from the early 1940s until 1973, DDT was largely responsible for increasing farm productivity in this country, but at what cost? In 1962, Rachel Carson's classic *Silent Spring* detailed the full range of DDT's hazards, including its persistence and deadly effects in the food chain, but it was another 10 years later before the federal government banned the use of this deadly compound. Unfortunately, although DDT has been banned for nearly 20 years, it is still found in the soil and in root vegetables such as carrots and potatoes. According to studies performed by the Natural Resources Defense Council, a public-interest environmental group, 17 percent of the carrots they analyzed still contained detectable traces of DDT.[42]

Pesticides in Use Today

Most pesticides currently used in the United States are probably less toxic than DDT and other banned pesticides (including aldrin, dieldrin, endrin, and heptachlor). However, many pesticides banned from use in the United States are shipped to other countries such as Mexico, which then sends food treated with them back to the United States. Although over 600 pesticides are currently used in the United States, most experts are most concerned about relatively few of these. The Environmental Protection Agency has identified 64 pesticides as potentially cancer-causing compounds (see Table 2.2), while the National Research Council found that 80 percent of our cancer risk from pesticides is due to 13 pesticides used widely in the production of 15 important foods.[43] The pesticides are linuron, permethrin, chlordimeform, zineb, captafol, captan, maneb, mancozeb, folpet, chlorothalonil, metiram, benomyl, and O-phenylphenol. These pesticides are used on many crops, but the affected foods of greatest concern (in descend-

Table 2.2 Pesticides Identified as Potentially Carcinogenic by the EPA

Acephate (Orthene)	Diallate	O-Phenylphenol
Acifluorfen (Blazer)	Diclofop methyl (Hoelon)	Oryzalin (Surflan)
Alachlor (Lasso)	Dicofol (Kelthane)	Oxadiazon (Ronstar)
Amitraz (Baam)	Ethalfluralin (Sonalan)	Paraquat (Gramoxone)
Arsenic acid	Ethylene oxide	Parathion
Asulam	Folpet	PCNB
Azinphos-methyl (Guthion)	Fosetyl Al (Aliette)	Permethrin (Ambush, Pounce)
Benomyl (Benlate)	Glyphosate (Roundup)	Pronamide (Kerb)
Calcium arsenate	Lead arsenate	Sodium arsenate
Captafol (Difolatan)	Lindane	Sodium arsenite
Captan	Linuron (Lorox)	Terbutryn
Chlordimeform (Galecron)	Maleic hydrazine	Tetrachlorvinphos
Chlorobenzilate	Mancozeb	Thiodicarb (Larvin)
Chlorothalonil (Bravo)	Maneb	Thiophanate-methyl
Copper arsenate	Methanearsonic acid	Toxaphene
Cypermethrin (Ammo, Cymbush)	Methomyl (Dual)	Trifluralin (Treflan)
Cyromazine (Larvadex)	Metiram	Zineb
Daminozide (Alar)	Metolachlor (Dual)	

ing order) are tomatoes, beef, potatoes, oranges, lettuce, apples, peaches, pork, wheat, soybeans, beans, carrots, chicken, corn, and grapes.

Pesticide residue levels in food are monitored by both state and federal regulatory agencies. Such monitoring provides an evidentiary basis for enforcing legal tolerance levels. However, there has been increasing public and governmental concern over the possible inadequacy of the residue monitoring programs. The monitoring system is designed to work as follows. The EPA establishes a tolerance level for pesticides in raw or unprocessed foods, utilizing key data as listed in Table 2.3. The Food and Drug Administration (FDA) is then responsible for enforcing the EPA limits. Individual state agencies, such as state departments of health and agriculture, may also be involved in monitoring food safety. This system falls short in several ways, beginning with the determination of the tolerance level. But even more important are weaknesses in three areas:

1. Probably less than 1 percent of our domestic food supply is screened by the FDA.
2. The FDA does not test for all pesticides.
3. The FDA does not prevent the marketing of foods that it finds contain illegal residues.

A number of pesticide poisoning epidemics have been reported over the years. The largest to date occurred in 1985. It involved the illegal use of aldicarb, an extremely toxic pesticide, on watermelons. Aldicarb is a systemic pesticide; this means that it permeates the entire fruit. Over 1,000 people in the western United States and Canada were struck. Resulting illnesses ranged from mild gastrointestinal upset to severe poisoning (vomiting, diarrhea, blurred vision, tremors, convulsions, and nerve damage).[44]

While the EPA and the FDA estimate that excessive pesticide residues are found on about 3 percent of domestic and 6 percent of foreign produce

Table 2.3 Key Data Elements for Determining Tolerance Levels for Pesticides

1. Chemistry of the pesticide
2. Expected quantity of residues present in food, based on field trials
3. Laboratory analytical procedures used to obtain residue data
4. Residues in animal feed derived from crop by-products and from forages and resulting residues (if any) in meat, milk, poultry, fish, and eggs
5. Toxicity data on parent compound and any major impurities, degradation products, or metabolites

and that detectable but acceptable residue levels are found on an additional 13 percent of domestic produce, other organizations report much higher estimates. For example, the Natural Resources Defense Council conducted a survey of fresh produce sold in San Francisco markets for pesticide residues and found that 44 percent of the 71 fruits and vegetables tested had detectable levels of one or more of 19 different pesticides, and that 42 percent of the produce with detectable pesticide residues had traces of more than one pesticide.[45] The sheer quantities of pesticides showered on certain foods are astounding. For example, over 50 different pesticides are used on broccoli, 110 on apples, 70 on bell peppers, and so on.[46] As many of these pesticides penetrate the entire fruit or vegetable and cannot be washed off, it is obviously best to buy organic.

Many supermarket chains and produce suppliers are employing their own testing measures for determining the pesticide content of produce and are refusing to stock foods that have been treated with relatively toxic pesticides such as alachlor, captan, or EBDCs (ethylene bisdithiocarbamates). In addition, many stores are asking growers to disclose all pesticides used on the foods as well as to phase out the use of the 64 pesticides suspected of being potentially cancer-causing. Ultimately, pressure from consumers influences food suppliers the most. Crop-yield studies support the desirability of organic farming, if risks to human health are added to the cost-benefit equation.

Waxes

In addition to avoiding pesticides, consumers must also be alert to the dangers of the waxes applied to many fruits and vegetables. Food producers apply these waxes to seal in the water that the produce contains, thereby keeping the produce fresh-looking. According to FDA law, grocery stores must display a sign identifying produce to which waxes or postharvest pesticides have been applied. Unfortunately most stores do not comply with the law, and the FDA lacks the manpower to enforce it. Currently, the FDA has approved six different wax compounds for use on produce, including shellac, paraffin, palm oil derivatives, and synthetic resins. These same items are used in furniture, floor, and car waxes. Foods to which these compounds can be applied include apples, avocados, bell peppers, cantaloupes, cucumbers, eggplants, grapefruits, lemons, limes, melons, oranges, parsnips, passionfruits, peaches, pineapples, pumpkins, rutabagas, squashes, sweet potatoes, tomatoes, and turnips.[47]

One main reason the waxes are added is to keep produce from spoiling during the (often long) period of time that elapses between harvest and arrival on grocery store shelves. If grocery store chains bought more local produce, the produce would not require chemical additives to keep it looking fresh. Instead, however, the large chains sign supply contracts with large produce suppliers, regardless of their location. This is why, for example, a grocery store in New York may be stocked with Washington state apples and California broccoli.

The waxes themselves probably pose little health risk. But most waxes have powerful pesticides or fungicides added to them. Since the waxes cannot be washed off with water, the fungicide or pesticide becomes cemented to the produce.

How to Reduce Your Exposure

Here are some recommendations for reducing your exposure to pesticides, as well as tips on removing surface pesticide residues, waxes, fungicides, and fertilizers from produce:

1. Buy organic produce. In the context of food and farming, the term *organic* indicates that the produce was grown without the aid of synthetic chemicals, including pesticides and fertilizers. In 1973, Oregon became the first state to pass laws defining labeling standards for organic produce. By 1989, 16 other states (California, Colorado, Iowa, Maine, Massachusetts, Minnesota, Montana, Nebraska, New Hampshire, North Dakota, Ohio, South Dakota, Texas, Vermont, Washington, and Wisconsin) had also adopted state laws governing organic agriculture. Consumers should ask their grocers whether produce advertised as organic is "certified organic." If so, by whom is it certified? Highly reputable certification organizations include California Certified Organic Farmers, Demeter, Farm Verified Organic, Natural Organic Farmers Association, and the Organic Crop Improvement Association. Although less than 3 percent of all produce grown in the United States is grown without the aid of pesticides, organic produce is widely available.
2. If organic produce is not readily available, develop a good relationship with your local grocery store produce manager. Explain to him or her your desire to reduce your exposure to pesticides and waxes. Ask what measures the store takes to ensure that pesticide residues fall within the government-mandated tolerance limits. Ask where the produce came from, since foreign produce is much more likely to contain excessive levels of pesticides or traces of pesticides that have been banned in the United States because of their suspected toxicity. Try to buy local produce that is in season.
3. To remove surface pesticide residues, waxes, fungicides, and fertilizers, soak produce in a mild solution of additive-free soap such as Ivory

or pure castile soap from a health-food store.

4. Peel off the skin or remove the outer layer of leaves. The down side of this technique is that many plants' nutritional benefits are concentrated in their skin and outer layers.

Water

Water is vital to our health. In fact, water is the most plentiful substance in our body, constituting over 60 percent of our body weight. Each day our body requires an intake of over 2 quarts of water to function optimally. About 1 quart of each day's requirement is supplied in the foods that we eat. This means that we need to drink at least 1 quart of liquids each day to maintain a good water balance. Drinking fresh fruit and vegetable juices (especially if derived from organic produce) is a fantastic way to give our body the natural pure water it desires. More liquids are needed by people who live in warmer climates or who are physically active. Not drinking enough liquids puts a great deal of stress on the body. Kidney function is likely to be affected, gallstones and kidney stones are likely to form, and the body's immune function will be impaired. Clearly, water is one of our most critical nutrients.

Many people today are expressing concern over our water supply, as pure water becomes increasingly difficult to find. Most of our water supply is full of chemicals, including not only chlorine and fluoride (which are routinely added) but a wide range of toxic organic compounds and chemicals such as PCBs, pesticide residues, nitrates, and heavy metals (including lead, mercury, and cadmium).[48] It has been estimated that lead alone may contaminate the water supplies of more than 40 million Americans.

Water Purification Units

In an effort to reduce exposure to these toxic compounds, some 2 million home water filtration units are purchased annually. What is the best filtration unit? According to Patrick Quillin, author of *Safe Eating*, the answer depends on the predominant local toxin.[49] For example, if the primary local toxin is lead, a carbon filter will provide very little benefit. This is significant, since carbon filters are the most popular water purification units sold. To determine the safety of your tap or well water, consult your local water company. Most cities have quality assurance programs that perform rou-

Table 2.4 Effectiveness of Various Water Filtration Methods

	Water Filtration Methods		
Water Impurities	*High-density Carbon Filter*	*Reverse Osmosis*	*Distillation*
Toxic heavy metals			
arsenic	leaves in	removes	removes
lead			
mercury			
cadmium			
Trihalomethanes			
chlorine	removes	probably removes	removes
chloroform			
Microbes			
Giardia	removes	removes	removes
E. coli			
most bacteria & worms			
Synthetic organic chemicals			
benzene	removes	removes	removes
pesticide/herbicide			
PCB, DDT			
petroleum distillates			
Asbestos	removes	removes	removes
Nitrates	probably removes	removes	removes
Useful minerals			
calcium	leaves in	removes	removes
magnesium			
fluoride			
Flavor	good	better	strange
Cost (purchase & maintain)	reasonable	high	high

tine analyses. Simply ask for the most recent analysis. Private water-testing companies like WaterTest (1-800-426-8378) and Suburban Water Testing (1-800-433-6595) will test your water for a fee. Table 2.4 compares the filtering abilities, water flavor, and cost of the three most effective filtration methods.

Granulated Activated Carbon Units These tend to be small units that attach to the faucet head. Carbon has been used for centuries as a filtering substance. Activated carbon is carbon that has been specially treated to increase its absorptive surface area. Impurities are bound by the carbon as the water passes through. The major problem with granulated carbon units is that the air spaces between the carbon particles can serve as a breeding ground for bacteria and other microorganisms. To counteract this problem, many companies impregnate the carbon with silver to kill the bacteria. However, this creates additional problems, including silver toxicity and reduced filtration capacity. Fortunately, better alternatives to this form of carbon filter are available.

Solid Carbon Block Units These units alleviate much of the concern over breeding microorganisms. They are quite effective at removing chlorine, bacteria, pesticides, and other organic chemicals, yet they allow desirable dissolved minerals (calcium, magnesium, and fluoride) to pass through. Unfortunately, harmful dissolved minerals such as lead, mercury, and arsenic are not filtered by these units either. The filters should be equipped with a prefiltration unit to remove sediment, and they should be replaced at a minimum of once every 6 months.

Reverse Osmosis Units These range from small home units to industrial-size. In reverse osmosis units, the water is filtered through small pores the size of water molecules in a special membrane. Often, a solid carbon unit is attached to remove any contaminates that might pass through the membrane. A reverse osmosis unit eliminates nearly all contaminants and all minerals. The disadvantages of reverse osmosis units are their cost, their water wastefulness (they lose up to 7 gallons of incoming water for every 1 gallon of drinking water obtained), their limited water output, and their bulky size.

Distilled Water Units The purest water is distilled water. The distillation process involves vaporizing water into steam and then cooling it in a separate chamber or through coils. When water is vaporized, the steam rises and the impurities remain behind. The steam then passes into the cooling chamber, where through condensation the water once again assumes its liquid form. Distillation is extremely effective at eliminating most impurities. The only possible exception may be volatile pollutants that could vaporize along with the water. Filtering the water through a carbon filter prior to distillation can overcome this problem.

Disadvantages of distillation are the electrical energy needs of the unit, the cost, and the slow output. In addition, since distillation removes all minerals from the water, drinking distilled water may eventually "leech out" beneficial minerals such as calcium, magnesium, and fluoride from the body.

Summary

More and more evidence is accumulating about the dangerous health effects of pesticides, food additives, and other contaminants in our food supply. To reduce intake of these potentially harmful substances, foods laden with empty calories, additives, and artificial sweeteners should be avoided, and their place in the diet taken by natural foods, preferably organically grown. As for our water supply, its safety is also coming under scrutiny. Fresh fruit and vegetable juices are a great way to supply the body's water requirements. Check your water supply to make sure it is safe. If it isn't, invest in a home water purification unit that will rid your water of the impurity.

3

Nutrients in Foods

Foods provide the nutrients we require in order to live. Specifically, foods provide the body with protein, carbohydrates, essential fatty acids, vitamins, and minerals. In addition to these nutrients, foods also provide numerous accessory food components known as anutrients or minor dietary constituents, including fiber, enzymes, pigments (such as carotenes, chlorophyll, and flavonoids), and numerous other beneficial compounds. The anutrients are discussed in the next chapter. This chapter describes the nutritional elements found in foods and discusses their importance to our health and their necessity as a part of our dietary intake.[1]

Protein

After water, proteins constitute the next most plentiful component of our body. The body manufactures proteins to make up hair, muscles, nails, tendons, ligaments, and other body structures. Proteins also function as enzymes, as hormones, and as important cell components such as genes. Adequate protein intake is essential to good health, and advertisers for the meat and dairy industry have spent a great deal of money educating us on the importance of protein. In fact, they have done such a good job that most Americans consume far more protein than their body actually requires. The recommended daily allowance for protein is about 1½ ounces (44 g) for the average woman and 2 ounces (56 g) for the average man, or approximately 8 to 9 percent of total daily calories. Most Americans consume more than twice this amount daily. A high-protein intake is linked to many chronic diseases, including osteoporosis, kidney disease, atherosclerosis, and cancer.

Proteins are composed of individual building blocks known as amino acids. The human body can manufacture most of the amino acids it needs for making body proteins. However, there are nine amino acids that the body cannot manufacture. These are termed "essential" amino acids. The essential amino acids required from our dietary intake are arginine, histadine, isoleucine, lysine, methionine, phenylalanine, threonine, tryptophan, and valine. The quality of a protein source depends on its level of these essential amino acids, along with its digestibility and ability to be utilized by the body.

A complete protein source is one that provides all nine essential amino acids in adequate amounts. Animal products—meat, fish, dairy, poultry, and so on—are examples of complete proteins. Plant foods, especially grains and legumes, often lack one or more of the essential amino acids, but they may become complete protein sources when they are combined. For example, combining grains with legumes (beans) results in a complete protein, as the two protein sources complement each other in their amino acid profiles. With a varied diet of grains, legumes, fruits, and vegetables, a person is virtually assured of having adequate amounts of complete proteins, as long as the calorie content of the diet is high enough. Nonetheless, when electing to reduce the amount of animal foods in the diet, we must take care to design the diet in a way that provides adequate amounts of protein. This is discussed in Chapter 11.

Animal Protein vs. Plant Protein

In the United States, an estimated 72 percent of all protein in the diet comes from animal products. Specifically, 49 percent comes from meat, fish, and poultry; 18 percent from dairy; and 4 percent from eggs. Plant foods account for only 28 percent of the protein intake, with fruits and vegetables providing about 8 percent, legumes about 3 percent, and grain products about 18 percent. Table 3.1 lists the protein content of various foods.

It is often difficult to separate the effects of animal protein from the effects of animal fats, because they are so highly correlated; that is, when animal protein intake is high, animal fat intake is typically also high. This makes it difficult for researchers to determine the effects of a high-protein diet, based on population studies. Despite this obstacle, much evidence indicates that relying on animal proteins to meet protein requirements increases the risk of developing several chronic degenerative diseases. Evidence also suggests that the body handles animal proteins differently from plant proteins. This is supported by population studies comparing vegetarians to omnivores, as well as by animal studies. The data indicate that the source of protein is as important as the quantity of protein.

Table 3.1 Protein Content (as a Percentage of Calories) of Selected Foods

Legumes		*Grains*	
Soybean sprouts	54%	Wheat germ	31%
Mung bean sprouts	43%	Rye	20%
Soybean curd (tofu)	43%	Wheat, hard red	17%
Soy flour	35%	Wild rice	16%
Soy sauce	33%	Buckwheat	15%
Broad beans	32%	Oatmeal	15%
Lentils	29%	Millet	12%
Split peas	28%	Barley	11%
Kidney beans	26%	Brown rice	8%
Navy beans	26%		
Lima beans	26%	*Nuts and Seeds*	
Garbanzo beans	23%	Pumpkin seeds	21%
		Peanuts	18%
Vegetables		Sunflower seeds	17%
Spinach	49%	Walnuts, black	13%
Kale	45%	Sesame seeds	13%
Broccoli	45%	Almonds	12%
Brussels sprouts	44%	Cashews	12%
Turnip greens	43%	Filberts	8%
Collards	43%		
Cauliflower	40%	*Fruits*	
Mushrooms	38%	Lemons	16%
Parsley	34%	Honeydew melons	10%
Lettuce	34%	Cantaloupe	9%
Green peas	30%	Strawberries	8%
Zucchini	28%	Oranges	8%
Green beans	26%	Blackberries	8%
Cucumbers	24%	Cherries	8%
Green peppers	22%	Grapes	8%
Artichokes	22%	Watermelons	8%
Cabbage	22%	Tangerines	7%
Celery	21%	Papayas	6%
Eggplant	21%	Peaches	6%
Tomatoes	18%	Pears	5%
Onions	16%	Bananas	5%
Beets	15%	Grapefruit	5%
Pumpkin	12%	Pineapple	3%
Potatoes	11%	Apples	1%

SOURCE: "Nutritive Value of American Foods in Common Units," U.S.D.A. Handbook No. 456.

A high intake of animal protein is linked to heart disease, many cancers, high blood pressure, kidney disease, osteoporosis, and kidney stones. The latter two conditions involve detrimental effects of calcium metabolism in a high-protein diet, which increases the excretion of calcium in the urine. Simply raising the intake of protein from 47 to 142 grams per day doubles the excretion of calcium in the urine. A diet this high in protein is common in the United States and is a significant factor in the increased number of people suffering from osteoporosis and kidney stones in this country. A vegetarian diet is associated with a reduced risk for the above-mentioned diseases and conditions.

Protein Supplements and Meal Replacement Formulas

A popular method of achieving weight loss involves reducing calories by consuming a "meal replacement formula" instead of a meal. The majority of these popular formulas, including Ultra SlimFast, contain a milk protein known as casein. Casein is often difficult for people to digest, and many people are allergic to it. Besides being used in many meal replacement formulas, casein is also used in glues, molded plastics, and paints.

More and more people are avoiding casein-containing meal replacement formulas and are instead looking to vegetarian alternatives, which provide significant advantages over casein. For example, experimental studies in animals and humans have shown that vegetarian protein sources (such as soy protein) tend to lower body cholesterol levels, while protein from animal sources (particularly casein) tend to raise body cholesterol levels. Casein has been shown to increase the likelihood of developing gallstones as well.

Carbohydrates

Carbohydrates provide us with the energy we need for body functions. There are two groups of carbohydrates: simple and complex. Simple carbohydrates, or sugars, are quickly absorbed by the body as a ready source of energy. The natural simple sugars in fruits and vegetables have an advantage over sucrose (white sugar) and other refined sugars in that they are balanced by a wide range of nutrients that aid in the utilization of the sugars. Problems with carbohydrates begin when they are refined and stripped of these nutrients. Virtually all of the natural vitamin content has been removed from white sugar, white breads and pastries, and many breakfast cereals.

When high-sugar foods are eaten alone, the blood-sugar level rises quickly, imposing a strain on blood-sugar controls. Too much of any simple sugar, including the sugars found in fruit and vegetable juices, can be harmful—especially if you are hypoglycemic, diabetic, or prone to candida infection. Since fruit juices have a higher sugar content than do vegetable juices, their use should be limited. Sources of refined sugar should be limited even more strictly. Read food labels carefully for clues on sugar content. If the words *sucrose, glucose, maltose, lactose, fructose, corn syrup,* or *white grape juice concentrate* appear on the label, extra sugar has been added.

Complex carbohydrates, or starches, are composed of many sugars (polysaccharides) joined together by chemical bonds. The body breaks down complex carbohydrates into simple sugars gradually, which permits better blood-sugar control. More and more research indicates that complex carbohydrates should form a major part of the diet. Vegetables, legumes, and grains are excellent sources of complex carbohydrates.

Fats and Oils

A great deal of research links a diet high in saturated fat to numerous cancers, to heart disease, and to strokes. Both the American Cancer Society and the American Heart Association have recommended a diet in which less than 30 percent of calories are from fat. As Table 3.2 makes clear, the easiest way for most people to achieve this goal is to eat fewer animal products and more plant foods. Other than nuts and seeds, most plant foods contain very little fat, but the fats they do contain are essential to human health.

In addition to providing the body with energy, the essential fatty acids—linoleic and linolenic acid—provided by plant foods function in our bodies as components of nerve cells, cellular membranes, and hormonelike substances known as prostaglandins. In addition, these polyunsaturated fats appear to be protective and therapeutic against heart disease, cancer, autoimmune diseases like multiple sclerosis and rheumatoid arthritis, many skin diseases, and many other diseases.

Reducing total fat intake is not the whole story. It is also important to reduce the amount of saturated fat in the diet. The typical saturated fat is an animal fat that is semisolid to solid at room temperature. Most vegetable fats are liquid at room temperature and are referred to as unsaturated fats or oils. Fats are usually found in foods as triglycerides. A triglyceride is composed of a glycerol molecule with three fatty acids attached (see Figure 3.1).

The triglyceride shown in Figure 3.1 is a saturated fat, because the fatty acids are saturated with all the hydrogen molecules they can carry. If some of the hydrogen molecules were removed, it would then be an unsaturated

Table 3.2 Fat Content (as a Percentage of Calories) of Selected Foods

Meats	
Sirloin steak, hipbone, lean w/fat	83%
Pork sausage	83%
T-bone steak, lean w/fat	82%
Porterhouse steak, lean w/fat	82%
Bacon, lean	82%
Rib roast, lean w/fat	81%
Bologna	81%
Country-style sausage	81%
Spareribs	80%
Frankfurters	80%
Lamb rib chops, lean w/fat	79%
Duck meat, w/skin	76%
Salami	76%
Liverwurst	75%
Rump roast, lean w/fat	71%
Ham, lean w/fat	69%
Stewing beef, lean w/fat	66%
Goose meat, w/skin	65%
Ground beef, fairly lean	64%
Veal breast, lean w/fat	64%
Leg of lamb, lean w/fat	61%
Chicken, dark meat w/skin, roasted	56%
Round steak, lean w/fat	53%
Chuck rib roast, lean only	50%
Chuck steak, lean only	50%
Sirloin steak, hipbone, lean only	47%
Turkey, dark meat w/skin	47%
Lamb rib chops, lean only	45%
Chicken, light meat w/skin, roasted	44%
Fish	
Tuna, chunk, oil-packed	63%
Herring, Pacific	59%
Anchovies	54%
Bass, black sea	53%
Perch, ocean	53%
Caviar, sturgeon	52%
Mackerel, Pacific	50%
Sardines, Atlantic, in oil, drained	49%
Salmon, sockeye (red)	49%

Vegetables	
Mustard greens	13%
Kale	13%
Beet greens	12%
Lettuce	12%
Turnip greens	11%
Mushrooms	8%
Cabbage	7%
Cauliflower	7%
Eggplant	7%
Asparagus	6%
Green beans	6%
Celery	6%
Cucumber	6%
Turnip	6%
Zucchini	6%
Carrots	4%
Green peas	4%
Artichokes	3%
Onions	3%
Beets	2%
Chives	1%
Potatoes	1%
Legumes	
Tofu	49%
Soybean	37%
Soybean sprouts	28%
Garbanzo bean	11%
Kidney bean	4%
Lima bean	4%
Mungbean sprouts	4%
Lentil	3%
Broad bean	3%
Mung bean	3%

Table 3.2 (*continued*)

Dairy Products		*Fruits*	
Butter	100%	Olive	91%
Cream, light whipping	92%	Avocado	82%
Cream cheese	90%	Grape	11%
Cream, light or coffee	85%	Strawberry	11%
Egg yolks	80%	Apple	8%
Half and half	79%	Blueberry	7%
Blue cheese	73%	Lemon	7%
Brick cheese	72%	Pear	5%
Cheddar cheese	71%	Apricot	4%
Swiss cheese	66%	Orange	4%
Ricotta cheese, whole-milk type	66%	Cherry	4%
Eggs, whole	65%	Banana	4%
Ice cream, 16%	64%	Cantaloupe	3%
Mozzarella cheese, part skim type	55%	Pineapple	3%
Goat's milk	54%	Grapefruit	2%
Cow's milk	49%	Papaya	2%
Yogurt, plain	49%	Peach	2%
Ice cream, regular	48%	Prune	1%
Cottage cheese	35%		
Low-fat milk (2%)	31%	*Grains*	
Low-fat yogurt (2%)	31%	Oatmeal	16%
Ice milk	29%	Buckwheat, dark	7%
Nonfat cottage cheese (1%)	22%	Rye, dark	7%
		Whole wheat	5%
Meat and Fish Products		Brown rice	5%
Hormel Spam luncheon meat	77%	Corn flour	5%
Mrs. Paul's Buttered Fish Filets	75%	Bulgur	4%
Del Monte Bonito	67%	Barley	3%
Morton Beef Tenderloin	64%	Buckwheat, light	3%
Mrs. Paul's Fried Shrimp	58%	Rye, light	2%
Mrs. Paul's Clam Crepes	55%	Wild rice	2%
Hormel Dinty Moore Corned Beef	53%		
Swanson Salisbury Steak	52%	*Nuts and Seeds*	
Nabisco Chicken in a Biskit	51%	Coconut	85%
Morton House Beef Stew	49%	Walnut	79%
Mrs. Paul's Flounder	48%	Sesame	76%
Swanson Veal Parmigiana	48%	Almond	76%
Swanson Fried Chicken	46%	Sunflower	71%
Hormel Dinty Moore Beef Stew	45%	Pumpkin seeds	71%
Morton Beef Pot Pie	45%	Cashew	70%
Mrs. Paul's Fish Au Gratin	43%	Peanut	69%
Morton Chicken Croquettes	40%	Chestnut	7%

SOURCE: "Nutritive Value of American Foods in Common Units," U.S.D.A. Handbook No. 456.

Figure 3.1 Glycerol + fatty acid.

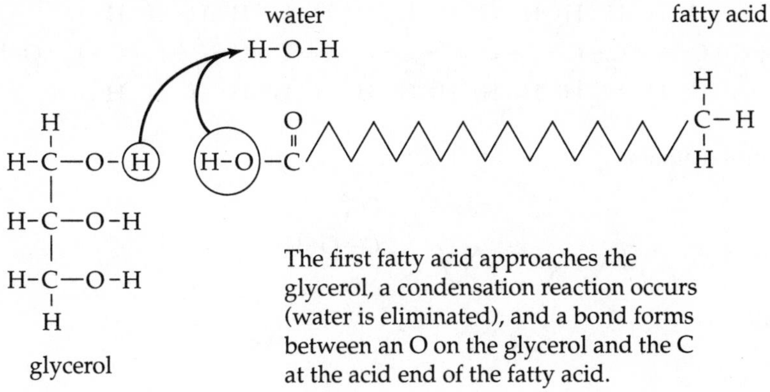

The first fatty acid approaches the glycerol, a condensation reaction occurs (water is eliminated), and a bond forms between an O on the glycerol and the C at the acid end of the fatty acid.

Later, 2 more fatty acids attach themselves to the glycerol by the same means; the resulting structure is a triglyceride.

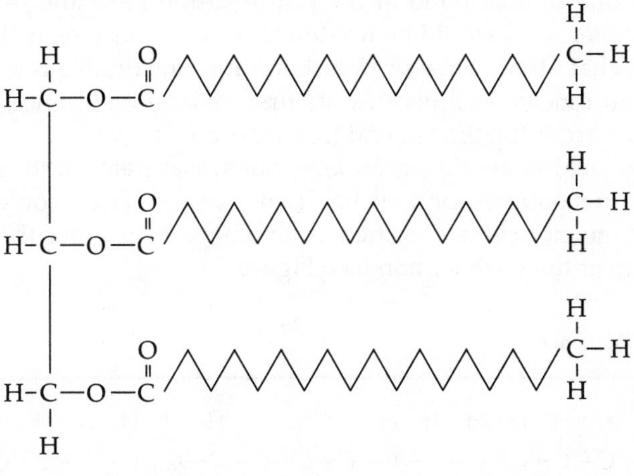

a fat (triglyceride) that might be found in butter.

fatty acid. To illustrate this further, let's look at the 18-carbon family of fatty acids.

Stearic acid is an 18-carbon-long saturated fatty acid (see Figure 3.2). This means that it is carrying as many saturated carbon molecules as it can.

Oleic acid is an 18-carbon-long monounsaturated fatty acid (see Figure 3.3). It is missing two hydrogen molecules, leaving two carbon

Figure 3.2 Stearic acid.

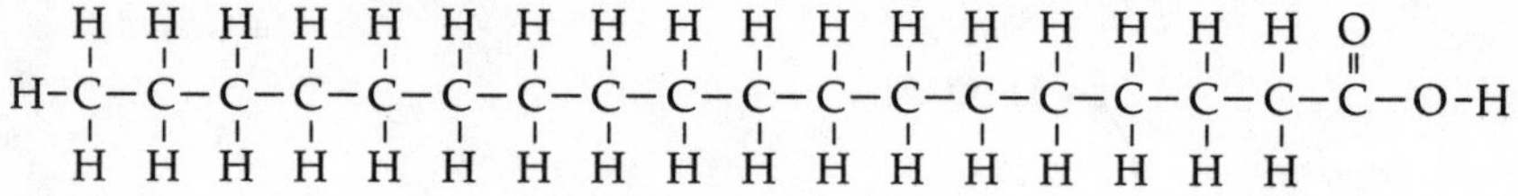

Simplified diagram:

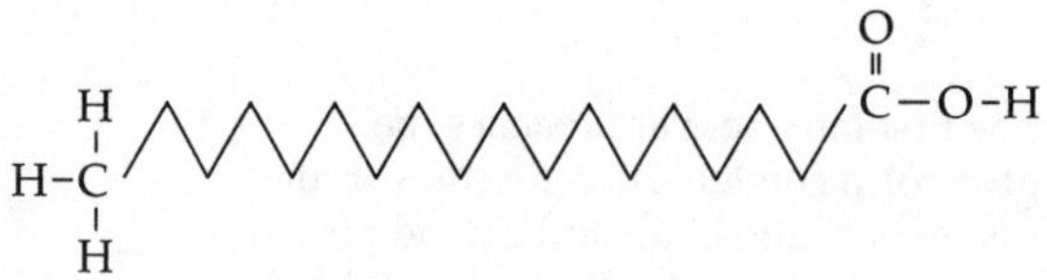

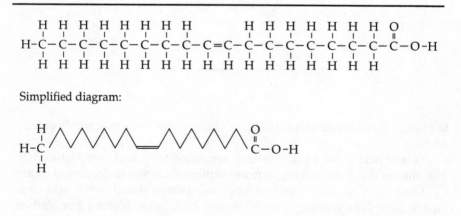

molecules unsaturated (see Figure 3.4). This causes the carbons to bind to each other to form a double bond. Oleic acid is monounsaturated because it contains one double bond at the ninth carbon molecule. In descriptive shorthand, oleic acid would be written C18:1ω9. This means that oleic acid is a carbon chain that contains 18 carbons and one double bond. Oleic acid is termed an omega-9 oil because its first unsaturated bond occurs at the ninth carbon from the omega end (see Figure 3.5).

Linoleic acid is an 18-carbon-long polyunsaturated fatty acid; instead of having one double bond, it has two. Linoleic acid would be written C18:2ω6. Linoleic acid is classified as an omega-6 oil, since the first double bond occurs at the sixth carbon (see Figure 3.6).

Figure 3.3 Oleic acid.

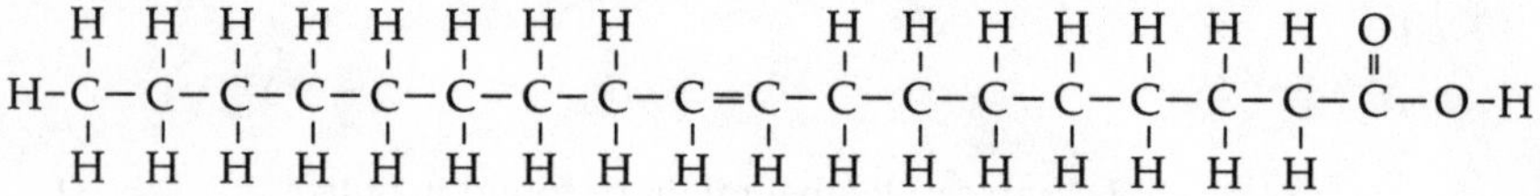

Simplified diagram:

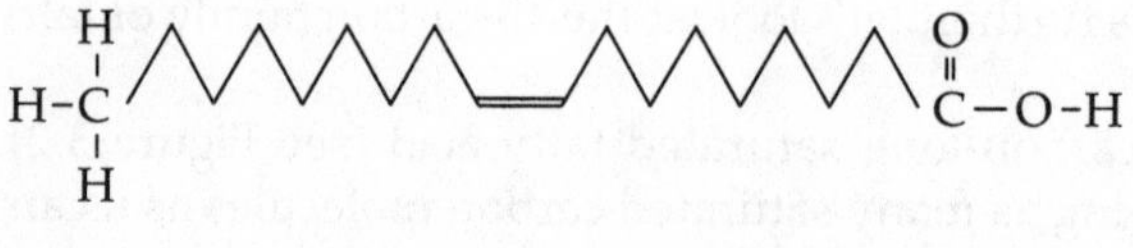

Figure 3.4 Unsaturated fatty acid.

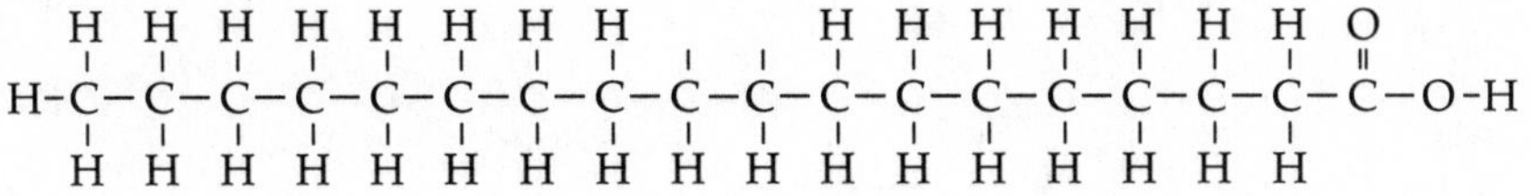

Figure 3.5 An omega-9 oil (oleic acid).

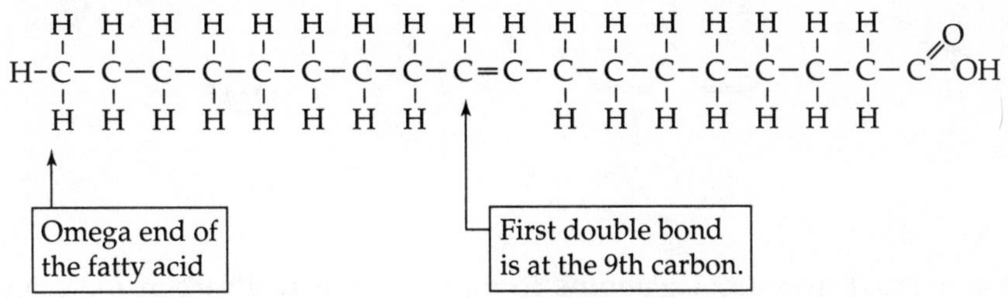

Linolenic acid is an 18-carbon-long polyunsaturated fatty acid with three double bonds, and would be written C18:3ω3. Linolenic acid is an omega-3 oil because its first double bond is at the third carbon (see Figure 3.7).

The balance of omega-6 to omega-3 oils is critical to proper prostaglandin metabolism (see Figure 3.8). Prostaglandins and related compounds are hormonelike molecules derived from 20-carbon-chain fatty acids that contain three, four, or five double bonds. Linoleic and linolenic acids can

Figure 3.6 An omega-6 oil (linoleic acid).

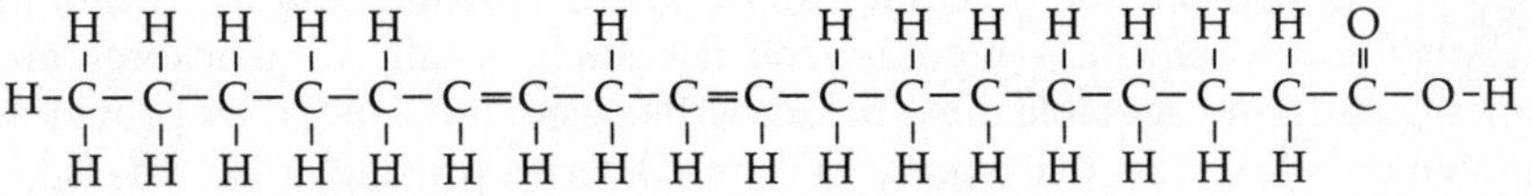

Simplified diagram:

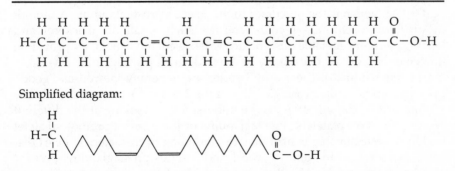

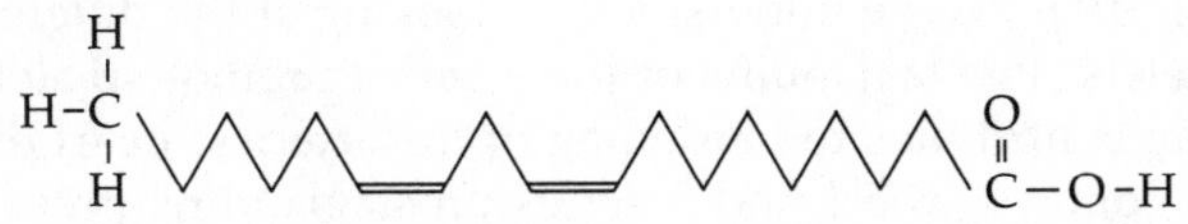

Figure 3.7 An omega-3 oil (linolenic acid).

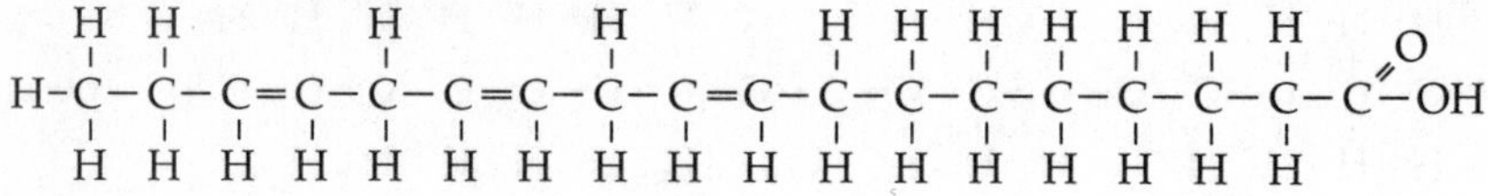

Simplified diagram:

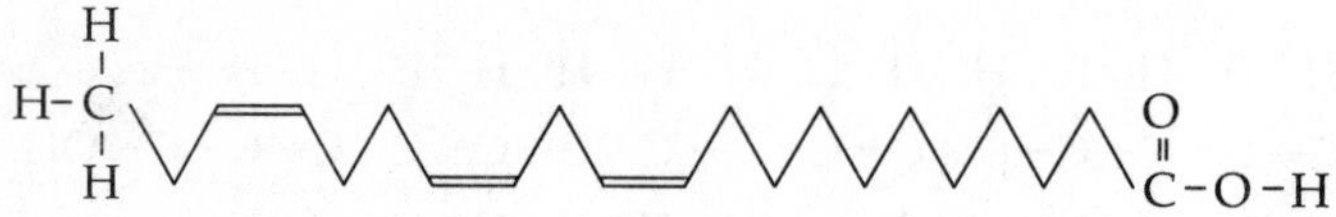

be converted into prostaglandins through adding two carbon molecules and removing hydrogen molecules (if necessary). The number of double bonds in the fatty acid determines the classification of the prostaglandin.

Series 1 and series 2 prostaglandins come from omega-6 fatty acids, with linoleic acid serving as the starting point. Linoleic acid is changed into gamma-linolenic acid and then into dihomo-gamma-linolenic acid, which contains three double bonds and is the precursor to prostaglandin of the 1 series. Dihomo-gamma-linolenic acid (DHGLA) can also be converted into arachidonic acid, which contains four double bonds and is precursor to the 2 series of prostaglandins. However, the enzyme (delta-5 desaturase) that converts DHGLA into arachidonic acid prefers to act on the omega-3 oils, as shown in Figure 3.8. Therefore, preformed arachidonic acid from the diet is the major source of arachidonic acid in the body.

The omega-3 prostaglandin pathway can begin with linolenic acid, an essential fatty acid that can eventually be converted into eicosapentaenoic acid (EPA), which is the precursor to the 3 series prostaglandins. Although EPA is found preformed in cold-water fish such as salmon, mackerel, and herring, certain vegetable oils, including flaxseed and canola, by providing linolenic acid, can increase body EPA and 3-series prostaglandin levels.

Prostaglandins of the 1 and 3 series are generally viewed as "good" prostaglandins, while prostaglandins of the 2 series are viewed as bad. The reason for this classification can be understood by looking at the different series' effects on platelets. Prostaglandins of the 2 series promote platelet stickiness, a factor that contributes to hardening of the arteries, heart disease, and strokes. In contrast, the 1 and 3 series prostaglandins prevent platelets from sticking together, improve blood flow, and reduce inflammation. Although the precursor to 2 series prostaglandins can be derived

Figure 3.8 Prostaglandin metabolism.

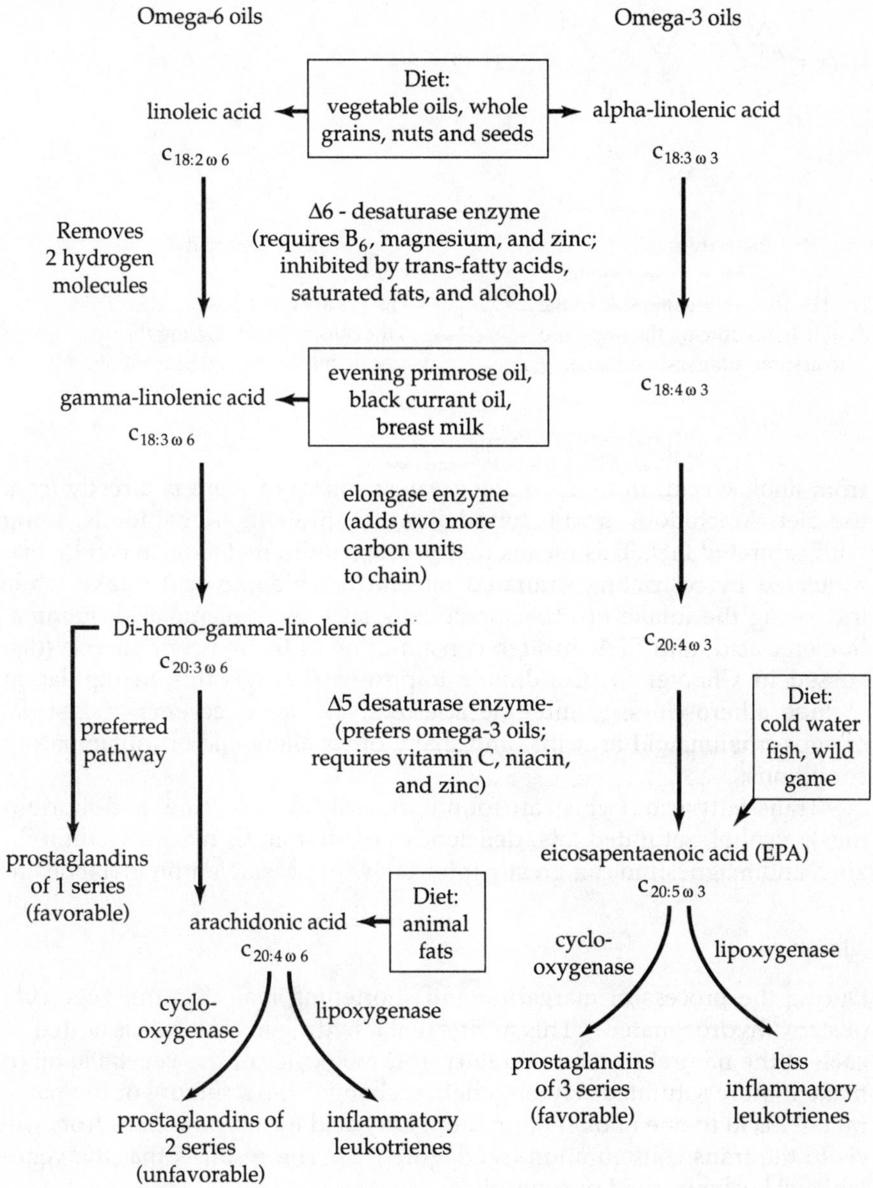

Figure 3.9 *Cis* vs. *trans* fatty acid configuration.

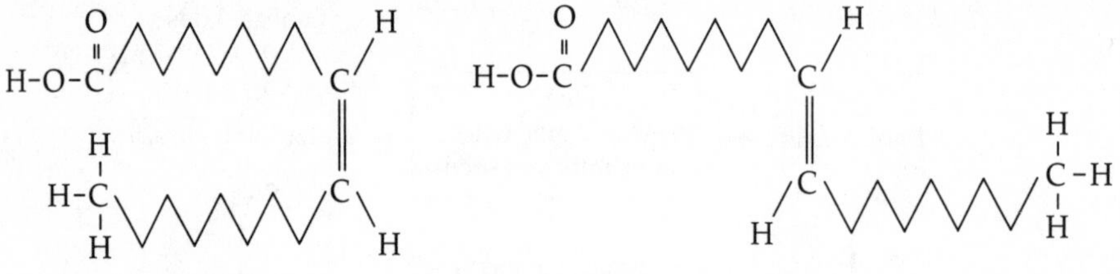

cis-fatty acid

The H's are on the same side of the double bond, forcing the molecule to assume a horseshoe shape.

trans-fatty acid

The H's are on opposite sides of the double bond, forcing the molecule into an extended position.

from linoleic acid, in humans the greatest source of them is directly from the diet. Arachidonic acid is found almost entirely in animal foods, along with saturated fats. This means that prostaglandin metabolism can be manipulated by restricting saturated fat and arachidonic acid intake while increasing the intake of other precursors such as linolenic acid, gamma-linolenic acid, and EPA through consumption of the appropriate oils (discussed in Chapter 9). Conditions improved through this manipulation include atherosclerosis, multiple sclerosis, psoriasis, eczema, menstrual cramps, rheumatoid arthritis, and many other allergenic or inflammatory conditions.

Trans-fatty acids (which are found primarily in margarines and shortenings), alcohol, saturated fats, deficiencies of vitamin C, niacin, vitamin B_6, zinc, and magnesium can greatly interfere with prostaglandin metabolism.

Margarine

During the process of margarine and shortening manufacture, vegetable oils are "hydrogenated." This means that a hydrogen molecule is added to each of the natural unsaturated fatty acid molecules of the vegetable oil to make it more saturated. Hydrogenation changes the structure of the natural fatty acid to one of many unnatural fatty acid forms, as well as from the cis to the trans configuration (see Figure 3.9). The result is that the vegetable oil becomes solid or semisolid.

Many researchers and nutritionists have been concerned about the health effects of margarine since it was first introduced. Although many Americans assume that they are doing their body good by consuming margarine rather than butter and saturated fats, they are actually doing more harm. Margarine and other hydrogenated vegetable oils not only raise LDL cholesterol, they also lower the protective HDL cholesterol level, interfere with essential fatty acid metabolism, and are suspected of being the cause of certain cancers. Although butter may be better than margarine, the bottom line is that they both need to be restricted in a healthful diet, while natural polyunsaturated oils—canola, safflower, soy, and flaxseed oils—should be used to meet essential fatty acid requirements. The requirement for essential fatty acids is not high, just 1 percent of the total caloric intake.

Vitamins

There are 13 different known vitamins, each with its own special role to play. The vitamins are classified into two groups: fat-soluble (A, D, E, and K) and water-soluble (the B-vitamins and vitamin C). Vitamins are essential to good health; without them, key body processes would halt. Low levels of vitamins and minerals in the body may prevent many people from achieving optimal health. Vitamins function along with enzymes in chemical reactions necessary for human bodily function, including energy production. Together, vitamins and enzymes work together as catalysts in speeding up the making or breaking of chemical bonds that join molecules together.

Fat-soluble Vitamins

Vitamin A Vitamin A was the first fat-soluble vitamin to be recognized. The initial discovery of vitamin A in 1913 was made almost simultaneously by two groups of research workers: McCollum and Davis at the University of Wisconsin, and Osborne and Mendel at Yale University. They found that young animals fed a diet deficient in natural fats became very unhealthy, as evidenced by their inability to grow and their poor immune function. These researchers also noted that the animals' eyes would become severely inflamed and infected on the restricted diet and that this could be quickly relieved by the addition to the diet of either butterfat or cod liver oil. Once known as the "anti-infective vitamin," vitamin A has recently regained recognition as a major determinant of the body's immune status.

The best-understood function of vitamin A relates to its effects on the visual system. The human retina has four kinds of vitamin A–containing compounds, which function in the visual process. Night blindness or poor dark adaptation is an early consequence of vitamin A deficiency. Vitamin A is also necessary for proper growth and development. Vitamin A is particularly important in maintaining the health and structure of the skin.

Table 3.3 Vitamin A Content of Selected Foods, in International Units (I.U.) per 3½-oz (100-g) Serving

Liver, beef	43,900	Sweet potatoes	8,800
Liver, calf	22,500	Parsley	8,500
Chili peppers	21,600	Spinach	8,100
Dandelion root	14,000	Mustard greens	7,000
Chicken liver	12,100	Mangoes	4,800
Carrots	11,000	Hubbard squash	4,300
Apricots, dried	10,900	Cantaloupe	3,400
Collard greens	9,300	Apricots	2,700
Kale	8,900	Broccoli	2,500

Many skin disorders, including acne and psoriasis, are responsive to vitamin A. Other body functions aided by vitamin A include reproduction, adrenal and thyroid hormone manufacture and activity, maintenance of nerve cell structure and function, general body immunity, and cell growth.

Vitamin A was originally measured in international units (I.U.). In 1967, an FAO/WHO Expert Committee recommended that vitamin A activity be referred to in terms of retinol (vitamin A) equivalents rather than in I.U., with 1 μg of retinol being equivalent to 1 retinol equivalent (R.E.). The amount of beta-carotene required for 1 R.E. is 6 μg, while the amount required for other provitamin A carotenoids is 12 μg. In 1980, the Food and Nutrition Board of the NRC/NAS adopted this recommendation, and the 1980 Recommended Dietary Allowance (RDA) for vitamin A is stated in μg and R.E. For an adult male, the RDA is set at 1,000 R.E. (750 as retinol and 250 as beta-carotene, or 5,000 I.U.) while the RDA for women is lower at 800 R.E. (4,000 I.U.). Children need 400 to 1,000 R.E. (2,000 to 5,000 I.U.) daily, increasing from infancy to 14 years.

The most concentrated sources of preformed vitamin A are liver, kidney, butter, whole milk, and fortified skim milk. Vitamin A can also be formed from beta-carotenes and other carotenes (see Table 3.3). This is fully discussed in Chapter 4. The leading sources of provitamin A carotenes are dark green leafy vegetables (collards and spinach) and yellow-orange vegetables (carrots, sweet potatoes, yams, and squash). Toxicity to vitamin A has been reported in people who supplement their natural intake with excessive doses or who eat large amounts of liver (6 to 24 pounds per week). In contrast, beta-carotene exerts no toxicity.

Vitamin D Since vitamin D can be produced in our bodies by the action of sunlight on the skin, many experts consider it to be more properly a hormone than a vitamin. Vitamin D is best known for its ability to stimulate the absorption of calcium. In the skin, sunlight changes the precursor to vitamin D, 7-dehydrocholesterol, into vitamin D_3 (cholecalciferol). It is then transported to the liver and converted by an enzyme into 25-hydroxycholecalciferol (25-OHD3), which is five times more potent than cholecalciferol (D_3). The 25-hydroxycholecalciferol is then converted by an enzyme in the kidneys into 1,25-dihydroxycholecalciferol (1,25-(OH)2D3), which is 10 times more potent than cholecalciferol and the most potent form of vitamin D_3. The metabolism sequence for vitamin D is shown in Figure 3.10.

Disorders of the liver or kidneys result in impaired conversion of cholecalciferol into more potent vitamin D compounds. Many patients with osteoporosis have high levels of 25-OHD3 but low levels of 1,25-(OH)2D3. This signifies an impairment of the conversion of 25-OHD3 into 1,25-(OH)2D3 in osteoporosis. Many theories have been proposed to account for this decreased conversion, including relationships to estrogen and magnesium deficiency. Recently, the trace mineral boron has been theorized to play a role in this conversion.

Vitamin D deficiency results in rickets in children and osteomalacia in adults. Rickets is characterized by an inability to calcify the bone matrix, causing softening of the skull bones, bowing of the legs, spinal curvature, and increased size of the joints. Once common, rickets and osteomalacia are now extremely rare.

Vitamin D is added to milk and other foods. Natural sources include cod liver oil, cold-water fish (mackerel, salmon, herring, and so on), butter, and egg yolks. Vegetables are generally low in vitamin D, but the best sources are dark green leafy vegetables. Vitamin D has the greatest potential to cause toxicity. Supplementation at amounts greater than 400 I.U. per day (the RDA for children) appears to be unwarranted.

Vitamin E Vitamin E is required by most animal species, including humans. It was discovered in 1922 when rats fed a purified diet lacking in vitamin E became unable to reproduce. Wheat germ oil added to their diet restored fertility. Later, vitamin E was isolated, and it was originally called the "antisterility" vitamin. Alphatocoperol is the chemical name for the most active form of vitamin E. The term *tocopherol* comes from the Greek words *tokos* (which means "offspring") and *phero* (which means "to bear"). Hence, *tocopherol* literally means to bear children.

Vitamin E functions primarily as an antioxidant in protecting against damage to cell membranes. Without vitamin E, the cells of the body would be quite susceptible to damage. Nerve cells would be particularly vulnerable. Severe vitamin E deficiency is quite rare, but various conditions have been associated with low levels of vitamin E, including acne, anemia, some cancers, gallstones, Lou Gehrig's disease, muscular dystrophy, Parkinson's disease, and Alzheimer's disease.

Figure 3.10 Vitamin D metabolism.

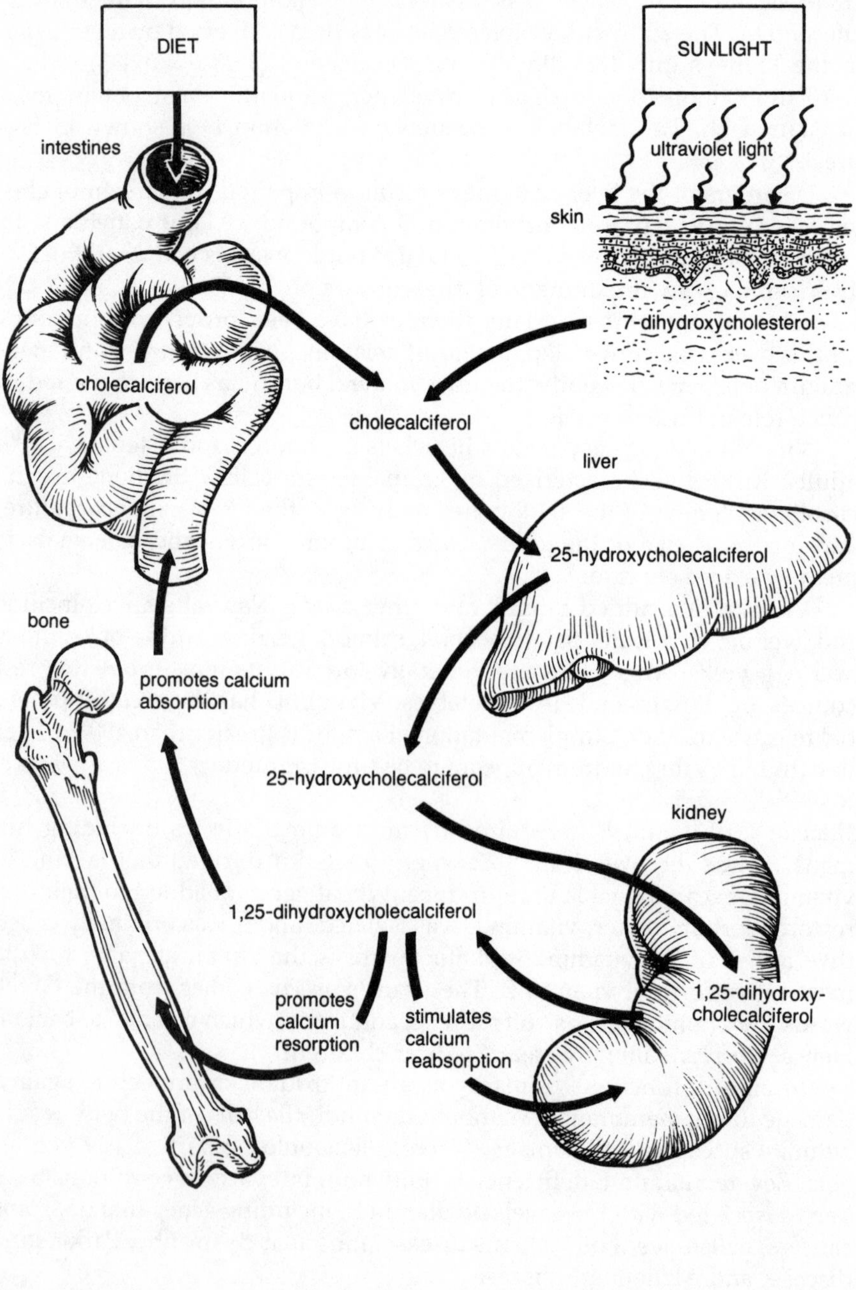

A diet high in vitamin E has been shown to exert a protective effect against many common health conditions, including heart disease, cancer, strokes, fibrocystic breast disease, and viral infections. Vitamin E, as an important antioxidant, helps support many body functions. Its clinical applications are quite extensive. Typically it is used at a dose of 400 to 600 I.U. per day. Vitamin E is extremely well tolerated, even at these high doses.

Although the RDA for vitamin E is set at 10 mg (roughly 15 I.U.), the amount of vitamin E actually required depends largely on the amount of polyunsaturated fats in the diet. The more polyunsaturated fats consumed, the greater the risk that they will be damaged. Since vitamin E prevents this damage, as the intake of polyunsaturated fatty acids increases, so does the need for vitamin E. Fortunately, in nature, where there are high levels of polyunsaturated fatty acids there are also higher levels of vitamin E. The best sources of vitamin E are polyunsaturated vegetable oils, seeds, nuts, and whole grains. Good sources include asparagus, avocados, berries, green leafy vegetables, and tomatoes.

Vitamin K One often neglected vitamin is vitamin K. Natural vitamin K from plants is termed vitamin K_1 or phylloquinone. Vitamin K_2 or menaquinone is derived from bacteria in the gut, and vitamin K_3 or menadione is a synthetic derivative.

The three vitamin K's function similarly in helping promote blood clotting, but for other important functions vitamin K_1 appears to be substantially superior. For example, vitamin K_1 plays an important role in bone health, as it is responsible for converting a bone protein from its inactive form to its active form. Osteocalcin is the major noncollagen protein found in our bones. As shown in Figure 3.11, vitamin K is necessary for allowing the osteocalcin molecule to join with the calcium and hold it in place within the bone.

A deficiency of vitamin K_1 leads to impaired mineralization of the bone, due to inadequate osteocalcin levels. Very low blood levels of vitamin K_1 have been found in patients with fractures due to osteoporosis. The severity of the fracture in each case strongly correlated with the level of circulating vitamin K. The lower the level of vitamin K, the greater the severity of the fracture. Vitamin K_1 is found in green leafy vegetables and may be one of the primary protective factors of a vegetarian diet against osteoporosis.

Rich sources of vitamin K include dark green leafy vegetables, broccoli, lettuce, cabbage, spinach, and green tea; good sources include asparagus, oats, whole wheat, and fresh green peas (see Table 3.4). The RDA for vitamin K is 1 μg per 2.2 pounds of body weight.

Figure 3.11 Activation of osteocalcin.

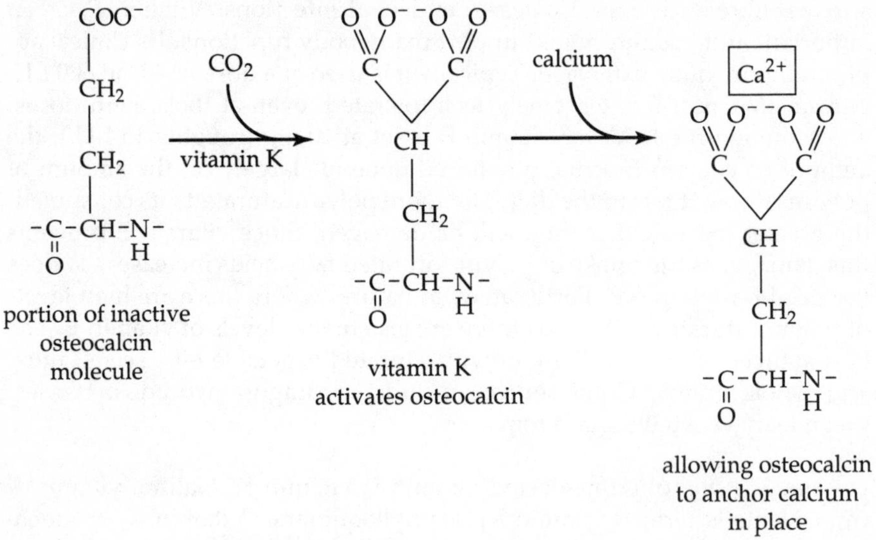

Water-soluble Vitamins

Thiamine Thiamine or vitamin B_1 was the first B-vitamin discovered. It has an interesting history (see pages 155–56). Thiamine functions as part of an enzyme (thiamine pyrophosphate or TPP) that is essential for energy production, carbohydrate metabolism, and nerve cell function. A deficiency of thiamine usually results initially in fatigue, depression, pins-and-needles sensations or numbness of the legs, and constipation. Severe thiamine deficiency results in a deficiency syndrome known as beriberi; symptoms include mental confusion, muscle wasting (dry beriberi), fluid retention (wet beriberi), high blood pressure, difficulty walking, and heart disturbances.

Table 3.4 Vitamin K Content of Selected Foods, in Micrograms (μg) per 3½-oz (100-g) Serving

Kale	729	Lettuce	129	Green peas	19
Green tea	712	Cabbage	125	Whole wheat	17
Turnip greens	650	Watercress	57	Green beans	14
Spinach	415	Asparagus	57		
Broccoli	200	Oats	20		

Table 3.5 Thiamine Content of Selected Foods, in Milligrams (mg) per 3½-oz (100-g) Serving

Yeast, brewer's	15.61	Lima beans, dry	.48
Yeast, torula	14.01	Hazelnuts	.46
Wheat germ	2.01	Wild rice	.45
Sunflower seeds	1.96	Cashews	.43
Rice polishings	1.84	Rye, whole-grain	.43
Pine nuts	1.28	Mung beans	.38
Peanuts, with skins	1.14	Cornmeal, whole-ground	.38
Soybeans, dry	1.10	Lentils	.37
Peanuts, without skins	.98	Green peas	.35
Brazil nuts	.96	Macadamia nuts	.34
Pecans	.86	Brown rice	.34
Soybean flour	.85	Walnuts	.33
Beans, pinto & red	.84	Garbanzos	.31
Split peas	.74	Garlic, cloves	.25
Millet	.73	Almonds	.24
Wheat bran	.72	Lima beans, fresh	.24
Pistachio nuts	.67	Pumpkin & squash seeds	.24
Navy beans	.65	Chestnuts, fresh	.23
Buckwheat	.60	Soybean sprouts	.23
Oatmeal	.60	Peppers, red chili	.22
Whole-wheat flour	.55	Sesame seeds, hulled	.18
Whole-wheat grain	.55		

Although severe thiamine deficiency is uncommon (except in alcoholics), many Americans do not consume the RDA of 1.5 mg. Rich plant sources of thiamine include soybeans, brown rice, sunflower seeds, and peanuts; good sources include whole wheat and nuts (see Table 3.5). Thiamine is extremely sensitive to alcohol and sulfites. In the presence of either, thiamine is destroyed or made useless. Thiamine is also sensitive to a factor in uncooked freshwater fish and shellfish, and in tea. There is no known toxicity due to thiamine.

Riboflavin Riboflavin or vitamin B_2 was first recognized as a yellow-green pigment in milk in 1879. Ingesting an excess of riboflavin results in an increased urine content of riboflavin, which can give urine a yellow-green fluorescent glow. Riboflavin functions in two important enzymes (FMN and FAD) that are involved in energy production.

Early riboflavin deficiency is characterized by cracking of the lips and corners of the mouth; an inflammed tongue; visual disturbances such as sensitivity to light and loss of visual acuity; cataract formation; burning and itching of the eyes, lips, mouth, and tongue; and other signs of disorders of mucous membranes. The RDA for riboflavin is 1.7 mg for males and

Table 3.6 Riboflavin Content of Selected Foods, in Milligrams (mg) per 3½-oz (100-g) Serving

Yeast, torula	5.06	Wheat bran	.35	Sunflower seeds	.23
Yeast, brewer's	4.28	Collards	.31	Navy beans	.22
Liver, calf	2.72	Soybeans, dry	.31	Beet & mustard greens	.22
Almonds	.92	Split peas	.29	Lentils	.22
Wheat germ	.68	Kale	.26	Prunes	.22
Wild rice	.63	Parsley	.26	Rye, whole grain	.22
Mushrooms	.46	Cashews	.25	Mung beans	.21
Millet	.38	Rice bran	.25	Beans, pinto & red	.21
Peppers, hot red	.36	Broccoli	.23	Blackeye peas	.21
Soy flour	.35	Pine nuts	.23		

1.3 mg for females. Rich sources of riboflavin are organ meats (liver, kidney, heart); good plant sources are almonds, mushrooms, whole grains, soybeans, and green leafy vegetables (see Table 3.6). Riboflavin is destroyed by light, but it is not destroyed by cooking.

Niacin Since niacin or vitamin B_3 can be made in the body by the conversion of tryptophan, many nutritionists do not consider niacin an essential nutrient as long as tryptophan intake is adequate. Niacin functions in the body as a component in the coenzymes NAD and NADP, which are involved in well over 50 different chemical reactions in the body. Niacin-containing enzymes play an important role in energy production; fat, cholesterol, and carbohydrate metabolism; and the manufacture of many body compounds, including sex and adrenal hormones.

Niacin was discovered in the course of research to find the cause of pellagra, a common disease in Spain and Italy in the eighteenth century. In Italian, *pellagra* means "skin that is rough." Pellagra is now known to be due to a severe deficiency of niacin and tryptophan. Pellagra is characterized by dermatitis, dementia, and diarrhea. The skin develops a cracked, scaly dermatitis; the brain does not function properly, leading to confusion and dementia; and diarrhea results from the impaired manufacture of the mucous lining of the gastrointestinal tract. Although the RDA for niacin is based on caloric intake, an intake of at least 18 mg per day is recommended by most authorities.

Additional niacin has been shown to exert a favorable effect on many health conditions. It is available either as nicotinic acid or as niacinamide. Each form has different applications. In its nicotinic acid form, it is effective at lowering blood cholesterol levels, while in its niacinamide form it is useful in combating arthritis. In the field of orthomolecular psychiatry, large doses of niacin are often prescribed in the treatment of schizophrenia.

Table 3.7 Niacin Content of Selected Foods, in Milligrams (mg) per 3½-oz (100-g) Serving

Yeast, torula	44.4	Wild rice	6.2	Whole-wheat grain	4.4
Yeast, brewer's	37.9	Sesame seeds	5.4	Whole-wheat flour	4.3
Rice bran	29.8	Sunflower seeds	5.4	Wheat germ	4.2
Rice polishings	28.2	Brown rice	4.7	Barley	3.7
Wheat bran	21.0	Pine nuts	4.5	Almonds	3.5
Peanuts, with skins	17.2	Buckwheat, whole-grain	4.4	Split peas	3.0
Peanuts, without skins	15.8	Peppers, red chili	4.4		

Doses in excess of 50 mg of niacin (as nicotinic acid) typically produce a transient flushing of the skin. High doses (2 to 6 g per day) of either niacin or niacinamide should be monitored by a physician, as they may cause liver disorders, peptic ulcers, and glucose intolerance.

Rich food sources of niacin include liver and other organ meats, eggs, fish, and peanuts. All of these foods are also rich sources of tryptophan. Good sources of niacin include legumes, whole grains (except corn), milk, and avocados (see Table 3.7).

Pantothenic Acid Pantothenic acid or vitamin B_5 is a component of coenzyme A (CoA), which plays a critical role in the utilization of fats and carbohydrates in energy production, as well as in the manufacture of adrenal hormones and red blood cells. Pantothenic acid is particularly important for optimum adrenal function, and it has long been considered the "anti-stress" vitamin because of its central role in adrenal function and cellular metabolism.

A deficiency of pantothenic acid is believed to be quite rare in humans, since pantothenic acid is found in a large number of foods. In fact, its name is derived from the Greek word *pantos,* which means "everywhere." Additional pantothenic acid is often used to support adrenal function; and pantethine, the most active stable form of pantothenic acid, is used to lower blood cholesterol and triglyceride levels.

Pantothenic acid is found in high concentrations in liver and other organ meats, milk, fish, and poultry. Good plant sources of pantothenic acid include whole grains, legumes, sweet potatoes, broccoli, cauliflower, oranges, and strawberries (see Table 3.8). There is no official RDA for pantothenic acid, but a daily intake of 4 to 7 mg is believed to be adequate.

Pyridoxine Pyridoxine or vitamin B_6 is an extremely important B vitamin. It is involved in the formation of body proteins and structural compounds, chemical transmitters in the nervous system, red blood cells, and

Table 3.8 Pantothenic Acid Content of Selected Foods, in Milligrams (mg) per 3½-oz (100-g) Serving

Yeast, brewer's	12.0	Oatmeal, dry	1.5	Hazelnuts	1.1
Yeast, torula	11.0	Buckwheat flour	1.4	Brown rice	1.1
Liver, calf	8.0	Sunflower seeds	1.4	Whole-wheat flour	1.1
Peanuts	2.8	Lentils	1.4	Peppers, red chili	1.1
Mushrooms	2.2	Rye flour, whole	1.3	Avocados	1.1
Soybean flour	2.0	Cashews	1.3	Blackeye peas, dry	1.0
Split peas	2.0	Garbanzos	1.2	Wild rice	1.0
Pecans	1.7	Wheat germ, toasted	1.2	Cauliflower	1.0
Soybeans	1.7	Broccoli	1.2	Kale	1.0

prostaglandins. Vitamin B_6 is also critical in maintaining hormonal balance and proper immune function.

Deficiency of vitamin B_6 is characterized by depression, convulsions (especially in children), glucose intolerance, and impaired nerve function.

Although extreme deficiency of vitamin B_6 is believed to be quite rare, numerous clinical studies have demonstrated the importance of vitamin B_6 in a number of health conditions that typically respond to B_6 supplementation, including asthma, premenstrual syndrome (PMS), carpal tunnel syndrome, depression, morning sickness, and kidney stones. Interestingly, the increased rate of these disorders since the 1950s parallels the increased levels of vitamin B_6 antagonists found in the food supply and used as drugs during the same period. Antagonists to vitamin B_6 include the hydrazine dyes (FD&C yellow #5), certain medicinal drugs (isoniazid, hydralazine, dopamine, and penicillamine), oral contraceptives, alcohol, and excessive protein. The intake of yellow dye #5 is often consumed in greater quantities (per capita intake of 15 mg per day) than the RDA for vitamin B_6 of 2.0 mg for males and 1.6 mg for females.

Good plant sources of vitamin B_6 include whole grains, legumes, bananas, seeds and nuts, potatoes, Brussels sprouts, and cauliflower (see Table 3.9). Vitamin B_6 levels inside the cells of the body appear to be intricately linked to the magnesium content of the diet as well.

Folic Acid Folic acid—also known as folate, folacin, and pteroylmonoglutamate—functions together with vitamin B_{12} in many body processes and is critical to cellular division because it is necessary in DNA synthesis. Without folic acid, cells do not divide properly. Folic acid is critical to the development of the nervous system of the fetus. Deficiency of folic acid during pregnancy has been linked to several birth defects, including neural tube defects like spina bifida.

Table 3.9 Pyridoxine Content of Selected Foods, in Milligrams (mg) per 3½-oz (100-g) Serving

Yeast, torula	3.00	Navy beans, dry	.56	Spinach	.28
Yeast, brewer's	2.50	Brown rice	.55	Turnip greens	.26
Sunflower seeds	1.25	Hazelnuts	.54	Peppers, sweet	.26
Wheat germ, toasted	1.15	Garbanzos, dry	.54	Potatoes	.25
Soybeans, dry	.81	Pinto beans, dry	.53	Prunes	.24
Walnuts	.73	Bananas	.51	Raisins	.24
Soybean flour	.63	Avocados	.42	Brussels sprouts	.23
Lentils, dry	.60	Whole-wheat flour	.34	Barley	.22
Lima beans, dry	.58	Chestnuts, fresh	.33	Sweet potatoes	.22
Buckwheat flour	.58	Kale	.30	Cauliflower	.21
Blackeye peas, dry	.56	Rye flour	.30		

In a case of folic acid deficiency, all cells of the body are affected, but rapidly dividing cells like red blood cells and cells of the gastrointestinal and genital tract are affected the most. Folic acid deficiency is characterized by poor growth, diarrhea, anemia, gingivitis, and an abnormal pap smear in women.

Despite folic acid's wide occurrence in food, folic acid deficiency is the most common vitamin deficiency in the world. The reason reflects food choices: animal foods, with the exception of liver, are poor sources of folic acid, while plant sources are rich sources but are not as frequently consumed. In addition, alcohol and many prescription drugs (including estrogens, sulfasalazine, and barbiturates) impair folic acid metabolism. Moreover, folic acid is extremely sensitive and easily destroyed by light or heat. The RDA for folic acid is 200 μg for males and 180 μg for females.

Folic acid received its name from the Latin word *folium* (which means "foliage"), because it is found in high concentrations in green leafy vegetables such as kale, spinach, beet greens, and chard. Other good sources of folic acid include legumes, asparagus, broccoli, cabbage, oranges, root vegetables, and whole grains (see Table 3.10).

Vitamin B_{12} Vitamin B_{12} or cobalamin was isolated from a liver extract in 1948 and subsequently identified as the nutritional factor in liver that prevented pernicious anemia. Vitamin B_{12} is a bright red crystalline compound with a high content of the mineral cobalt. Vitamin B_{12} works with folic acid in many body processes, including the synthesis of DNA. Since vitamin B_{12} works to reactivate folic acid, a deficiency of B_{12} will result in a folic acid deficiency if folic acid levels are only marginal. On its own, a vitamin B_{12} deficiency leads to impaired nerve function, which can cause in the feet

Table 3.10 Folic Acid Content of Selected Foods, in Micrograms (μg) per 3½-oz (100-g) Serving

Yeast, brewer's	2,022	Lentils	105	Whole-wheat flour	38
Blackeye peas	440	Walnuts	77	Oatmeal	33
Rice germ	430	Spinach, fresh	75	Cabbage	32
Soy flour	425	Kale	70	Dried figs	32
Wheat germ	305	Filbert nuts	65	Avocado	30
Liver, beef	295	Beet & mustard greens	60	Green beans	28
Soy beans	225	Peanuts, roasted	56	Corn	28
Wheat bran	195	Peanut butter	56	Coconut, fresh	28
Kidney beans	180	Broccoli	53	Pecans	27
Mung beans	145	Barley	50	Mushrooms	25
Lima beans	130	Split peas	50	Dates	25
Navy beans	125	Whole-wheat cereal	49	Blackberries	14
Garbanzos	125	Brussels sprouts	49	Orange	5
Asparagus	110	Almonds	45		

numbness, pins-and-needles sensations, or a burning feeling, as well as causing impaired mental function that in the elderly can mimic Alzheimer's disease. Vitamin B_{12} deficiency is thought to be quite common in the elderly. Symptoms include depression or mental confusion; anemia; a smooth, beefy red tongue; and diarrhea.

Vitamin B_{12} is necessary in very small quantities. The RDA is 2.0 μg. Vitamin B_{12} is found in significant quantities only in animal foods. The richest sources are liver and kidney, followed by eggs, fish, cheese, and meat (see Table 3.11). Strict vegetarians (vegans) are often told that fermented foods like tempeh and miso are excellent sources of vitamin B_{12}. However, apart from the tremendous variation in B_{12} content of fermented foods, there is some evidence that the form of B_{12} in these foods is not exactly the form that meets our body requirements. Although the vitamin B_{12} content of certain cooked sea vegetables is in the same range as that of beef, it is not known whether this form is utilized in the same manner. Therefore, at this time it appears to be an extremely good idea for vegetarians to supplement their diets with vitamin B_{12}.

Biotin Biotin is a B vitamin that functions in the manufacture and utilization of fats and amino acids. Without biotin, metabolism is severely impaired. Since biotin is manufactured in the intestines by gut bacteria, it is not frequently discussed. A vegetarian diet has been shown to alter the intestinal bacterial flora in such a manner as to enhance the synthesis of biotin and to promote its absorption.

A biotin deficiency in adults is characterized by dry, scaly skin; nausea;

Table 3.11 Vitamin B_{12} Content of Selected Foods, in Micrograms (μg) per 3½-oz (100-g) Serving

Liver, lamb	104	Salmon, flesh	4.0	Blue cheese	1.4
Clams	98	Tuna, flesh	3.0	Haddock, flesh	1.3
Liver, beef	80	Lamb	2.1	Flounder, flesh	1.2
Kidneys, lamb	63	Eggs	2.0	Scallops	1.2
Liver, calf	60	Whey, dried	2.0	Cheddar cheese	1.0
Kidneys, beef	31	Beef, lean	1.8	Cottage cheese	1.0
Liver, chicken	25	Edam cheese	1.8	Mozzarella cheese	1.0
Oysters	18	Swiss cheese	1.8	Halibut	1.0
Sardines	17	Brie cheese	1.6	Perch, filets	1.0
Trout	5.0	Gruyère cheese	1.6	Swordfish, flesh	1.0

anorexia; and seborrhea. In infants under 6 months of age, the symptoms are seborrheic dermatitis (cradle cap) and alopecia (hair loss). In fact, the underlying factor for cradle cap—a common condition that may be associated with excessive oiliness (seborrhea) and scales—in infants appears to be a biotin deficiency, due to the absence of normal intestinal flora. A number of studies have demonstrated successful treatment of cradle cap with supplements of biotin in both the nursing mother and the infant.

The best sources of biotin are cheese, organ meats, and soybeans; good sources are cauliflower, eggs, mushrooms, nuts, peanuts, and whole wheat (see Table 3.12). Raw egg whites contain avidin, a protein that binds biotin and prevents its absorption. There is no official RDA for biotin, but a daily intake of 30 to 100 μg is believed to be adequate.

Vitamin C Vitamin C is perhaps the most publicized vitamin. The primary role of vitamin C is in the manufacture of collagen, the main protein substance of the human body. Specifically, vitamin C is involved in joining a portion of a molecule of water to the amino acid proline to form

Table 3.12 Biotin Content of Selected Foods, in Micrograms (μg) per 3½-oz (100-g) Serving

Yeast, brewer's	200	Peanut butter	39	Split peas	18
Liver, beef	96	Walnuts	37	Almonds	18
Soy flour	70	Peanuts, roasted	34	Cauliflower	17
Soybeans	61	Barley	31	Mushrooms	16
Rice bran	60	Pecans	27	Whole-wheat cereal	16
Rice germ	58	Oatmeal	24	Lentils	13
Rice polishings	57	Blackeye peas	21	Brown rice	12

hydroxyproline. The result is a very stable collagen structure. Since collagen is such an important protein in the structures that hold our body together (connective tissue, cartilage, tendons, and so on), vitamin C is vital for wound repair, healthy gums, and the prevention of easy bruising. In cases of scurvy or severe vitamin C deficiency, the classic symptoms are bleeding gums, poor wound healing, and extensive bruising. In addition to these symptoms, susceptibility to infection, hysteria, and depression are hallmark features. In addition to its role in collagen metabolism, vitamin C is also critical to immune function, the manufacture of certain neural transmitting substances and hormones, and the absorption and utilization of other nutritional factors. Vitamin C is also a very important nutritional antioxidant.

Numerous experimental, clinical, and population studies have shown that increased vitamin C intake produces a number of beneficial effects, including reducing cancer rates, boosting immunity, protecting against pollution and cigarette smoke, enhancing wound repair, increasing life expectancy, and reducing the risk for cataracts. Many claims have also been made about the role of vitamin C (ascorbic acid) in enhancing the immune system, especially with regard to preventing and treating the common cold. Despite numerous positive clinical and experimental studies, however, this effect remains hotly debated. From a biochemical viewpoint, considerable evidence indicates that vitamin C plays a vital role in many immune mechanisms. The high concentration of vitamin C in white blood cells, particularly lymphocytes, is rapidly depleted during infection, and a relative vitamin C deficiency may ensue if vitamin C is not regularly replenished.

Vitamin C has been shown to increase many different immune functions, including enhancing white blood cell function and activity and increasing interferon levels, antibody responses, antibody levels, secretion of thymic hormones, and integrity of ground substance. Vitamin C also possesses many biochemical effects very similar to interferon, the body's natural antiviral and anticancer compound.

During times of chemical, emotional, psychological, or physiological stress, the urinary excretion of vitamin C increases, signifying an increased need for vitamin C during these times. Examples of chemical stressors include cigarette smoke, pollutants, and allergens. Extra vitamin C in the form of supplementation or increased intake of vitamin C–rich foods is often recommended to keep the immune system working properly during times of stress. In certain instances, vitamin C supplementation is the only way to meet the concentrations needed for particular health conditions. For example, it is a good idea for cancer patients to supplement their diet with additional vitamin C (usually 3 to 8 grams daily), as well as to consume vitamin C–rich foods—especially vegetable juices, because they are also rich sources of carotenes. Other conditions for which extra vitamin C is often recommended include infections, allergies, cataracts, high cholesterol levels, high blood pressure, diabetes, and hepatitis. It is important that flavonoids be administered at the same time.

The debate over how much vitamin C is required by humans is ongoing. At one end of the spectrum, two-time Nobel Prize winner Linus Pauling and his followers recommend an intake somewhere between 2 and 9 grams a day during periods of health and even higher doses during times of stress or illness. At the other end of the spectrum, the RDA has been established at 60 mg for adults. While I lean toward Pauling's recommendation, I must stress that you should not rely on supplements to meet all your vitamin C requirements. Vitamin C–rich foods are rich in compounds such as flavonoids and carotenes that enhance the effects of vitamin C and exert favorable effects of their own.

While most people think of citrus fruits as being the best source of vitamin C, vegetables also contain high levels, especially broccoli, peppers, potatoes, and Brussels sprouts (see Table 3.13). Vitamin C is destroyed by exposure to air, so eating fresh foods as quickly as possible is the very best. Although a salad from a salad bar is a relatively healthful choice, the vitamin C content of the fruits and vegetables is only a fraction of what it would have been if the salad had just been made fresh. For example,

Table 3.13 Vitamin C Content of Selected Foods, in Milligrams (mg) per 3½-oz (100-g) Serving

Acerola	1,300	Strawberries	59	Okra	31
Peppers, red chili	369	Papayas	56	Tangerines	31
Guavas	242	Spinach	51	New Zealand spinach	30
Peppers, red sweet	190	Oranges & juice	50	Oysters	30
Kale leaves	186	Cabbage	47	Lima beans, young	29
Parsley	172	Lemon juice	46	Black-eyed peas	29
Collard leaves	152	Grapefruit & juice	38	Soybeans	29
Turnip greens	139	Elderberries	36	Green peas	27
Peppers, green sweet	128	Liver, calf	36	Radishes	26
Broccoli	113	Turnips	36	Raspberries	25
Brussels sprouts	102	Mangoes	35	Chinese cabbage	25
Mustard greens	97	Asparagus	33	Yellow summer squash	25
Watercress	79	Cantaloupe	33	Loganberries	24
Cauliflower	78	Swiss chard	32	Honeydew melons	23
Persimmons	66	Green onions	32	Tomatoes	23
Cabbage, red	61	Liver, beef	31	Liver, pork	23

SOURCE: "Nutritive Value of American Foods in Common Units," U.S.D.A. Agriculture Handbook No. 456.

freshly sliced cucumbers, if left standing, lose between 41 and 49 percent of their vitamin C content within the first 3 hours. A sliced cantaloupe, if left uncovered in the refrigerator, loses 35 percent of its vitamin C content in less than 24 hours.

Minerals

At least 22 different minerals are important in human nutrition. Along with vitamins, minerals function as components of body enzymes. Minerals are also needed for proper composition of bone and blood and for maintenance of normal cell function. Minerals are classified into two categories—major and minor—based on intake level, not on necessity. If a mineral is required at an intake level of greater than 100 mg per day, it is considered a major mineral. The major minerals include calcium, phosphorus, potassium, sodium, chloride, magnesium, and sulfur. The minor (or trace) minerals include boron, chromium, cobalt, copper, fluoride, iodine, iron, manganese, molybdenum, selenium, silicon, vanadium, and zinc. Figure 3.12 shows the quantities of the 11 most common minerals in the body.

Plants incorporate minerals from the soil into their own tissues. For this reason, fruits, vegetables, grains, legumes, nuts, and seeds are often excellent sources of minerals. The minerals, as they occur in the earth, are inorganic—lifeless. In plants, however, most minerals are complexed with organic molecules. This usually results in better mineral absorption, although some plant compounds complex minerals so tightly that they cannot be absorbed. Juicing is thought to allow even better mineral absorption compared to the intact fruit or vegetable because it liberates the minerals into a highly bio-available medium and separates the minerals from fiber constituents that can interfere with absorption. Green leafy vegetables are the best source for many minerals, especially calcium.

Major Minerals

Calcium Calcium is the most abundant mineral in the body. It constitutes from 1.5 to 2 percent of the total body weight, with more than 99 percent of this calcium being present in the bones. In addition to its major function in building and maintaining bones and teeth, calcium is also important in the activity of many enzymes in the body. Contraction of muscles, release of neurotransmitters, regulation of heartbeat, and clotting of blood all depend on calcium.

The current RDA for calcium is 1,000 mg for adults. There has been

Figure 3.12 Total body mineral content.

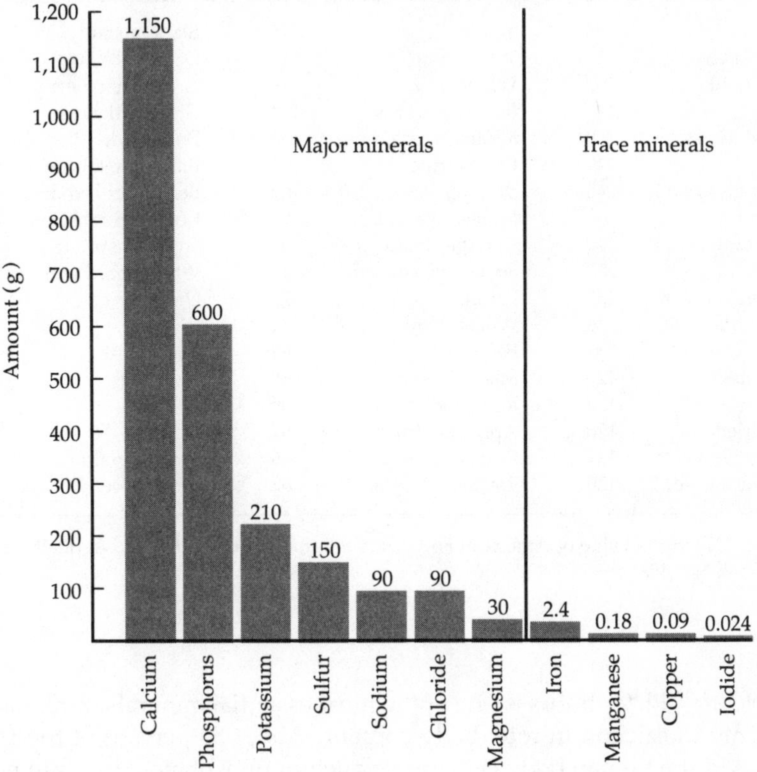

considerable concern that this recommendation may be inadequate to maintain the integrity of the bone, especially during periods of growth, pregnancy, and lactation. Preadolescent growing children may need even more calcium than an adult. The recommendation for this group is 1,200 mg of calcium per day. During pregnancy and lactation, the recommendation is also 1,200 mg per day.

Calcium deficiency in children may lead to rickets, resulting in bone deformities and growth retardation. In adults, calcium deficiency may lead to osteomalacia or softening of the bone. Extremely low levels of calcium in the blood may result in muscle spasms and leg cramps. It is also generally well accepted that low calcium intake contributes greatly to high blood pressure and osteoporosis (see pages 310 and 327–330 respectively). Table 3.14 lists the calcium content of some selected foods.

Table 3.14 Calcium Content of Selected Foods, in Milligrams (mg) per 3½-oz (100-g) Serving

Kelp	1,093	Yogurt	120	Black currant	60
Cheddar cheese	750	Wheat bran	119	Dates	59
Carob flour	352	Whole milk	118	Green snap beans	56
Dulse	296	Buckwheat, raw	114	Globe artichoke	51
Collard leaves	250	Sesame seeds, hulled	110	Prunes, dried	51
Kale	249	Olives, ripe	106	Pumpkin/squash seeds	51
Turnip greens	246	Broccoli	103	Beans, cooked dry	50
Almonds	234	English walnuts	99	Common cabbage	49
Yeast, brewer's	210	Cottage cheese	94	Soybean sprouts	48
Parsley	203	Soybeans, cooked	73	Wheat, hard winter	46
Dandelion greens	187	Pecans	73	Orange	41
Brazil nuts	186	Wheat germ	72	Celery	41
Watercress	151	Peanuts	69	Cashews	38
Goat's milk	129	Miso	68	Rye grain	38
Tofu	128	Romaine lettuce	68	Carrot	37
Figs, dried	126	Apricots, dried	67	Barley	34
Buttermilk	121	Rutabaga	66	Sweet potato	32
Sunflower seeds	120	Raisins	62	Brown rice	32

SOURCE: "Nutritive Value of American Foods in Common Units," U.S.D.A. Agriculture Handbook No. 456.

Phosphorus Phosphorus is one of the most essential minerals, ranking second only to calcium in total body content. About 80 percent of the phosphorus in the human body is found as calcium phosphate crystals in bones and teeth. However, phosphorus participates in many other body functions as well. Specifically, phosphorus is required for use in energy metabolism, DNA synthesis, and calcium absorption and utilization.

Phosphorus is readily available in most foods, especially high-protein foods. More important than the total phosphorus intake in a diet is the ratio of calcium to phosphorus. A diet with too little calcium and too much phosphorus has been linked to osteoporosis. Foods low in calcium but high in phosphorus include red meats, poultry, and soft drinks. The ratio of calcium to phosphorus in red meats and poultry is generally 1 to 20 while the level of phosphorus per serving in soft drinks is typically 500 mg, with virtually no calcium. The RDA for phosphorus is equal to the RDA of calcium.

Magnesium Magnesium is an extremely important mineral. Next to potassium, it is the second most common mineral in our cells. Magnesium functions very closely with calcium and phosphorus. Approximately 60 percent of the magnesium in the body is found in bone; 26 percent in muscle; and the remainder in soft tissue and body fluids. The functions of magnesium primarily center on its ability to activate many enzymes. Like potassium, it is also involved in maintaining the electrical charge of cells, particularly of muscle and nerve cells. Magnesium is involved in many cellular functions, including energy production, protein formation, and cellular replication.

Magnesium deficiency is characterized by symptoms quite similar to those of potassium deficiency: mental confusion, irritability, weakness, heart disturbances, and problems in nerve conduction and muscle contraction. Other symptoms of magnesium deficiency may include muscle cramps, loss of appetite, insomnia, and a predisposition toward stress.

Magnesium deficiency is extremely common in the geriatric population and in women during the premenstrual period. Magnesium deficiency is often secondary to factors that reduce absorption or increase secretion, such as high calcium intake, alcohol, surgery, diuretics, liver disease, kidney disease, and oral contraceptive use.

The RDA for magnesium is 350 mg per day for adult males and 300 mg per day for adult females. For pregnant and lactating women, the recommended allowance is 450 mg per day. Many nutritional experts feel that the ideal intake for magnesium should be based on body weight (6 mg/kg body weight). For a 110-pound person, the recommendation would be 300 mg; for a 154-pound person, 420 mg; and for a 200-pound person, 540 mg.

The average intake of magnesium by healthy adults in the United States ranges between 143 and 266 mg per day. This is obviously far below the RDA. Food choices are the main reason. Since magnesium occurs abundantly in whole foods, most nutritionists and dieticians assume that most Americans get enough magnesium in their diet. But most Americans do not eat whole, natural foods; instead, they consume large quantities of processed foods. Since food processing refines out a very large portion of the natural magnesium content, most Americans do not get the RDA for magnesium. Low levels of magnesium in the diet and in our bodies increase our susceptibility to various ailments, including heart disease, high blood pressure, kidney stones, cancer, insomnia, PMS, and menstrual cramps.

Magnesium's role in preventing heart disease and kidney stones is the most widely accepted by medical experts. Individuals dying suddenly of heart attacks have been shown to have very low levels of magnesium in their heart. Magnesium is extremely important to the heart, both in terms of energy production and contraction of heart muscle. A magnesium deficiency may cause a heart attack by producing a spasm of the coronary arteries, thereby reducing the flow of blood and oxygen to the heart. Magnesium also increases the solubility of calcium in the urine, thereby

Table 3.15 Magnesium Content of Selected Foods, in Milligrams (mg) per 3½-oz (100-g) Serving

Kelp	760	Soybeans, cooked	88	Potato with skin	34
Wheat bran	490	Brown rice	88	Crab	34
Wheat germ	336	Figs, dried	71	Banana	33
Almonds	270	Apricots, dried	62	Sweet potato	31
Cashews	267	Dates	58	Blackberry	30
Molasses, blackstrap	258	Collard leaves	57	Beets	25
Yeast, brewer's	231	Shrimp	51	Broccoli	24
Buckwheat	229	Corn, sweet	48	Cauliflower	24
Brazil nuts	225	Avocado	45	Carrot	23
Dulse	220	Cheddar cheese	45	Celery	22
Filberts	184	Parsley	41	Beef	21
Peanuts	175	Prunes, dried	40	Asparagus	20
Millet	162	Sunflower seeds	38	Chicken	19
Wheat grain	160	Common beans, cooked	37	Green pepper	18
Pecan	142	Barley	37	Winter squash	17
English walnuts	131	Dandelion greens	36	Cantaloupe	16
Rye	115	Garlic	36	Eggplant	16
Tofu	111	Raisins	35	Tomato	14
Coconut meat, dry	90	Green peas, fresh	35	Milk	13

preventing stone formation. Supplementing magnesium in the diet has been demonstrated to be effective in preventing recurrences of kidney stones.

The best dietary sources of magnesium are tofu, legumes, seeds, nuts, whole grains, and green leafy vegetables (see Table 3.15). Fish, meat, milk, and most commonly eaten fruits are quite low in magnesium. Most Americans consume a low-magnesium diet because their diet is high in refined foods, meat, and dairy products.

Potassium, Sodium, and Chloride Potassium, sodium, and chloride are electrolytes—mineral salts that can conduct electricity when they are dissolved in water. They are so intricately related that they are usually discussed together in nutrition textbooks. Electrolytes are always found in pairs; a positive ion like sodium or potassium is always accompanied by a negative ion like chloride. Electrolytes function in the maintenance of water balance and distribution, acid–base balance, muscle and nerve cell function, heart function, and kidney and adrenal function.

Over 95 percent of the potassium in the body is found within cells. In contrast, most of the sodium in the body is located outside the cells—in the blood and in other fluids. How does this happen? Cells actually pump sodium out and potassium in via the "sodium–potassium pump." This pump is found in the membranes of all cells in the body. One of its most important functions is to prevent the swelling of cells. If sodium is not pumped out, water accumulates within the cell, causing it to swell and ultimately burst.

The sodium–potassium pump also functions to maintain the electrical charge within the cell. This is particularly important to muscle and nerve cells. During nerve transmission and muscle contraction, potassium exits the cell and sodium enters, resulting in a change in electrical charge that triggers a nerve impulse or muscle contraction. It is not surprising that a potassium deficiency affects muscles and nerves first.

The balance of sodium, potassium, and chloride is extremely important to human health. Too much sodium in the diet can lead to disruption of this balance. Numerous studies have demonstrated that a low-potassium, high-sodium diet plays a major role in the development of cancer and cardiovascular disease (heart disease, high blood pressure, strokes, and so on). Conversely, a diet high in potassium and low in sodium protects against these diseases, and in the case of high blood pressure it can be therapeutic.

Excessive consumption of dietary sodium chloride (table salt), coupled with diminished dietary potassium, is a common cause of high blood pressure. Numerous studies have shown that sodium restriction alone does not improve blood-pressure control in most people; it must be accompanied by a high potassium intake. In our society only 5 percent of sodium intake comes from the natural ingredients in food. Prepared foods contribute 45 percent of our sodium intake, another 45 percent is added in cooking, and a final 5 percent is added as a condiment. All that the body requires in most instances is the salt that is supplied in the food.

Most Americans have a potassium-to-sodium (K:Na) ratio of less than 1:2. This means that most people ingest twice as much sodium as they do potassium. Researchers recommend a dietary potassium-to-sodium ratio of greater than 5:1 to maintain health. This represents a potassium intake 10 times higher than the average intake. However, even this may not be optimal. A natural diet rich in fruits and vegetables can produce a K:Na ratio greater than 100:1, since most fruits and vegetables have a K:Na ratio of at least 50:1. For example, as Table 3.16 indicates, here are the average K:Na ratios for several common fresh fruits and vegetables:

Carrots 6:1
Potatoes 130:1
Apples 91:1
Bananas 440:1
Oranges 263:1.

Table 3.16 Potassium/Sodium Content of Selected Foods, in Milligrams (mg) per Serving

Food	*Portion Size*	*Potassium (mg)*	*Sodium (mg)*
Fresh Vegetables			
Asparagus	½ cup	165	1
Avocado	½	680	5
Carrot, raw	1	225	38
Corn	½ cup	136	trace
Lima beans, cooked	½ cup	581	1
Potato	1 medium	782	6
Spinach, cooked	½ cup	292	45
Tomato, raw	1 medium	444	5
Fresh Fruits			
Apple	1 medium	182	2
Apricots, dried	¼ cup	318	9
Banana	1 medium	440	1
Cantaloupe	¼ melon	341	17
Orange	1 medium	263	1
Peach	1 medium	308	2
Plums	5	150	1
Strawberries	½ cup	122	trace
Unprocessed Meats			
Chicken, light meat	3 ounces	350	54
Lamb, leg	3 ounces	241	53
Roast beef	3 ounces	224	49
Pork	3 ounces	219	48
Fish			
Cod	3 ounces	345	93
Flounder	3 ounces	498	201
Haddock	3 ounces	297	150
Salmon	3 ounces	378	99
Tuna, drained solids	3 ounces	225	38

Although sodium and chloride are important, potassium is the most important dietary electrolyte. In addition to functioning as an electrolyte, potassium is essental for the conversion of blood sugar into glycogen—the storage form of blood sugar found in the muscles and in the liver. A potassium shortage results in lower levels of stored glycogen. Because glycogen is used by exercising muscles for energy, a potassium deficiency will produce great fatigue and muscle weakness. These are typically the first signs of potassium deficiency.

A potassium deficiency is also characterized by mental confusion, irritability, heart disturbances, and problems in nerve conduction and muscle contraction. Dietary potassium deficiency is typically caused by a diet low in fresh fruits and vegetables but high in sodium. It is more common to see dietary potassium deficiency in the elderly. Dietary potassium deficiency is less common than deficiency due to excessive fluid loss (sweating, diarrhea, or urination) or due to the use of diuretics, laxatives, aspirin, and other drugs.

The amount of potassium lost in sweat can be quite significant, especially if the exercise is prolonged in a warm environment. Athletes or people who regularly exercise have higher potassium needs. Because up to 3 g of potassium can be lost in one day by sweating, a daily intake of at least 4 g of potassium is recommended for these individuals.

The estimated safe and adequate daily dietary intake of potassium, as set by the Committee on Recommended Daily Allowances, is 1.9 to 5.6 g. If body potassium requirements are not being met through diet, supplementation is essential to good health. This is particularly true for the elderly and for athletes. Potassium salts are commonly prescribed by physicians in the dosage range of 1.5 to 3.0 g per day. However, potassium salts can cause nausea, vomiting, diarrhea, and ulcers. These effects are not seen when potassium levels are increased entirely through the diet. This highlights the advantages of using juices, foods, or food-based potassium supplements to meet the human body's high potassium requirements.

Can you take too much potassium? Of course, but most people can handle any excess of potassium. The exception is people with kidney disease. These people do not handle potassium in the normal way and are likely to experience heart disturbances and other consequences of potassium toxicity. Individuals with kidney disorders usually need to restrict their potassium intake and should follow the dietary recommendations of their physicians.

Sulfur Sulfur, as a component of four amino acids (methionine, cysteine, cystine, and taurine), performs a number of important functions. It is found in high concentrations in the protein structure of the joints, hair, nails, and skin. The hormone insulin is rich in sulfur-containing amino acids. The detoxifying compound glutathione is also a sulfur-containing compound.

Although there is no official RDA for sulfur, it is a critical nutrient. Certain health conditions, such as arthritis and liver disorders, may be improved by increasing the intake of such sulfur-rich foods as legumes, whole grains, garlic, onions, Brussels sprouts, and cabbage.

Minor (Trace) Minerals

Boron It has already been mentioned that vegetarians are at lower risk for osteoporosis. In addition to vitamin K_1 and the high levels of many major minerals found in plant foods, the high content of the trace mineral boron in a vegetarian diet may be partly responsible for this protective effect. Boron has been shown to have a positive effect on calcium and active estrogen levels in postmenopausal women, the group at highest risk for developing osteoporosis. In one study, supplementing the diet of postmenopausal women with 3 mg of boron per day reduced urinary calcium excretion by 44 percent and dramatically increased the levels of 17-beta-estradiol, the most biologically active estrogen. It appears that boron is required to activate certain hormones, including estrogen and vitamin D. Since fruits and vegetables are the main dietary sources of boron, diets low in these foods may be deficient in boron. Boron has also been shown to be of benefit in arthritis.

Chromium Chromium functions in the "glucose tolerance factor," a critical enzyme system involved in blood-sugar regulation. Either a lack or an excess of blood sugar (glucose) in the body can be devastating. For this reason, the body strives to maintain blood-sugar levels within a narrow range, with the help of homones like insulin and glucagon. Considerable evidence now indicates that chromium levels are a major determinant of insulin sensitivity. If chromium levels are low, blood-sugar levels may remain high due to a lack of sensitivity to insulin. Insulin promotes the absorption and utilization of glucose by the cells. Insulin insensitivity is a classic feature in obesity and diabetes.

Reversing a chromium deficiency by supplementing the diet with chromium has been demonstrated to lower overall body weight, increase lean body mass, improve glucose tolerance, and decrease total cholesterol and triglyceride levels. All these effects appear to be due to increased insulin sensitivity.

Although there is no RDA for chromium, we seem to need at least 200 μg per day in our diet. Chromium levels can be depleted by consumption of refined sugars and white flour products, and by a lack of exercise. Table 3.17 lists the chromium content of various foods.

Copper Copper functions as an important factor in the manufacture of hemoglobin, collagen structures (including joints and arteries), and en-

Table 3.17 Chromium Content of Selected Foods, in Micrograms (μg) per 3½-oz (100-g) Serving

Yeast, brewer's	112	Green pepper	19	Carrots	9
Liver, calf's	55	Apple	14	Navy beans, dry	8
Whole-wheat bread	42	Butter	13	Orange	5
Wheat bran	38	Parsnips	13	Blueberries	5
Rye bread	30	Cornmeal	12	Green beans	4
Potatoes	24	Banana	10	Cabbage	4
Wheat germ	23	Spinach	10		

ergy. Copper deficiency is characterized by anemia, fatigue, poor wound healing, elevated cholesterol levels, and poor immune function.

Since a deficiency of copper produces a marked elevation of cholesterol, copper deficiency has been suggested to play a major role in the development of atherosclerosis. Evidence indicates that copper levels are typically marginal in U.S. diets, and recent surveys show that less than 25 percent of Americans appear to be meeting the RDA of 2 mg. On the other hand, there is also conflicting evidence that, because of copper-lined water pipes, many Americans are getting too much copper. Excessive copper levels have been linked to schizophrenia, learning disabilities, premenstrual syndrome, and anxiety.

Many of the potential problems of copper can be offset by zinc, since zinc and copper compete for absorption sites. If there is too much zinc, copper absorption will be decreased, and vice versa. In nature, foods rich in copper are typically even higher in zinc; nuts and legumes are good examples of this (see Table 3.18).

Table 3.18 Copper Content of Selected Foods, in Milligrams (mg) per 3½-oz (100-g) Serving

Brazil nuts	2.3	Butter	0.4	Corn oil	0.2
Almonds	1.4	Rye grain	0.4	Ginger root	0.2
Hazelnuts	1.3	Barley	0.4	Molasses	0.2
Walnuts	1.3	Olive oil	0.3	Turnips	0.2
Pecans	1.3	Carrot	0.3	Green peas	0.1
Split peas, dry	1.2	Coconut	0.3	Papaya	0.1
Buckwheat	0.8	Garlic	0.3	Apple	0.1
Peanuts	0.8	Millet	0.2		
Sunflower oil	0.5	Whole wheat	0.2		

Iodine The thyroid gland adds iodine to the amino acid tyrosine to create thyroid hormones. A deficiency of iodine results in the development of an enlarged thyroid gland, commonly referred to as a goiter. When the level of iodine is low in the diet and in the blood, it causes the cells of the thyroid gland to become quite large; and eventually the entire gland swells at the base of the neck.

Goiters are estimated to affect over 200 million people worldwide. In all but 4 percent of these cases, the goiter is caused by an iodine deficiency. Iodine deficiency is now quite rare in the United States and other industrialized countries, because of the addition of iodine to table salt. Adding iodine to table salt began in Michigan, where in 1924 the goiter rate was an incredible 47 percent.

Few people in the United States are now considered iodine deficient, and yet the rate of goiter is still relatively high (5 to 6 percent) in certain high-risk areas. The goiter in these people is probably a result of excessive ingestion of certain foods that block iodine utilization. These foods are known as goitrogens and include such foods as turnips, cabbage, mustard, cassava root, soybean, peanuts, pine nuts, and millet. Cooking usually inactivates goitrogens.

The recommended dietary allowance (RDA) for iodine in adults is quite small, 150 μg. Seafoods, including seaweeds like kelp, are nature's richest sources of iodine. However, in the United States the majority of iodine is derived from the use of iodized salt (70 μg of iodine per gram of salt). Sea salt in comparison has little iodine. Due to the high level of consumption in the United States, the average American intake of iodine is estimated to be over 600 μg per day.

Too much iodine can actually inhibit thyroid gland synthesis. For this reason and because the only function of iodine in the body is for thyroid hormone synthesis, dietary levels or supplementation of iodine should not exceed 1 mg (1,000 μg) per day for any length of time.

Iron Iron is critical to human life. It plays a central role in the hemoglobin molecule of our red blood cells (RBC), where it functions in transporting oxygen from the lungs to the body's tissues and in transporting carbon dioxide from the tissues to the lungs. Iron also participates in energy production and metabolism, including DNA synthesis, by several key enzymes.

Iron deficiency is the most common nutrient deficiency in the United States. The groups at highest risk for iron deficiency are infants under 2 years of age, teenage girls, pregnant women, and the elderly. Studies have found evidence of iron deficiency in as many as 30 to 50 percent of people in these groups. For example, some degree of iron deficiency occurs in 35 to 58 percent of young, healthy women. During pregnancy, the percentage is even higher.

Iron deficiency may be due to an increased iron requirement, decreased dietary intake, diminished absorption or utilization of iron, blood loss, or a combination of these factors. Increased requirements for iron occur during the growth spurts of infancy and adolescence, and during pregnancy and lactation. Currently, the vast majority of pregnant women are routinely given iron supplements during their pregnancy, since the dramatically increased need for iron during pregnancy cannot usually be met through diet alone. Inadequate intake of iron is common in many parts of the world, especially in areas where people consume primarily a vegetarian diet. Typical infant diets in developed countries (high in milk and cereals) are also low in iron. An adolescent who subsists on a "junk food" diet is at high risk for iron deficiency. However, the population at greatest risk for a diet deficient in iron is the low-income elderly population, in particular because of decreased absorption of iron. Decreased absorption of iron is often due to a lack of hydrochloric acid secretion in the stomach, an extremely common condition in the elderly. Other causes of decreased absorption include chronic diarrhea or malabsorption, surgical removal of the stomach, and antacid use. Blood loss is the most common cause of iron deficiency in women of childbearing age. This is most often due to excessive menstrual bleeding. Interestingly, iron deficiency is itself a common cause of excessive menstrual blood loss. Other common causes of blood loss include bleeding from peptic ulcers, hemorrhoids, and donating blood.

The negative effects of iron deficiency are due largely to the impaired delivery of oxygen to the tissues and the impaired activity of iron-containing enzymes in various tissues. Iron deficiency can lead to anemia, excessive menstrual blood loss, learning disabilities, impaired immune function, and decreased energy levels and physical performance.

Anemia refers to a condition in which the blood is deficient in red blood cells or in the hemoglobin (iron-containing) portion of red blood cells. The primary function of the red blood cell is to transport oxygen from the lungs to the tissues of the body and to exchange it for carbon dioxide. The symptoms of anemia, such as extreme fatigue, reflect insufficient oxygen being delivered to tissues and a resulting buildup of carbon dioxide.

Although iron deficiency is the most common cause of anemia, anemia is the last stage of iron deficiency. Iron-dependent enzymes involved in energy production and metabolism are the first to be affected by low iron levels. Serum ferritin is the best laboratory test for determining the body's iron stores.

Several researchers have clearly demonstrated that even slight iron-deficiency anemia leads to a reduction in a person's physical work capacity and productivity. Nutrition surveys done in the United States have indicated that iron deficiency is a major impairment of health and work capacity and consequently a source of economic loss to the individual and the country. Dietary supplementation with iron has yielded rapid improvements in work capacity in previously iron-deficient individuals. Impaired physical performance due to iron deficiency does not depend on fully developed anemia. Again, the iron-dependent enzymes involved in energy production and metabolism are impaired long before anemia occurs.

The RDA for iron is 10 mg for males and 15 mg for females. There are two forms of dietary iron: "heme" iron and "nonheme" iron. Heme iron is iron bound to hemoglobin and myoglobin. It is found in animal products and is the most efficiently absorbed form of iron. Nonheme iron is found in plant foods. Compared to heme iron, it is poorly absorbed by the body. Table 3.19 lists the iron content of selected foods.

Manganese Manganese functions in many enzyme systems, including enzymes involved in blood-sugar control, energy metabolism, and thyroid hormone function. Manganese also functions in the antioxidant enzyme superoxide dismutase or SOD. This enzyme is responsible for preventing the deleterious effects of the superoxide free radical from destroying cellular components. Without SOD, cells are highly susceptible to damage and inflammation. Manganese supplementation has been shown to increase SOD activity, indicating increased antioxidant activity. Clinically,

Table 3.19 Iron Content of Selected Foods, in Milligrams (mg) per 3½-oz (100-g) Serving

Kelp	100.0	Cashews	3.8	Peanuts	2.1
Yeast, brewer's	17.3	Raisins	3.5	Tofu	1.9
Molasses, blackstrap	16.1	Jerusalem artichoke	3.4	Green peas	1.8
Wheat bran	14.9	Brazil nuts	3.4	Brown rice	1.6
Pumpkin & squash seeds	11.2	Beet greens	3.3	Olives, ripe	1.6
Wheat germ	9.4	Swiss chard	3.2	Artichoke	1.3
Liver, beef	8.8	Dandelion greens	3.1	Mung bean sprouts	1.3
Sunflower seeds	7.1	English walnuts	3.1	Broccoli	1.1
Millet	6.8	Dates	3.0	Currants	1.1
Parsley	6.2	Beans, cooked dry	2.7	Whole-wheat bread	1.1
Clams	6.1	Sesame seeds, hulled	2.4	Cauliflower	1.1
Almonds	4.7	Pecans	2.4		
Prunes, dried	3.9	Lentils	2.1		

Table 3.20 Manganese Content of Selected Foods, in Milligrams (mg) per 3½-oz (100-g) Serving

Pecans	3.5	Walnuts	0.8	Brussels sprouts	0.3
Brazil nuts	2.8	Spinach, fresh	0.8	Oatmeal	0.3
Almonds	2.5	Peanuts	0.7	Cornmeal	0.2
Barley	1.8	Oats	0.6	Millet	0.2
Rye	1.3	Raisins	0.5	Carrots	0.16
Buckwheat	1.3	Turnip greens	0.5	Broccoli	0.15
Split peas, dry	1.3	Rhubarb	0.5	Brown rice	0.14
Whole wheat	1.1	Beet greens	0.4	Whole-wheat bread	0.14

manganese is used to treat strains, sprains, and inflammation. Evidence suggests that patients with rheumatoid arthritis and (presumably) other chronic inflammatory diseases have an increased need for manganese. No trials have yet been done with manganese and RA, but supplementation appears to be indicated.

A low level of manganese has also been linked to epilepsy. This link was first suggested in 1963, when it was observed that manganese-deficient rats were more susceptible to seizures than were manganese-replete animals, and that manganese-deficient animals exhibited epileptic-like brain wave tracings. This prompted researchers to look at manganese concentrations in epileptics. Low manganese levels in whole blood and in hair have been found in epileptics, and patients who have the lowest levels typically have the highest rates of seizure activity.

Manganese plays a significant role in cerebral function, as it is a critical metal for glucose utilization within the neuron, for adenylate cyclase activity, and for neurotransmitter control. Obviously, for optimal central nervous system function, proper manganese levels must be maintained. A high-manganese diet or manganese supplementation may be helpful in controlling seizure activity for some patients.

Although there is no specific RDA for manganese, most people are thought to require between 2 and 5 mg per day. This can easily be met by regularly consuming nuts and whole grains, which are the best natural sources of manganese (see Table 3.20).

Molybdenum Molybdenum functions as a component in several enzymes, including those involved in alcohol detoxification, uric acid formation, and sulfur metabolism. A molybdenum deficiency has been suggested as a cause for sulfite sensitivities, because sulfite oxidase, the enzyme that detoxifies sulfites, is molybdenum-dependent. The average diet contains

Table 3.21 Molybdenum Content of Selected Foods, in Milligrams (mg) per 3½-oz (100-g) Serving

Lentils	155	Rye bread	50	Molasses	19
Split peas	130	Corn	45	Cantaloupe	16
Cauliflower	120	Barley	42	Apricots	14
Green peas	110	Whole wheat	36	Raisins	10
Yeast, brewer's	109	Whole-wheat bread	32	Butter	10
Wheat germ	100	Potatoes	30	Strawberries	7
Spinach	100	Onions	25	Carrots	5
Brown rice	75	Peanuts	25	Cabbage	5
Garlic	70	Coconut	25		
Oats	60	Green beans	21		

between 50 and 500 μg of molybdenum per day. Legumes and whole grains are the richest sources of this element (see Table 3.21).

Selenium Selenium, as a component of the antioxidant enzyme, glutathione peroxidase, works with vitamin E in preventing free-radical damage to cell membranes. Low levels of selenium put people at higher risk for cancer, cardiovascular disease, inflammatory diseases, and other conditions associated with increased free-radical damage, including premature aging and cataract formation. Selenium supplementation is often used in treating these disorders.

Although there is no specific RDA for selenium, a daily intake of 200 μg is often recommended. At high intake levels (daily intake in excess of 2,000 μg), selenium can produce toxicity. Table 3.22 identifies the selenium content of selected foods.

Silicon Silicon is responsible for crosslinking collagen strands, which contribute greatly to the strength and integrity of the connective tissue matrix of bone. Since silicon concentrations are increased at calcification sites in growing bone, this process may depend on the presence of adequate levels

Table 3.22 Selenium Content of Selected Foods, in Micrograms (μg) per 3½-oz (100-g) Serving

Wheat germ	111	Bran	63	Turnips	27
Brazil nuts	103	Red Swiss chard	57	Garlic	25
Barley	66	Oats	56	Barley	24
Whole-wheat bread	66	Brown rice	39	Orange juice	19

of silicon. It is not known whether the typical American diet provides adequate amounts of silicon. In patients with osteoporosis or in situations where accelerated bone regeneration is desired, silicon requirements may be increased. An increased need for silicon is best met by increasing the consumption of unrefined whole grains, because they are a rich source of absorbable silicon (silicic acid).

Vanadium Vanadium was named after an appellation of Freyja, the Norse goddess of beauty, fertility, and luster. Researchers disagree about whether vanadium is an essential trace mineral in human nutrition. Although it has been suggested to function in hormone, cholesterol, and blood-sugar metabolism, no specific deficiency signs have been reported. Some researchers have speculated that vanadium deficiency may contribute to elevated cholesterol levels and faulty blood-sugar control, manifested as either diabetes or hypoglycemia. Making things more difficult is the fact that vanadium exists in the body in five different forms, the most biologically significant of which are vanadyl and vanadate.

Since vanadium can be a relatively toxic mineral and since it has no obvious role as yet discovered in humans, there appears to be no need at this time to supplement the dietary intake of vanadium, despite the fact that vanadium supplementation has produced impressive results in rats with diabetes. Until more is known about this mineral, consumers should be wary of vanadium-containing supplements. The major concern is that excessive levels of vanadium have been suspected as a factor in manic-depressive illness, since increased levels of vanadium are found in hair samples from manic patients, and these values fall toward normal levels with recovery. Vanadium, as the vanadate ion, is a strong inhibitor of the sodium–potassium pump. Lithium, the drug of choice for manic-depressive illness, has been reported to reduce this inhibition.

Although Table 3.23 lists the vanadium content of some selected foods,

Table 3.23 Vanadium Content of Selected Foods, in Micrograms (μg) per 3½-oz (100-g) Serving

Buckwheat	100	Corn	15	Onions	5
Parsley	80	Green beans	14	Whole wheat	5
Soybeans	70	Peanut oil	11	Beets	4
Safflower oil	64	Carrots	10	Apples	3
Sunflower seed oil	41	Cabbage	10	Plums	2
Oats	35	Garlic	10	Lettuce	2
Olive oil	30	Tomatoes	6	Millet	2
Sunflower seeds	15	Radishes	5		

it is unclear how meaningful these data are; some studies have shown that greater than 95 percent of ingested vanadium is not absorbed.

Zinc Zinc is a component of over 200 enzymes in our bodies. In fact, zinc functions in more enzymatic reactions than does any other mineral. Although severe zinc deficiency is very rare in developed countries, many individuals in the United States have marginal zinc deficiency. This is particularly true in the elderly population. It may be reflected by increased susceptibility to infection, poor wound healing, a decreased sense of taste or smell, and skin disorders.

Adequate tissue zinc levels are necessary for proper immune system function. Zinc deficiency results in an increased susceptibility to infection. Zinc also appears to be vital for normal thymus gland functioning in the synthesis and secretion of thymic hormones and in the protection of the thymus from cellular damage. Several defects in immune function related to aging are reversible with zinc supplementation—again highlighting the importance of this nutrient to the elderly. Besides stimulating the body's immune system, zinc displays virus-inhibiting activity. In one double-blind clinical study, zinc supplementation reduced the average duration of colds by 7 days.

Zinc is essential for the maintenance of vision, taste, and smell. A zinc deficiency leads to impaired functioning of these special senses. Night-blindness is often due to a zinc deficiency. Loss of the sense of taste and/or smell is a common complaint in the elderly. Zinc supplementation has been shown to improve taste and/or smell acuity in some individuals.

Zinc is required for protein synthesis and cell growth, and therefore for wound healing. Zinc supplementation has been shown to decrease the time needed for wound healing, while a zinc deficiency prolongs it. A high zinc intake is indicated to aid protein synthesis and cell growth following any sort of trauma (burns, surgery, wounds, or the like).

Zinc is critical to healthy male sex hormone and prostate function. Widespread zinc deficiency may contribute to the high rate of prostate enlargement in this country. It is estimated that 50 to 60 percent of men between the ages of 40 and 59 years of age have prostatic enlargement. Zinc supplementation has been shown to reduce the size of the prostate and the associated symptoms in most patients. Male infertility may be caused by a zinc deficiency that leads to a decreased sperm count.

The importance of zinc in normal skin function is well known. Typically serum zinc levels are lower in 13- to 14-year-old males than in any other age group. This group is also the most susceptible to acne. During puberty, the requirement for zinc increases as a result of the increased hormonal production. Some researchers believe that low levels of zinc are re-

Table 3.24 Zinc Content of Selected Foods, in Milligrams (mg) per 3½-oz (100-g) Serving

Oysters, fresh	148.7	Oats	3.2	Turnips	1.2
Pumpkin seeds	7.5	Peanuts	3.2	Parsley	0.9
Ginger root	6.8	Lima beans	3.1	Potatoes	0.9
Pecans	4.5	Almonds	3.1	Garlic	0.6
Split peas, dry	4.2	Walnuts	3.0	Carrots	0.5
Brazil nuts	4.2	Buckwheat	2.5	Whole-wheat bread	0.5
Whole wheat	3.2	Hazel nuts	2.4	Black beans	0.4
Rye	3.2	Green peas	1.6		

sponsible for acne during puberty. Several double-blind studies have confirmed this hypothesis, as zinc supplementation has been shown to be as effective as tetracycline in combating acne, but without the side effects. Zinc appears to be able to normalize some of the hormonal factors responsible for acne.

Optimal zinc levels must be attained for optimum health. Although severe zinc deficiency is quite rare in this country, many individuals consume a diet that is low in zinc. The RDA is 15 mg for men and 12 mg for women. In addition to its presence in oysters, shellfish, fish, and red meats, zinc is found in good amounts in whole grains, legumes, nuts, and seeds (see Table 3.24).

4

Anutrients in Foods

Foods, especially plant foods, contain a wide range of substances often collectively referred to as *anutrients.* Nutrients are classically defined as substances that either provide nourishment or are necessary for body functions or structures. The designation *anutrient* signifies that these compounds are without nutritional benefit. However, although these substances are thought to possess little or no real nutritional value, they do offer profound health benefits. Indeed, anutrients provide many of the known and the unknown benefits of foods. Included in this category are dietary fiber; enzymes; pigments such as carotenes, chlorophyll, and flavonoids; vitamin-like compounds; and minor dietary constituents.

Dietary Fiber

Originally, the definition of *dietary fiber* was restricted to the sum of plant compounds that are not digestible by the secretions of the human digestive tract. But this definition is vague, since it depends on an exact understanding of what exactly is not digestible. For our purposes the term *dietary fiber* refers to the components of plant cell walls as well as to the indigestible residues.

The composition of the plant cell wall varies according to the species of plant. Most plant cell walls contains 35 percent insoluble fiber, 45 percent soluble fiber, 17 percent lignans, 3 percent protein, and 2 percent ash (see Table 4.1). Dietary fiber is a complex of these constituents, and for this reason supplementation of a single component does not substitute for a diet rich in high-fiber foods (see Tables 4.2 and 4.3).

Insoluble Fibers

The best example of an insoluble fiber is wheat bran. Wheat bran is rich in cellulose; and although wheat bran is relatively insoluble in water, it has

Table 4.1 Classification of Dietary Fiber

Fiber Class	*Chemical Structure*	*Sources*	*Physiological Effect*
Cellulose	Unbranched 1-4-beta-D-glucose polymer	Principal plant wall component; wheat bran	Increases fecal weight and size
Noncellulose polysaccharides:			
Hemicellulose	Mixture of pentose and hexose molecules in branching chains	Plant cell walls; oat bran	Same as above; binds bile acids; lowers cholesterol
Gums	Branched-chain uronic acid containing polymers	Karaya; gum arabic	Same as above
Mucilages	Similar to hemicelluloses	Found in endosperm of plant seeds; guar; legumes; psyllium	Hydrocolloids that bind steroids and delay gastric emptying; heavy metal chelation
Pectins	Mixture of methylesterified galacturan, galactan, and arabinose in varying proportions	Citrus rind; apple; onion skin	Same as above
Algal polysaccharides	Polymerized D-mannuronic and L-glucuronic acids	Algin; carrageenan	Same as above
Lignans	Noncarbohydrate polymeric phenylpropene	Woody part of plant: Wood (40–50%) Wheat (25%) Apple (25%) Cabbage (6%)	Antioxidants; anticarcinogenic

Table 4.2 Dietary Fiber Constituents of the Food Groups

Food Group	*Fiber Constituents*
Fruits and vegetables	cellulose, hemicellulose, lignan, pectin substances, cutin, waxes
Grains	cellulose, hemicellulose, lignan, phenolic esters
Nuts, seeds, and legumes	cellulose, hemicellulose, pectin substances, guar gum

Table 4.3 Dietary Fiber Content of Selected Foods

Food	*Serving*	*Calories*	*Fiber (in g)*
Fruits			
Apple (with skin)	1 medium	81	3.5
Banana	1 medium	105	2.4
Cantaloupe	¼ melon	30	1.0
Cherries, sweet	10	49	1.2
Grapefruit	½ medium	38	1.6
Orange	1 medium	62	2.6
Peach (with skin)	1	37	1.9
Pear (with skin)	½ large	61	3.1
Prunes	3	60	3.0
Raisins	¼ cup	106	3.1
Raspberries	½ cup	35	3.1
Strawberries	1 cup	45	3.0
Vegetables, Raw			
Bean sprouts	½ cup	13	1.5
Celery, diced	½ cup	10	1.1
Cucumber	½ cup	8	0.4
Green Pepper	½ cup	9	0.5
Lettuce	1 cup	10	0.9
Mushrooms	½ cup	10	1.5
Spinach	1 cup	8	1.2
Tomato	1 medium	20	1.5
Vegetables, Cooked			
Asparagus, cut	1 cup	30	2.0
Broccoli	1 cup	40	4.4
Brussels sprouts	1 cup	56	4.6
Cabbage, red	1 cup	30	2.8
Carrots	1 cup	48	4.6
Cauliflower	1 cup	28	2.2
Corn	½ cup	87	2.9
Green beans	1 cup	32	3.2
Kale	1 cup	44	2.8
Parsnip	1 cup	102	5.4
Potato (with skin)	1 medium	106	2.5
Potato (without skin)	1 medium	97	1.4

Food	Serving	Calories	Fiber (in g)
Vegetables, Cooked (continued)			
Spinach	1 cup	42	4.2
Sweet potatoes	1 medium	160	3.4
Zucchini	1 cup	22	3.6
Legumes			
Baked beans	½ cup	155	8.8
Kidney beans, cooked	½ cup	110	7.3
Lima beans, cooked	½ cup	64	4.5
Lentils, cooked	½ cup	97	3.7
Navy beans, cooked	½ cup	112	6.0
Peas, dried, cooked	½ cup	115	4.7
Rice, Breads, and Pastas			
Bran muffins	1 muffin	104	2.5
Bread, white	1 slice	78	0.4
Bread, whole-wheat	1 slice	61	1.4
Crisp bread, rye	2 crackers	50	2.0
Rice, brown, cooked	½ cup	97	1.0
Rice, white, cooked	½ cup	82	0.2
Spaghetti, reg., cooked	½ cup	155	1.1
Spaghetti, whole-wheat, cooked	½ cup	155	3.9
Breakfast Cereals			
All-Bran	⅓ cup	71	8.5
Bran Chex	⅔ cup	91	4.6
Corn Bran	⅔ cup	98	5.4
Cornflakes	1¼ cup	110	0.3
Grape-Nuts	¼ cup	101	1.4
Oatmeal	¾ cup	108	1.6
Raisin Bran (type)	⅔ cup	115	4.0
Shredded Wheat	⅔ cup	102	2.6
Nuts			
Almonds	10 nuts	79	1.1
Filberts	10 nuts	54	0.8
Peanuts	10 nuts	105	1.4

the ability to bind water. This ability accounts for its effect of increasing fecal size and weight, thus promoting regular bowel movements. Although cellulose cannot be digested by humans, it is partially digested by the microflora of the gut. This natural fermentation process, which occurs in the colon, results in the degradation of about 50 percent of the cellulose and is an important source of short-chain fatty acids that nourish our intestinal cells.

Soluble Fibers

The majority of fiber in most plant cell walls consists of water-soluble compounds. Included in this class are hemicelluloses, mucilages, gums, and pectin substances. These fiber compounds exert the most beneficial effects. For example, hemicelluloses like those found in oat bran promote regular bowel movements and provide short-chain fatty acids just as cellulose does; but in addition they can lower cholesterol levels.

Mucilages Structurally, mucilages resemble the hemicelluloses, but they are not classed as such due to their unique location in the seed portion of the plant. They are generally found within the inner layer (endosperm) of grains, legumes, nuts, and seeds. Guar gum, found in most legumes (beans), is the most widely studied plant mucilage. Commercially, guar gum is used as a stabilizing, thickening, and film-forming agent in the production of cheese, salad dressings, ice cream, soups, toothpaste, pharmaceutical jelly, lotion, skin cream, and tablets. Guar gum is also used as a laxative.

Guar gum and other mucilages, including psyllium seed husk and glucomannan, are perhaps the most potent cholesterol-lowering agents of gel-forming fibers. In addition, mucilage fibers have been shown to reduce fasting and after-meal glucose and insulin levels in both healthy and diabetic subjects; and they have decreased body weight and hunger ratings when taken with meals by obese subjects.

Pectin and Pectinlike Substances Pectins are found in all plant cell walls, as well as in the outer skin and rind of fruits and vegetables. For example, the rind of an orange contains 30 percent pectin; an apple peel 15 percent; and onion skins 12 percent. The gel-forming properties of pectin are well known to anyone who has made jelly or jam. These same gel-forming qualities are responsible for the cholesterol-lowering effects of pectins. Pectins lower cholesterol by binding it and bile acids in the gut and promoting their excretion.

Lignans Lignans are compounds found in high-fiber foods that show important properties, such as anticancer, antibacterial, antifungal, and antiviral activity. Plant lignans are changed by the gut flora into enterolactone and enterodiol, two compounds that are believed to protect against cancer—particularly breast cancer. Flaxseeds are the most abundant source of lignans. Other good sources are other seeds, grains, and legumes.

Physiological Effects of Dietary Fiber

It is beyond the scope of this chapter to detail all the known effects of dietary fiber on humans. Instead, we will concentrate on the effects of greatest significance (stool weight, transit time, digestion, lipid metabolism, short-chain fatty acids, and colon flora) and a selection of diseases highly correlated with lack of dietary fiber (colon diseases, obesity, and diabetes). Table 4.4 summarizes the beneficial effects of dietary fiber.

Stool Weight and Transit Time Fiber has long been used in the treatment of constipation. Dietary fiber—particularly water-insoluble forms such as cellulose (found, for example, in wheat bran)—increases stool weight as a result of their water-holding properties.[1] Transit time (the time taken for passage of material from the mouth to the anus) is greatly reduced on a high-fiber diet.

Cultures that consume a high-fiber diet (100 to 170 grams/day) usually have a transit time of 30 hours and a fecal weight of 500 grams. In contrast, Europeans and Americans who eat a typical, low-fiber diet (20 grams/day) have a transit time of greater than 48 hours and a fecal weight of only 100 grams.[2] The increased intestinal transit time associated with the Western

Table 4.4 Beneficial Effects of Dietary Fiber

- Decreased intestinal transit time
- Delayed gastric emptying, resulting in reduced after-meal elevations of blood sugar
- Increased satiety
- Increased pancreatic secretion
- Increased stool weight
- More advantageous intestinal microflora
- Increased production of short-chain fatty acids
- Decreased serum lipids
- More soluble bile

diet results in prolonged exposure to various cancer-causing compounds within the intestines.[3]

Fiber should not be thought of only in relation to the treatment of constipation; it is also extremely useful for treating diarrhea due to irritable bowel syndrome. When fiber is added to the diets of subjects who have abnormally rapid transit times (less than 24 hours), it slows the transit time. Dietary fiber thus acts to normalize bowel movements.

Dietary fiber's effect on transit time is apparently directly related to its effect on stool weight and size. A larger, bulkier stool passes through the colon more easily and requires less pressure (and straining) to be expelled during defecation. This puts less stress on the colon wall and thereby avoids the ballooning effect that causes diverticuli. It also prevents the formation of hemorrhoids and varicose veins.

Digestion Although dietary fiber increases the rate of transit through the gastrointestinal tract, it slows gastric emptying. As a result, food is released more gradually into the small intestine and blood glucose levels rise more gradually. Pancreatic enzyme secretion and activity also increase in response to fiber.

A number of research studies have examined the effects of fiber on mineral absorption. Although the results are somewhat contradictory, it appears that large amounts of dietary fiber may impair absorption and/or produce negative balance of some minerals. Fiber as a dietary component does not appear to interfere with the minerals in other foods; however, supplemental fiber (especially wheat bran) may result in a mineral deficiencies.

Lipid Metabolism Water-soluble gels and mucilagenous fibers such as oat bran, guar gum, and pectin are capable of lowering serum lipid (cholesterol and triglyceride) levels by greatly increasing fecal excretion of these lipids and preventing their manufacture in the liver. Water-insoluble fibers such as wheat bran have much less effect on reducing serum lipid levels.[4]

Short-chain Fatty Acids (SCFA) Fermentation of dietary fiber by the intestinal flora produces three main end products: short-chain fatty acids, various gases, and energy. The SCFAs—acetic, proprionic, and butyric acids—have many important physiological functions.

Proprionate and acetate are transported directly to the liver and utilized for energy production, while butyrate provides an important energy source for cells that line the colon. In fact, butyrate is the preferred source for energy metabolism in the colon. Butyrate production may be responsible for the anticancer properties of dietary fiber. Butyrate has been shown to perform impressive anticancer activity and is being used in enemas for ulcerative colitis.

Certain fibers appear to be more effective than others in increasing the levels of SCFAs in the colon. Pectins (both apple and citrus), guar gum, and other legume fibers produce more SCFAs than beet fiber, corn fiber, or oat bran.[5]

Intestinal Bacterial Flora Dietary fiber improves all aspects of colon function. Of central importance is the role it plays in maintaining a suitable bacterial flora in the colon. A low-fiber intake is associated with an overgrowth of endotoxin-producing bacteria (bad guys) and with a lower percentage of lactobacillus (good guys) and other acid-loving bacteria.[6] A diet high in dietary fiber promotes the growth of acid-loving bacteria through the increased synthesis of short-chain fatty acids, which reduce the colon's pH.

Enzymes

Fresh juice is referred to as a "live" food because it contains active enzymes. As mentioned earlier, enzymes often work with vitamins to speed up chemical reactions. Without enzymes, there would be no life in our cells. Enzymes are found in substantially higher amounts in raw foods because they are extremely sensitive to heat and are destroyed during cooking and pasteurization.

The two major types of enzymes are synthetases and hydrolases. The synthetases help build body structures by making or synthesizing larger molecules. The synthetases are also referred to as metabolic enzymes. The hydrolases work to break down large molecules into smaller ones by adding water to the larger molecule—a process known as hydrolysis. The hydrolases are also known as digestive enzymes.

The best example of the beneficial effects of plant enzymes is perhaps offered by bromelain, an enzyme found in the pineapple plant (see Table 4.5). Bromelain was introduced as a medicinal agent in 1957, and since that

Table 4.5 Conditions in Which Bromelain Has Documented Clinical Efficacy

Angina	Dysmenorrhea	Scleroderma
Arthritis	Ecchymosis	Sinusitis
Athletic injury	Edema	Sports injuries
Bronchitis	Maldigestion	Staphylococcal infection
Burn debridement	Pancreatic insufficiency	Surgical trauma
Cellulitis	Pneumonia	Thrombophlebitis

time over 200 scientific papers on its therapeutic applications have appeared in the medical literature.[7]

Bromelain has been reported in these scientific studies to exert a wide variety of beneficial effects, including the following:

- Assisting digestion
- Reducing inflammation in cases of arthritis, sports injury, or trauma
- Preventing swelling (edema) after trauma or surgery
- Inhibiting blood platelet aggregation and enhancing antibiotic absorption
- Relieving sinusitis
- Inhibiting appetite
- Enhancing wound healing

Although most studies have utilized commercially prepared bromelain, it is conceivable that drinking fresh pineapple juice exerts similar, if not superior, benefits. One question that often comes up in relation to enzymes like bromelain is whether or not the body actually the absorbs enzymes in their active form. There is definite evidence that, in both animals and man, up to 40 percent of bromelain given by mouth is absorbed intact, without being broken down.[8] This provides some evidence that other plant enzymes may also be absorbed intact and exert beneficial effects as well.

Pigments

Carotenes

Carotenes or carotenoids represent the most widespread group of naturally occurring pigments in nature. They are a highly colored (red to yellow) group of fat-soluble compounds that function in plants to protect against damage caused during photosynthesis.[9] Carotenes are best known for their capacity for conversion into vitamin A; for their antioxidant activity; and for their correlation with the maximum life-span potential of humans, other primates, and mammals.

Over 400 carotenes have been characterized, but only about 30 to 50 of these are believed to have vitamin A activity. These are referred to as "provitamin A carotenes." The biological effects of a carotene have historically been based on its corresponding vitamin A activity. In fact, beta-carotene has been considered the most active of the carotenes, due to its having a higher provitamin A activity than other carotenes. However, recent research suggests that these vitamin A activities have been overemphasized, since other, non-vitamin-A carotenes exhibit far greater antioxidant and anticancer activities.[10]

The conversion of a provitamin A carotene into vitamin A is dependent on several factors: the level of vitamin A in the body, protein status, thyroid hormones, zinc, and vitamin C. The conversion diminishes as carotene intake increases, and when serum vitamin A levels are adequate. If vitamin A levels are sufficient, the carotene is not converted into vitamin A. Instead it is delivered to body tissues for storage.[11]

Unlike vitamin A, which is stored primarily in the liver, unconverted carotenes are stored in fat cells, epithelial cells, and other organs (the adrenals, testes, and ovaries have the highest concentrations). Epithelial cells are found in the skin and in the linings of our internal organs (including the respiratory tract, gastrointestinal tract, and genitourinary tract). Population studies have demonstrated a strong correlation between carotene intake and various cancers involving epithelial tissues (lung, skin, uterine cervix, gastrointestinal tract, and so on).[12] The higher the carotene intake, the lower the risk for cancer. Scientific studies show that carotenes also have antitumor and immune-enhancing activity.[13]

Cancer and aging share a number of common characteristics, including an association with free-radical damage, which has led to the idea that preventing cancer should also promote longevity. Some evidence supports this claim, since it appears that tissue carotene content has a better correlation with the maximal life-span potential (MLSP) of mammals (including humans) than does any other factor that has been studied.[14] For example, the human MLSP of approximately 120 years correlates with serum carotene levels of 50 to 300 μg/dl, while another primate, the rhesus monkey, has a MLSP of approximately 34 years, correlating with serum carotene levels of 6 to 12 μg/dl.

Since tissue carotenoids appear to be the most significant factor in determining a species' maximal life-span potential, individuals within the species that have the highest carotene levels in their tissues could be expected to live the longest. Tissue carotene contents can best be increased by eating a juiced diet high in mixed carotenes.

The leading sources of carotenes are dark green leafy vegetables (kale, collards, and spinach), and yellow-orange fruits and vegetables (apricots, cantaloupes, carrots, sweet potatoes, yams, and squash). Table 4.6 lists the carotene content of various fruits and vegetables. The carotenes present in green plants are found in the chloroplasts in association with chlorophyll, usually in complexes with a protein or a lipid. Beta-carotene is the predominant form in most green leaves; and in general, the greater the intensity of the green color, the greater the concentration of beta-carotene.

Orange-colored fruits and vegetables (carrots, apricots, mangoes,

Table 4.6 Carotene Levels of Some Common Raw Fruits and Vegetables, in Micrograms (μg) per 3½-oz (100-g) Serving

Apples		Kale	75,000
Unpeeled	5,500–12,600	Melons	2,100–6,200
Peeled	100–500	Oranges	2,400–2,700
Apricots	3,500	Papaya	1,100–3,000
Beet greens	10,000	Peaches	2,700
Blackberries	600	Spinach	37,000
Broccoli	5,200	Squash	
Brussels sprouts	7,000	Acorn	3,900
Carrots	11,100	Butternut	17,700
Collard greens	20,000	Yellow	1,400
Grapes	200	Zucchini	900
Green bell peppers	900–1,100	Tomatoes	7,200

yams, squash, and so on) typically have higher concentrations of provitamin A carotenes. Again, the provitamin A content parallels the intensity of the color.

In the orange and yellow fruits and vegetables, beta-carotene concentrations are high, but other carotenes are present as well, including many with more potent antioxidant and anticancer effects than beta-carotene itself. The red and purple vegetables and fruits (such as tomatoes, red cabbage, berries, and plums) contain a large number of non-vitamin-A-active pigments, including flavonoids and carotenes. Legumes, grains, and seeds are also significant sources of carotenes.[15]

Juicing carotene-rich foods may provide greater benefit than taking beta-carotene supplements or eating intact carotene-rich foods because juicing ruptures cell membranes, thereby liberating important nutritional compounds (like carotenes) for easier absorption than would be possible with intact foods.

Beta-carotene supplementation, while beneficial, only provides one particular type of carotene. In contrast, juicing a wide variety of carotene-rich foods provides a broad range of carotenes, many of which have properties more advantageous than beta-carotene.

Unlike vitamin A, carotenes cannot be overconsumed. Studies done with beta-carotene have not shown it to possess any significant toxicity, even when used in very high doses to treat various medical conditions.[16] However, increased carotene consumption can result in the appearance of slightly yellow- to orange-colored skin, due to the storage of carotenes in epithelial cells. This is known as carotenodermia and is nothing to be alarmed about. In fact, it is probably a very beneficial sign. It simply indicates that the body has a good supply of carotenes.

Flavonoids

The flavonoids are another group of plant pigments that provide remarkable protection against free-radical damage. These compounds are largely responsible for the colors of fruits and flowers. However, they serve more than an aesthetic function. In plants, flavonoids protect against environmental stress. In humans, flavonoids seem to function as "biological response modifiers."

Flavonoids appear to modify the body's reaction to other compounds such as allergens, viruses, and carcinogens, as evidenced by their anti-inflammatory, antiallergic, antiviral, and anticarcinogenic properties.[17] Flavonoid molecules are unique in being active against a wide variety of oxidants and free radicals.

Recent research suggests that flavonoids may be useful in supporting many health conditions.[18] In fact, many of the medicinal actions of foods, of juices, of herbs, of pollens, and of propolis are now known to be directly related to their flavonoid content. Over 4,000 flavonoid compounds have been characterized and classified according to chemical structure.

Different fruits, vegetables, and juices provide different flavonoids and different benefits (see Table 4.7). For example, the flavonoids responsible for the red to blue colors of blueberries, blackberries, cherries, grapes, hawthorn berries, and many flowers are termed *anthocyanidins* and *proanthocyanidins*. These flavonoids are found in the flesh of the fruit as well as in the skin and possess very strong "vitamin P" activity.[19] Among their effects are abilities to increase vitamin C levels within our cells, to decrease the leakiness and breakage of small blood vessels, to protect against free-radical damage, and to support our joint structures.

Flavonoids also have a very beneficial effect on collagen. Collagen, the most abundant protein of the body, is responsible for maintaining the integrity of "ground substance," which in turn is responsible for holding together the tissues of the body. Collagen is also found in tendons, ligaments, and cartilage; it is destroyed during inflammatory processes that occur in rheumatoid arthritis, periodontal disease, gout, and other inflammatory conditions involving bones, joints, cartilage, and other connective tissue. Anthocyanidins and other flavonoids affect collagen metabolism in many ways:

- They can actually crosslink collagen fibers, resulting in reinforcement of the natural crosslinking of collagen that forms the so-called collagen

Table 4.7 Flavonoid Content of Selected Foods, in Milligrams (mg) per 3½-oz (100-g) Serving

Foods	*4-Oxo-flavonoids*[1]	*Anthocyanins*	*Catechins*[2]	*Biflavans*
Fruits				
Grapefruit	50			
Grapefruit juice	20			
Oranges, Valencia	50–100			
Orange juice	20–40			
Apples	3–16	1–2	20–75	50–90
Apple juice				15
Apricots	10–18		25	
Pears	1–5		5–20	1–3
Peaches		1–12	10–20	90–120
Tomatoes	85–130			
Blueberry		130–250	10–20	
Cherries, sour		45		25
Cherries, sweet			6–7	15
Cranberries	5	60–200	20	100
Cowberries		100	25	100–150
Currants, black	20–400	130–400	15	50
Currant juice		75–100		
Grapes, red		65–140	5–30	50
Plums, yellow		2–10		
Plums, blue		10–25	200	
Raspberries, black		300–400		
Raspberries, red		30–35		
Strawberries	20–100	15–35	30–40	
Hawthorn berries			200–800	
Vegetables				
Cabbage, red		25		
Onions	100–2,000	0–25		
Parsley	1,400			
Rhubarb		200		
Miscellaneous				
Beans, dry		10–1,000		
Sage	1,000–1,500			
Tea	5–50		10–500	100–200
Wine, red	2–4	50–120	100–150	100–250

[1]4-Oxo-flavonoids: the sum of flavanones, flavones, and flavanols (including quercetin).

[2]Catechins include proanthocyanins.

SOURCE: J. Kuhnau, "The Flavonoids: A Class of Semi-essential Food Components: Their role in Human Nutrition." *World Review of Nutrition and Diet* 24: 117–91 (1976).

matrix of connective tissue (ground substance, cartilage, tendon, and so on).

- They prevent free-radical damage with their potent antioxidant and free-radical scavenging action.
- They inhibit destruction of collagen structures by enzymes secreted by our own white blood cells during inflammation.
- They prevent the release and synthesis of compounds that promote inflammation, such as histamine.

Their remarkable effects on collagen structures and their potent antioxidant activity make the flavonoid components of berries extremely useful in treating arthritis and hardening of the arteries. Cherry juice has been shown to be of great benefit in treating gout, while feeding proanthocyanidin flavonoids from grape seeds to animals has reversed plaques of atherosclerosis (hardening arteries) and decreased serum cholesterol levels.[20] Since atherosclerotic processes remain major killers of Americans, foods rich in anthocyanidins and proanthocyanidins appear to offer significant preventive effects as well as a potential reversal of the process.

Still other flavonoids are remarkable antiallergic compounds, modifying and reducing all phases of the allergic response.[21] Specifically, they inhibit the formation and secretion of potent inflammatory compounds that produce the allergic response. Several prescription medications developed for allergic conditions (asthma, eczema, hives, and so on) were actually patterned after flavonoid molecules. An example of an antiallergic flavonoid is quercetin, which is contained in many fruits and vegetables. Quercetin is a potent antioxidant that inhibits the release of histamine and other allergic compounds.

Chlorophyll: Nature's Cleansing Agent

Chlorophyll is the green pigment of plants found in the chloroplast compartment of plant cells. In the chloroplast, electromagnetic energy (light) is converted into chemical energy through the process known as photosynthesis. The chlorophyll molecule is essential for this reaction to occur.

The natural chlorophyll found in green plants is fat-soluble. Most of the chlorophyll products found in health food stores, however, contain water-soluble chlorophyll. Because water-soluble chlorophyll is not absorbed from the gastrointestinal tract, its practical use is limited to treating ulcerative conditions of the skin and gastrointestinal tract.[22] Its beneficial effect is largely due to its astringent qualities, coupled with its ability to stimulate wound healing. These healing effects have also been noted from the topical administration of water-soluble chlorophyll in the treatment of skin wounds. Water-soluble chlorophyll is also used medically to help control body, fecal, and urinary odor.[23]

In order to produce water-soluble chlorophyll, the natural chlorophyll molecule must be altered chemically. The fat-soluble form—the natural form of chlorophyll as found in fresh juice—offers several advantages over water-soluble chlorophyll. This is particularly true with regard to chlorophyll's abilities to stimulate hemoglobin and red blood cell production and to relieve excessive menstrual blood flow.[24] In fact, the chlorophyll molecule is noticeably similar to the heme portion of the hemoglobin molecule of our red blood cells.

Unlike water-soluble chlorophyll, fat-soluble chlorophyll is absorbed easily by the rest of the body, and contains other components of the chloroplast complex (including beta-carotene and vitamin K_1) that possess significant health benefits. Water-soluble chlorophyll does not provide these additional benefits.

Like the other plant pigments, chlorophyll also produces significant antioxidant and anticancer effects.[25] It has been suggested that chlorophyll be added to certain beverages, foods, chewing tobacco, and tobacco snuff to reduce cancer risk. A better recommendation would be to include fresh green vegetable juices regularly in the diet. Greens such as parsley, spinach, kale, and beet greens are rich in chlorophyll as well as in carotenes and minerals such as calcium. Parsley or some other green should be consumed whenever fried, roasted, or grilled foods are eaten, as parsley has been shown to reduce the cancer-causing risk of fried foods in human studies.[26] Presumably other greens would offer similar protection.

Vitamin-like Compounds

Many compounds in foods act similarly to vitamins as catalysts of chemical reactions in the body. The reason these compounds are not considered vitamins is that they are viewed as "nonessential" food components, because they can be made in the body from other food components. Nonetheless, deficiency states for several of these vitamin-like compounds have been described. In this chapter we will consider the role and food sources of carnitine, choline, coenzyme Q10, and inositol.

Carnitine

Carnitine, a vitamin-like compound, stimulates the breakdown of long-chain fatty acids by mitochondria (energy-producing units in cells). Carnitine is essential in the transport of fatty acids into the mitochondria. A deficiency in carnitine results in a decrease in fatty acid concentrations in the mitochondria and reduced energy production for the cell.

Carnitine is synthesized from the amino acid lysine in the liver, kidney, and brain. It also requires adequate levels of iron and vitamin C. A deficiency of any of these factors leads to a deficiency of carnitine.

The normal heart stores more carnitine than it needs, but if the heart does not have a good supply of oxygen, carnitine levels quickly decrease. Supplementation with carnitine normalizes heart carnitine levels and allows the heart muscle to utilize its limited oxygen supply more efficiently.

Carnitine has been shown to offer significant support to people with heart disease. Since long-chain fatty acids are the preferred energy source in well-oxygenated heart tissue, normal heart function depends on adequate concentrations of carnitine within the heart. Carnitine also increases HDL (good) cholesterol levels, while decreasing triglyceride and LDL (bad) cholesterol levels.[27]

Carnitine deficiency is linked to a large number of heart disorders (familial endocardial fibroelastosis, cardiac enlargement, congestive heart failure, and cardiac myopathies), all of which respond to carnitine supplementation.[28]

Dietary sources richest in carnitine are red meats (lamb and beef in particular) and dairy products. Vegetables, fruits, and grains contain little or no carnitine, but our body can make carnitine from the amino acid lysine. A good dietary source of lysine is legumes. The most effective dose for carnitine supplementation is 300 mg three times daily.[29]

Choline

Choline performs the vital function of making the main components of our cell membranes, such as phosphatidylcholine (lecithin) and sphingomyelin. Choline is also required for the proper metabolism of fats. Without choline, fats become trapped in the liver, where they block metabolism. Although choline can be manufactured by humans from either of two amino acids—methionine and serine—there is much debate over whether it should be considered an essential nutrient. When animals are fed a choline-deficient diet, they develop liver and kidney disorders. This suggests that humans may also require dietary choline. For a long time, however, choline was never considered as a potentially essential nutrient for humans, primarily because no one tried to feed a choline-deficient diet to humans and observe the effects. A recent study demonstrated that humans fed a choline-deficient diet develop liver disorders and other signs of choline deficiency. Additional evidence supporting the role of choline as an essential nutrient relates to the fact that choline is an essential nutrient for human cells in cell cultures; moreover, humans who require intravenous feeding with solutions low in choline also develop signs of choline deficiency. Choline is found in grains and legumes as lecithin (phosphatidylcholine) and as free choline in vegetables, especially cauliflower and lettuce.[30]

Choline supplementation—as choline bitartrate, choline chloride, or phosphatidylcholine—is used in the treatment of liver disorders, elevated cholesterol levels, and Alzheimer's disease and other neurological disorders.

Coenzyme Q10

Coenzyme Q10 (CoQ10), also known as ubiquinone, is an essential component of our cells, where it plays a major role in energy production. Like carnitine, CoQ10 can be synthesized within the body. Nonetheless, deficiency states have been reported. Deficiency could result from impaired CoQ10 synthesis due to nutritional deficiencies, a genetic or acquired defect in CoQ10 synthesis, or increased tissue needs. Although CoQ10 is widely available in foods, CoQ10 deficiency is best met through supplementation, because of the higher levels that can be provided. A number of clinical conditions also raise an increased need for CoQ10.[31]

CoQ10 deficiency is common in individuals with heart disease. Heart tissue biopsies in patients with various heart diseases have shown a CoQ10 deficiency in 50 to 75 percent of cases. Being one of the most metabolically active tissues in the body, the heart may be unusually susceptible to the effects of CoQ10 deficiency. Accordingly, treatment with CoQ10 has shown great promise in supporting individuals with heart disease and high blood pressure. And like carnitine, CoQ10 has been shown to lower total cholesterol and triglyceride levels while raising the HDL cholesterol level.[32]

Various cardiovascular diseases, including angina, hypertension, mitral valve prolapse, and congestive heart failure, require increased tissue levels of CoQ10. In addition, the elderly in general may have increased CoQ10 requirements, since the decline of CoQ10 levels that occurs with age may be partly responsible for age-related deterioration of the immune system.[33]

CoQ10 is also indicated for individuals with diabetes mellitus and periodontal disease. Research also suggests that CoQ10 may be of value in diseases associated with immunodeficiency, to help promote the healing of gastric ulcers, to improve physical performance and endurance, and to accelerate weight loss in some obese patients.[34]

CoQ10 is also an antioxidant and may be used when a nutritional antioxidant program is indicated. CoQ10 supplements are typically recommended at a daily dosage of 60 mg.

Inositol

Inositol functions quite closely with choline. It, too, is a primary component of cell membranes where it is bound as phosphatidylinositol. Although inositol has not been shown to be essential in the human diet, it is recognized to exert some beneficial effects, especially in cases of liver disorders and diabetes. Inositol, like choline, exerts a "lipotropic" effect, promoting the flow of fat to and from the liver. This is critical to the health of the liver, because stagnation of fat and bile is associated with the likelihood of developing more serious liver disorders such as cirrhosis.

Inositol is showing some promise as a treatment in diabetic neuropathy, a nerve disease caused by diabetes.[35] Diabetic neuropathy is the most frequent complication of long-term diabetes. Much of the decreased nerve function is due to loss of inositol from the nerve cell. Inositol supplementation improves nerve conduction velocities in both diabetic rats and diabetic humans. Inositol is widely available in both animals foods (as myoinositol) and plant foods (as phytic acid). Good plant sources include citrus fruits, whole grains, nuts, seeds, and legumes.

Minor Dietary Constituents

Other plant compounds promote health, too. Many of these compounds, as well as several described earlier, have been categorized as "minor dietary consitutents." This term was coined by Lee Wattenberg, M.D., of the University of Minnesota Medical School, after his isolation of compounds in cabbage that acted to prevent cancer in animals.

Many minor dietary constituents are being investigated as researchers try to understand better why population studies have consistently shown that consuming higher levels of fresh fruits and vegetables is associated with a reduced risk of cancers at most body sites.[36] Fruits, vegetables, grains, and legumes are known to contain many potential anticancer substances, including both nutrients and anutrients. These plant substances have been shown to exert complementary and overlapping actions in reducing risk of cancer. The actions include producing antioxidant effects; inducing the manufacture of enzymes in the body that detoxify cancer-causing chemicals; blocking the chemical effects of cancer-causing compounds; and enhancing the immune system.[37]

A recent review on the role of fruits and vegetables in cancer prevention, published in the medical journal *Cancer Causes and Control,* concluded that humans appear to require a diet with a high intake of fruits and vegetables.[38] These plant foods supply substances crucial to maintaining normal body functions, but only some of these substances are thought of as "essential nutrients." Cancer is viewed by many experts as a "maladaptation" to a reduced level of intake of compounds in foods (anutrients) that are required by our body's metabolism for reasons other than their nutritive effects. In other words, they see cancer as being the result of a deficiency of plant foods in the diet. The review's final words are especially poignant, "Vegetables and fruit contain the anticarcinogenic cocktail to which we are adapted. We abandon it at our peril."

More and more experts are realizing that "essential nutrients" are not the only important food compounds. In fact, anutrients may possess even greater effect in protecting against cancer. Although some of the most potent antioxidants provided by fruits and vegetables are nutrients, the protective effects of fruits and vegetables go far beyond antioxidant effects. For example, one of the American Cancer Society's key dietary recommendations to reduce the risk of cancer is to include cruciferous vegetables, such as cabbage, broccoli, Brussels sprouts, and cauliflower in the diet.[39] Consuming these foods has been shown to exert a protective influence against the development of many types of cancer that exceeds the protective influence of their known nutrient content. The anticancer compounds in cabbage-family vegetables include phenols, indoles, isothiocyanates, and various sulfur-containing compounds. These compounds contain no real nutritional activity and are therefore classified as anutrients; however, these cabbage-family compounds stimulate the body to detoxify and eliminate cancer-causing chemicals—a very profound and powerful effect in the war against cancer.

Fresh fruits and vegetables contain many compounds that perform significant anticancer actions. Research demonstrates that many of these compounds are found in much higher concentrations in fresh fruits and vegetables than in their cooked counterparts. For example, the compounds ellagic acid, chlorogenic acid, and caffeic acid, which are found in fresh apples and other soft fruits and vegetables as well as in nuts, have exhibited significant anticancer properties. Fresh whole apples and fresh apple juice contain approximately 100 to 130 mg per 100 g (roughly 3½ ounces) of these valuable compounds. However, the content of these compounds in cooked or commercial apple products is at or near zero. The same is true

Table 4.8 Comparison of Glutathione Amounts in Fresh vs. Cooked Foods, in Milligrams (mg) per 3½-oz (100-g) Serving

	Glutathione Amount (dry weight)	
Food	*Fresh*	*Cooked*
Apples	21	0.0
Carrots	74.6	0.0
Grapefruit	70.6	0.0
Spinach	166	27.1
Tomatoes	169	0.0

of many of the anticancer compounds in cabbage-family vegetables as well. These are strong cases for eating fresh fruits and vegetables.

Ellagic acid has been referred to as representing a "new breed of anticancer drugs." A great deal of exciting research has been done on ellagic acid. One of the compound's primary actions is to protect against damage to our chromosomes and to block the cancer-causing actions of many pollutants.[40] Specifically, ellagic acid has been shown to block the cancer-causing effects of several compounds in cigarette smoke known collectively as polycyclic aromatic hydrocarbons (PAH) and including such toxic chemicals as benzopyrene. Ellagic acid is a potent antioxidant and has also shown an ability to increase many of the body's antioxidant compounds, including glutathione.[41] Ellagic acid is just one more example of an anutrient with powerful anticancer properties that exists in fresh foods.

Many fresh fruits and vegetables contain glutathione, an important antioxidant in our body. Glutathione is also an important anticancer agent and aids in detoxifying heavy metals like lead as well as in eliminating pesticides and solvents. It is a very important substance in all body tissues. When researchers measured the glutathione levels in foods, what do you suppose they found? Fresh fruits and vegetables provided excellent levels of glutathione, but cooked foods contained far less (see Table 4.8).[42] Again this evidence clearly points out that, to get the greatest benefit from our foods, we should consume them in their freshest form.

The study of foods is a dynamic and exciting field, especially in the area of anutrients. Every year, additional anutrients are discovered in foods that produce remarkable health-promoting effects (see Table 4.9). This emphasizes the importance of not relying on vitamin and mineral

Table 4.9 Health Benefits of Minor Dietary Constituents

Anutrient	*Health Benefits*	*Food Sources*
Allium compounds	Lower cholesterol levels; antitumor properties	Garlic and onions
Carotenes	Antioxidant; enhance immune system; anticancer properties	Dark-colored vegetables such as carrots, squash, spinach, kale, parsley; also cantaloupe, apricots, and citrus fruits
Coumarins	Antitumor properties; immune enhancement; stimulate antioxidant mechanisms	Carrots, celery, beets, citrus fruits
Dithiolthiones	Block the reaction of cancer-causing compounds with our cells	Cabbage-family vegetables
Flavonoids	Antioxidant, antiviral, and anti-inflammatory properties	Fruits, particularly darker fruits like cherries and blueberries; also vegetables, including tomatoes, peppers, and broccoli
Glucosinolates & Indoles	Stimulate enzymes that detoxify cancer-causing compounds	Cabbage, Brussels sprouts, kale, radishes, mustard greens
Isothiocyanates & Thiocyanates	Inhibit damage to genetic material (DNA)	Cabbage-family vegetables
Limonoids	Protect against cancer	Citrus fruits
Phthalides	Stimulate detoxification enzymes	Parsley, carrots, celery
Sterols	Block the production of cancer-causing compounds	Soy products, whole grains, cucumbers, squash, cabbage-family vegetables

supplements to supply all of your nutritional needs. Vitamin and mineral supplements are designed as "supplements" to a healthful diet. A healthful diet must not only include adequate levels of known nutrients, it must also contain large amounts of fresh fruits and vegetables to take advantage of their high content of "unknown" anutrients and accessory healing components.

5

The Healing Power of Vegetables

Vegetables provide the broadest range of nutrients and anutrients of any food class. They are rich sources of vitamins, minerals, carbohydrates, and protein. The little fat they contain is in the form of essential fatty acids. Vegetables provide large quantities of valuable anutrients, especially fiber and carotenes. In Latin, the word *vegetable* means "to enliven or animate." Vegetables give us life. More and more evidence shows that vegetables can prevent as well as treat many diseases.

The U.S. Department of Agriculture has established voluntary grade standards for fruits and vegetables. The official USDA grades are as follows:

U.S. Fancy – Premium quality, the top quality range.
U.S. No. 1 – The chief trading grade; represents good quality.
U.S. No. 2 – Represents intermediate quality.
U.S. No. 3 – Represents low quality.

The grading is largely visual, based on both external qualities and internal appearance. Models, color guides, and color photographs are available for graders to use in checking samples for shape, degree of coloring, and degree of defects or damage.

What is the difference between a vegetable and a fruit? In 1893, this question came before the U.S. Supreme Court, which ruled that a *vegetable* refers to a plant grown for an edible part that is generally eaten as part of the main course, while a *fruit* refers to a plant part that is generally eaten as an appetizer, as a dessert, or out of hand. Typical parts of plants used as vegetables include bulbs (garlic and onion), flowers (broccoli and cauliflower), fruits (pumpkins and tomatoes), leaves (spinach and lettuce), roots (carrots and beets), seeds (legumes, peas, and corn), stalks (celery), stems (asparagus), and tubers (potatoes and yams). Figure 5.1 lists the origins of various modern vegetables.

Figure 5.1 The origins of our modern vegetables.

Northern Europe	Mediterranean	Africa	Middle East	India	China	Central Asia	North America	Central America	South America
Beet	Artichoke	Fava bean	Fava bean	Eggplant	Bok choy	Beet	Jerusalem artichoke	Common bean	Corn
Broccoli	Asparagus	Cowpea	Cabbage	Mung bean	Eggplant	Chives		Corn	Lima bean
Brussels sprouts	Celery	Okra	Carrot		Soybean	Carrot		Jicama	Pepper
Cabbage	Chard	Yam	Cauliflower		Waterchestnut	Garlic		Peppers	Potato
Chives	Chickpea		Cress			Leek		Pumpkin	Sweet potato
Collards	Endive		Cucumber			Onion		Squash	Tomato
Fennel	Kale		Lentil			Pea		Sweet potato	
Horseradish	Kohlrabi		Lettuce			Shallot		Tomato	
Mustard greens	Olive		Mustard greens			Turnip			
Peas	Parsley		Radish						
Rutabaga	Parsnip		Spinach						
Turnip			Watercress						
Watercress			Yam						

How Should We Eat Vegetables?

Vegetables should play a major role in the diet. The U.S. National Academy of Science, the U.S. Department of Health and Human Services, and the National Cancer Institute recommend that Americans consume a minimum of three to five servings of vegetables per day. Table A.1 in the Appendix identifies the nutritive value of edible parts of selected vegetables.

The best way to consume many vegetables is in their fresh, raw form. Vegetables provide a broad range of important nutrient and anutrients; and in their fresh form, these compounds are present in much higher concentrations. For example, many beneficial anutrients in cabbage-family vegetables are destroyed by heat. Drinking fresh vegetable juices is an excellent way to make sure that you achieve your daily quota of vegetables.

When cooking vegetables, you must be careful not to overcook them. Overcooking destroys important nutrients and alters the vegetable's flavor. Light steaming, baking, and quick stir-frying are the best ways to cook vegetables. Do not boil vegetables unless you are making soup, as much of the surviving nutrients will be left in the water. If fresh vegetables are not available, frozen vegetables are preferable to canned vegetables.

Although pickled vegetables are quite popular, they may not be healthful choices. Not only are they high in salt, they may also be high in cancer-causing compounds. Several population studies in China have suggested an association between consumption of pickled vegetables and cancer of the esophagus. Pickled vegetables contain high concentrations of N-nitroso compounds. Once ingested, these compounds can form potent cancer-causing nitrosamines.

A recent study of Hong Kong Chinese sought to determine the relative risk of a number of different factors linked to esophageal cancer.[1] In addition to consumption of pickled vegetables, consumption of very hot drinks or soup, infrequent consumption of green leafy vegetables and citrus fruits, and tobacco smoking have all been linked to esophageal cancer. Green leafy vegetables and citrus fruits are rich sources of vitamin C. Since vitamin C has been shown to prevent nitrosamine formation, these foods are thought to protect against esophageal cancer. The results of the study are the first to show a direct link between consumption of pickled vegetables and esophageal cancer. However, individuals who ate citrus fruits daily (compared to those who ate them less than once a year) experienced an astonishing protective effect. The study appears to indicate that consumption of pickled vegetables should be limited and that, when they are consumed, high-vitamin-C foods should accompany them.

Artichoke

The globe artichoke (*Cynara scolymus*) is a member of the daisy family that originated somewhere between North Africa and the eastern end of the Mediterranean. The edible flower bud is enclosed by green leaflike scales or bracts. Both the bracts and the base of the flower or "heart" are edible. Most of the world's production (80 percent) comes from Italy, Spain, and France. California is the biggest producer in the United States.

Key Benefits

Fresh artichokes are very low in calories because most of the carbohydrate is in the form of inulin, a polysaccharide or starch that the body handles differently from other sugars. In fact, inulin is not utilized by the body for energy metabolism. This makes artichokes extremely beneficial to diabetics, because inulin has actually been shown to improve blood-sugar control in diabetes.[2] However, the artichoke must be as fresh as possible, since inulin is broken down into other sugars when artichokes are stored for any length of time.

The artichoke has a long folk history in treating many liver diseases. Recent evidence supports this longtime use.[3] The active ingredients in artichoke are caffeylquinic acids (such as cynarin). These compounds are found in highest concentrations in the leaves, but they are also found in the bracts and in the heart. Artichoke leaf extracts have demonstrated significant liver-protecting and -regenerating effects.[4] They also possess a choleretic effect, meaning that they promote the flow of bile and fat to and from the liver. This is a very important property: if bile is not transported adequately to the gallbladder, the liver is at increased risk of damage. Choleretics are very useful in the treatment of hepatitis and other liver diseases because of this "decongesting" effect.

Choleretics typically lower cholesterol levels, since they increase the excretion of cholesterol and decrease the synthesis of cholesterol in the liver. Consistent with their choleretic effect, artichoke extracts have been shown to lower blood cholesterol and triglyceride levels in both human and animal studies.[5]

Selection and Preparation

The best artichokes are compact, with tight-clinging bracts. Size does not determine quality or ripeness. Freshness is indicated by the vibrant green color. Overmature artichokes have hard-tipped leaf scales that are opening or spreading. They are typically tough and bitter. Avoid overripe artichokes as well as those with signs of bruising, discoloration, or mold.

Artichokes are quite easy to prepare. Simply boil them, tops down, in water with the aid of a steamer. They are done when a fork can easily penetrate the base of the artichoke. Artichokes can be served hot or cold. The bracts can be plucked off, and the tender part of each eaten. The center formation (the fuzzy part) is scooped out and discarded to expose the edible heart. The following recipes in *The Healing Power of Foods Cookbook* utilize artichokes: Medley of Artichoke and Asparagus; Marinated Artichokes; and Spring Green Pasta.

Asparagus

The asparagus is a member of the lily family. Native to the Mediterranean, asparagus is now grown all over the world. Although it is often expensive, fresh asparagus is a delicious addition to most plates.

Key Benefits

Asparagus is low in calories and carbohydrates, but very rich in protein. Asparagus is also a good source of many vitamins and minerals, including vitamin C, riboflavin, and folic acid. Historically asparagus has been used in the treatment of arthritis and rheumatism, and as a diuretic. Asparagus contains the amino acid asparagine, which when excreted in the urine has a strong odor. Don't be alarmed; the effect is only temporary.

Selection and Preparation

The best-quality asparagus is firm and fresh, with the tips closed. The greener the stalk, the higher the concentration of nutrients. Asparagus can be used in vegetable juices, but it is most often prepared by lightly steaming the entire spear or by cutting diagonally and stir-frying. Before cooking, snap off the tough stem-end by holding a spear in both hands and bending it. It will break where the tender and tough parts meet. The following recipes in *The Healing Power of Foods Cookbook* utilize asparagus: Medley of Artichoke and Asparagus; Carrot and Parsnip Soup with Vegetables; and Spring Green Pasta.

Beets

Beets belong to the same family as spinach and chard. Both the root and the leaves are eaten. Beets were originally cultivated in Europe and Asia, but they are now cultivated worldwide, for fresh food and as a source for sugar production.

Key Benefits

Beet greens are higher in nutritional value than beet roots, because they are much higher in calcium, iron, vitamin A, and vitamin C. Beet roots have long been used for medicinal purposes, primarily focusing on disorders of the liver. Beets have gained recognition for their reported anticancer properties.[6] Beet fiber has been shown to have a favorable effect on bowel function and cholesterol levels.[7]

Selection and Preparation

Good-quality beets should have their greens intact. The greens should be fresh-looking, with no signs of spoilage. Slightly flabby greens can be restored to freshness if stored in the refrigerator in water; if it is too late, simply cut off the greens. The beet roots should be firm, smooth, and vibrant red-purple (versus soft, wrinkled, and dull-colored). Fresh beets with the greens attached can be stored for 3 to 5 days in the refrigerator, but beets with the greens removed can be stored in the refrigerator for 2 to 4 weeks.

The smaller beets are generally better for juicing, while the larger varieties are best cooked. Beets are typically prepared by steaming. Their mild flavor makes them popular as a way to add color to vegetable dishes. One of the more popular beet dishes is borscht, a thick beet soup that is served hot or cold. For a deliciously nutritious borscht recipe, consult *The Healing Power of Foods Cookbook.*

Bell (Sweet) Peppers

Peppers are members of the Solanaceae or nightshade family of vegetables, which also includes potatoes, eggplant, and tomatoes. Peppers are native to Central and South America. Sweet or bell peppers are available in red, green, yellow, purple, black, and brown varieties. Red bell peppers are actually green peppers that have been allowed to ripen on the vine; hence they are much sweeter. Chili peppers are more pungent (hot) and are used in much smaller quantities in the diet (see pages 200, 201).

Key Benefits

Peppers are among the most nutrient-dense of foods and are good sources of many nutrients, including vitamin C. The red variety has significantly higher levels of nutrients than the green. Peppers contain substances that have been shown to prevent clot formation and to reduce the risks of heart attacks and strokes. Although not as rich in these compounds as chili peppers, sweet peppers should nonetheless be consumed regularly by individuals with elevated cholesterol levels. Nightshade-family vegetables may aggravate arthritis is some individuals.

Selection and Preparation

Peppers should be fresh, firm, and bright in appearance. Avoid peppers that appear dry, wrinkled, or decayed in spots. Raw peppers can be used in vegetable juices, salads, and vegetable trays. Peppers can be stuffed and baked, or used in casseroles, stir-fries, and other recipes. Here are some of the recipes in *The Healing Power of Foods Cookbook* that utilize peppers: Stuffed Peppers; Mediterranean Salad; Polenta Puttanesca; Ratatouille over Pasta; Curried Garbanzos with Peppers; and Tofu-Stuffed Peppers.

Bitter Melon

Bitter melon, also known as balsam pear, is a tropical fruit widely cultivated in Asia, Africa, and South America. Usually the bitter-flavored unripe fruit is used as a vegetable. In addition to being consumed as part of the diet, unripe bitter melon has been used extensively in folk medicine as a remedy for diabetes. The ripe fruit is showing promise in the treatment of leukemia, but the ripe fruit is not readily available in the United States. Unripe bitter melon is available primarily at Asian grocery stores.

Key Benefits

The blood-sugar-lowering action of the fresh juice of the unripe bitter melon has been confirmed in scientific studies in animals and humans. Bitter melon contains a compound known as charantin that is more potent than the drug tolbutamide, which is often used in the treatment of diabetes to lower blood-sugar levels. Bitter melon also contains an insulin-like compound referred to as polypeptide-P or vegetable insulin. Since polypeptide-P and bitter melon appear to have fewer side effects than insulin, they have been suggested as replacements for insulin in some patients. It may not even be necessary to inject the material, since oral administration of as little as 2 ounces of the juice has shown good results in clinical trials in patients with diabetes.[8] The ripe fruit of bitter melon has been shown to exhibit some rather profound anticancer effects, especially in leukemia.[9]

Selection and Preparation

The bitter melon is a green cucumber-shaped fruit with gourdlike bumps all over it. It looks like an ugly, light green cucumber. The fruit should be firm, like a cucumber. Bitter melon is, in my opinion, very difficult to make palatable. As its name implies, it is quite bitter. If you desire the medicinal effects, it is best simply to take a 2-ounce shot of the juice.

Broccoli

Broccoli is a member of the cruciferous or cabbage family of vegetables. Broccoli developed from wild cabbage native to Europe, was improved by the Romans and later-day Italians, and is now cultivated throughout the world.

Key Benefits

Broccoli is one of the most nutrient-dense foods. It is especially rich in vitamin C. A 1-cup serving of broccoli provides about the same amount of protein as 1 cup of corn or rice, but less than one-third the number of calories. Like the other members of the cabbage family, broccoli has demonstrated remarkable anticancer effects (see page 108), particularly in breast cancer. Compounds in broccoli known as indoles (specifically, indole-3-carbinol) increase the excretion of the form of estrogen (2-hydroxyestrone) linked to breast cancer.

Selection and Preparation

Broccoli should be dark-green, deep sage-green, or purplish-green, depending on the variety. The stalks and stems should be tender and firm. Yellowed or wilted leaves indicate the loss of much of the nutritional value.

Avoid wilted, soft, and noticeably aged broccoli. Broccoli can be juiced with other vegetables, lightly steamed (9 to 12 minutes), or stir-fried. The following recipes in *The Healing Power of Foods Cookbook* feature broccoli: No-Cream of Broccoli Soup; Carrot and Parsnip Soup with Vegetables; Farfalle with Broccoli; and Stir-Fried Vegetables.

Brussels Sprouts

Like broccoli, Brussels sprouts developed from the wild cabbage. The vegetable was developed to its present form near Brussels, Belgium, hence its name. It is cultivated throughout the world. In the United States, almost all Brussels sprouts come from California.

Key Benefits

Brussels sprouts are similar in nutritional quality to broccoli. As a member of the cabbage family, Brussels sprouts are being investigated for their anticancer properties (see page 108).

Selection and Preparation

Brussels sprouts should be firm and fresh in appearance, with a good green color. Avoid dull, wilted, or yellow Brussels sprouts. Brussels sprouts are best prepared by lightly steaming them for 5 to 7 minutes. For a deliciously nutritious Brussels sprouts recipe, try the Country Brussels Sprouts recipe in *The Healing Power of Foods Cookbook.*

Cabbage

The cabbage or cruciferous family of vegetables includes cabbage, broccoli, cauliflower, Brussels sprouts, kale, collard, mustard, radishes, rutabaga, turnips, and other common vegetables. This family of vegetables is receiving much attention for its members' impressive anticancer properties.

The modern-day cabbage developed from wild cabbage brought to Europe from Asia by roving bands of Celtic people around 600 B.C. Cabbage spread as a food crop throughout northern Europe (Germany, Poland, Russia, Austria, and so on) because it was well adapted to growing in cooler climates, had high yields per acre, and could be stored over the winter in cold cellars.

Table 5.1 Anutrient Compounds in Cabbage That Have Anticancer Properties

Compound	*Method of Action*
Dithiolthiones	Induce antioxidant and detoxification mechanisms
Glucosinolates	Induce antioxidant and detoxification mechanisms
Indoles	Induce antioxidant and detoxification mechanisms; improve metabolism of estrogen
Isothiocyanates	Inhibit cancer development and tumor growth
Coumarins	Block reaction of cancer-causing compounds at key sites
Phenols	Induce detoxification enzymes and prevent the formation of carcinogens

There are numerous types of cabbage, including different varieties of red and green cabbage. Varieties of cabbage are now cultivated throughout much of the northern latitudes of the Northern Hemisphere.

Key Benefits

The cabbage family of vegetables provides numerous health benefits. From a nutrient standpoint, cabbage provides excellent levels of vitamin C, potassium, iron, and calcium. But, perhaps more important than the nutrient content of cabbage is the anutrient level. The cabbage family contains more anutrients with demonstrable anticancer properties than any other vegetable family (see Table 5.1). In fact, one of the American Cancer Society's key dietary recommendations to reduce the risk of cancer is to include cruciferous vegetables, such as cabbage, broccoli, Brussels sprouts, and cauliflower, on a regular basis in the diet.

The anticancer effects of cabbage-family vegetables have been noted in population studies. Consistently, the higher the intake of cabbage-family vegetables, the lower the rates of cancer, particularly colon and breast cancer.[10] As is evident from Table 5.1, the anutrient components in cabbage work primarily by increasing antioxidant defense mechanisms and by improving the body's ability to detoxify and eliminate harmful chemicals and hormones.

Cabbage has also been shown to be extremely effective in treating peptic ulcers. Dr. Garnett Cheney, from Stanford University's School of Medicine, and other researchers in the 1950s clearly demonstrated that fresh cabbage juice is extremely effective in treating peptic ulcers—usually in less than 7 days.[11]

Cabbage-family vegetables contain goitrogens, compounds that can interfere with thyroid hormone action in certain situations (low iodine levels, primarily). The goitrogens are largely isothiocyanates, which block the utilization of iodine; however, there is no evidence that these compounds in cruciferous vegetables interfere with thyroid function to any significant degree when dietary iodine levels are adequate. Therefore, if large quantities of cruciferous vegetables (more than four servings per day) are being consumed in the diet, it is a good idea to include adequate amounts of iodine in the diet, too. Iodine is found in kelp and other seaweeds, in vegetables grown near the sea, in seafood, in iodized salt, and in food supplements. Rutabagas and turnips contain the highest concentrations of the goitrogens.

Selection and Preparation

Cabbage should appear fresh and crisp, with no evidence of decay or worm injury. Raw cabbage can be juiced, shredded and made into coleslaw, or chopped and added to salads. Cabbage can also be cooked in various ways. The following recipes in *The Healing Power of Foods Cookbook* utilize cabbage: Curried Coleslaw and Stir-Fried Vegetables.

Carrots

Carrots are believed to have originated in the Middle East and Asia. Earlier varieties were not orange; they were mostly purple and black. Apparently the modern-day carrot was originally a mutant variety lacking certain purple or black pigments. Carrots are now cultivated worldwide.

Key Benefits

The carrot is the king of the vegetables. It is the richest source of provitamin-A carotenes among the commonly consumed vegetables. Two carrots provide roughly 4,050 retinol equivalents, or roughly four times the RDA for vitamin A. But, unlike vitamin A, beta-carotene and other carotenes in carrots do not cause toxicity. Carrots are full of many other nutrients and anutrients, as well, but their carotene content receives the most attention. Based on extensive human studies, a diet including as little as one carrot per day could conceivably cut the rate of lung cancer in half.[12]

Selection and Preparation

Carrots should be fresh looking, firm, smooth, and vibrantly colored. Avoid carrots that have cracks, are bruised, or have mold growing on them.

Carrot juice is perhaps the most popular vegetable juice prepared on home juice extractors. Its sweetness and flavor blend well with other vegetables. Grated carrots can be added to many fruit salads, such as one with chopped apples, raisins, and pineapple. Chopped or sliced carrots can be added to vegetable salads. Carrots are delicious when lightly steamed on their own, or they can be added to baked goods (carrot cakes and muffins), soups, casseroles, or other recipes. The following recipes in *The Healing Power of Foods Cookbook* feature carrots: Carrot and Parsnip Soup with Vegetables; Apple Carrot Muffins; and Vegetable Curry.

Cauliflower

Like broccoli and Brussels sprouts, cauliflower developed from the wild cabbage. The original variety may have originated in Asia, but cauliflower developed to its present form in Italy. Because cauliflower is susceptible to both frost and hot weather, over 80 percent of the U.S. crop is produced in California.

Key Benefits

Cauliflower is not as nutrient-dense as many of the other cabbage-family vegetables. Its white color is a sign that it contains far less of the beneficial carotenes and chlorophyll. Cauliflower is a good source of boron and does not grow well in boron-deficient soil. For the anticancer properties of cauliflower, see page 108.

Selection and Preparation

Cauliflower should be fresh looking, with clean, white-colored flower heads, and crisp fresh leaves. Avoid cauliflower with wilted leaves, dirty flower heads, or obvious signs of decay. Cauliflower can be prepared in ways similar to broccoli. The following recipes in *The Healing Power of Foods Cookbook* utilize cauliflower: Cauliflower with Pasta Soup; Cauliflower Creole; and Stir-Fried Vegetables.

Celery

Celery is a member of the umbelliferous family, along with carrots, parsley, and fennel. The modern celery originated from wild celery native to the Mediterranean, where its seeds were once widely used as a medicine, particularly as a diuretic.

Key Benefits

Celery is rich in potassium and sodium. After a workout, celery-containing juices make a great electrolyte replacement drink. Celery contains anutrient compounds known as coumarins that appear to be useful in cancer prevention and to enhance the activity of certain white blood cells. Coumarin compounds also tone the vascular system, lower blood pressure, and may be useful in cases of migraines.

Two researchers at the University of Chicago Medical Center have performed studies on a coumarin compound found in celery, 3-n-butyl phthalide; they found that it can indeed lower blood pressure. In animals, a very small amount of 3-n-butyl phthalide lowered blood pressure by 12 to 14 percent and also lowered cholesterol by about 7 percent. The equivalent dose in humans can be supplied in about 4 ribs of celery. The research was prompted by the father of one of the researchers, who, after eating ¼ pound of celery every day for 1 week, observed that his blood pressure dropped from 158 over 96 to a normal reading of 118 over 82.

Selection and Preparation

The best celery is light green, fresh-looking, and crisp. The ribs should snap, not bend. Limp, pliable celery should be avoided. Raw celery can be eaten whole, juiced, or used in salads. Celery can be served on its own after lightly steaming, and it is an excellent addition to soups, stews, and vegetable stir-fries.

Cucumbers

The cucumber is a tropical plant that originated in Southeast Asia. Cucumbers are refreshing vegetables in their fresh form; unfortunately, over 70 percent of the U.S. cucumber crop is used to make pickles.

Key Benefits

Fresh cucumbers are composed primarily of water. The hard skin of the cucumber is an excellent source of some important minerals, including silica, which contributes to the strength of our body's connective tissue. Without silica, connective tissue—which includes intracellular cement, muscles, tendons, ligaments, cartilage, and bone—could not be properly constructed, leaving it impaired. Cucumber juice is often recommended as a source of silicon and as a way to improve the complexion and health of the skin.

Selection and Preparation

Cucumbers should be fresh-looking, well-shaped, and medium to dark green in color. Avoid withered, shriveled, and yellow cucumbers. Try to buy cucumbers that have not been waxed. The cucumber should be washed if it is organic, or soaked or sprayed with a biodegradable wash and then rinsed if it is nonorganic. If waxed, the cucumber should be peeled. Cucumbers are often converted into pickles; however, pickled vegetables are very high in salt, and intake of them should be limited. Most people consume cucumbers raw in salads or appetizers. For a refreshing summer soup, try the Cold Cucumber and Watercress Soup recipe in *The Healing Power of Foods Cookbook.*

Dandelion

The dandelion is a perennial plant with almost worldwide distribution. While many people consider the dandelion to be an unwanted weed, herbalists all over the world have revered this valuable herb. Its common name, *dandelion,* is a corruption of the French for "tooth-of-the-lion" (*Dent-de-Lion*), which describes the jagged toothlike lobes on the herb's leaves. Its scientific genus name, *Taraxacum,* comes from the Greek word *taraxos* (disorder) and *akos* (remedy). This alludes to dandelion's ability to correct a multitude of disorders.

Although generally regarded as a liver remedy, dandelion has enjoyed long and varied folk use throughout the world. In Europe, dandelion was used in the treatment of fevers, boils, eye problems, diarrhea, fluid retention, liver congestion, heartburn, and various skin problems. In China, dandelion has been used to treat breast problems (cancer, inflammation, lack of milk flow, and so on), liver diseases, appendicitis, and digestive ailments. Its use in India, Russia, and other parts of the world has revolved primarily around its action on the liver.

Key Benefits

Dandelion is a rich source of nutrients and other compounds that may improve liver functions, promote weight loss, and support diuretic activity. The dandelion contains greater nutritional value than many other vegetables. It is particularly high in vitamins and minerals, protein, choline, inulin, and pectins. Its carotenoid content is extremely high, as reflected by its higher vitamin A content than carrots (dandelion has 14,000 I.U. of vitamin A per 100 grams, compared to 11,000 I.U. for carrots). Dandelion should be thought of as an extremely nutritious food and as a rich source of medicinal compounds that have a "toning" effect on the body. Both the greens and the roots can be used for this purpose.

Dandelion root is regarded as one of the finest liver remedies, both as a food and as a medicine. Studies in humans and laboratory animals have shown that dandelion root enhances the flow of bile, improving such conditions as liver congestion, bile-duct inflammation, hepatitis, gallstones, and jaundice. Dandelion's action in increasing bile flow is twofold: it has a direct effect on the liver, causing an increase in bile production and flow to the gallbladder (choleretic effect); and it has a direct effect on the gallbladder, causing contraction and release of stored bile (cholagogue effect). Dandelion's historical use in treating so many different conditions is probably closely related to its ability to improve the functional ability of the liver.[13]

Dandelion has also been used historically as a weight-loss aid in the treatment of obesity. This fact prompted researchers to investigate the dandelion's effect on the body weight of experimental animals. When these animals were administered a fluid extract of dandelion greens for one month, they lost as much as 30 percent of their initial weights. Much of the weight loss appeared to be the result of significant diuretic activity.[14]

Selection and Preparation

Wild dandelion is plentiful in most parts of the United States. Dandelion greens are often available commercially as well, especially at open markets and health-food stores. The fresher the dandelion, the better. While dandelion greens can be added to salads, the whole dandelion is best consumed in juiced form along with other vegetable juices, such as carrot juice.

Eggplant

The modern eggplant (*Solanum melongena*) was originally cultivated in China, where it has grown since the fifth century B.C. Although the eggplant is now cultivated worldwide, China is still the world's leading producer, followed by Japan, Turkey, and Italy. The eggplant is underappreciated in the United States compared to these other countries. The leading American producer is Florida.

Key Benefits

The eggplant is low in calories and contains virtually no fat. Eggplant has been used as a medicinal food for thousands of years. Modern studies of eggplant have shown that it lowers blood cholesterol and improves digestion. Like other members of the nightshade family, eggplant may aggravate arthritis in some individuals.

Selection and Preparation

A good-quality eggplant is firm, heavy in relation to its size, and rich purple in color. Avoid eggplants that show signs of damage (cuts, scrapes, bruises, and so on); are wilted, shriveled, or soft; or show evidence of decay. Eggplants are most often used in Mediterranean and Asian dishes. The following recipes in *The Healing Power of Foods Cookbook* utilize eggplant: Baked Eggplant, Chickpeas, and Tomatoes; Eggplant Curry; Eggplant Caviar; and Eggplant and Tomatoes over Pasta.

Fennel

Fennel is a member of the umbelliferous family, along with celery, carrots, and parsley. Like many vegetables, modern-day fennel was developed in Italy. Fennel has a long history of use as a medicinal plant in the Mediterranean region. Fennel has a licorice flavor.

Key Benefits

Fennel offers some good nutrition, but it is largely used for its more medicinal effects. Among herbalists, fennel is viewed in several ways: (1) as an intestinal antispasmodic for relieving intestinal spasms or cramps; (2) as a carminative for relieving or expelling gas; (3) as a stomachic for toning and strengthening the stomach; and (4) as an anodyne for relieving or soothing pain. Fennel also contains substances known as "phytoestrogens," which make it useful in treating many female complaints, especially menopause. Fennel is even higher in coumarin compounds than is celery or carrots.

Selection and Preparation

Fennel should be bought with both the bulb and the stems attached. The fennel should be fresh-looking; and as with celery, its branches should snap (not bend) with pressure. Fresh fennel has a pretty overpowering flavor on its own, unless you really love licorice. When juicing fennel, mix it with carrots, apples, pears, or celery to cut down on its intensity. The leaves and stems are typically used in salads, while the bulb can be steamed or sautéed. The following recipes in *The Healing Power of Foods Cookbook* utilize fennel: Orange and Fennel Salad; Fennel and Mushrooms; and Insalata Mista.

Garlic

Garlic is a member of the lily family that is cultivated worldwide. The garlic bulb is composed of individual cloves enclosed in a papery white skin. Garlic has been used throughout history for treating a wide variety of conditions. Its usage predates written history. Sanskrit records document the use of garlic remedies approximately 5,000 years ago, while the Chinese have been using it for at least 3,000 years. The Codex Ebers, an Egyptian medical papyrus dating to about 1550 B.C., mentions garlic as an effective remedy for various ailments. Hippocrates, Aristotle, and Pliny cited numerous therapeutic uses for garlic. In general, garlic has been used throughout the world to treat coughs, toothache, earache, dandruff, hypertension, atherosclerosis, hysteria, diarrhea, dysentery, diphtheria, vaginitis, and many other conditions.[15]

Stories, verse, and folklore (such as its alleged ability to ward off vampires) offer historical documentation of garlic's power. Sir John Harrington, in *The Englishman's Doctor,* written in 1609, summarized garlic's virtues and faults:

> Garlic then have power to save from death
> Bear with it though it maketh unsavory breath,
> And scorn not garlic like some that think
> It only maketh men wink and drink and stink.

Key Benefits

It is beyond the scope of this book to detail all of the wonderful properties of this truly remarkable medicinal plant (see Table 5.2). Whole books are

Table 5.2 Beneficial Effects of Garlic

- Lowers cholesterol
- Lowers high blood pressure
- Lowers blood-sugar levels in diabetes
- Helps eliminate heavy metals like lead
- Promotes detoxification reactions
- Enhances the immune system
- Protects against cancer
- Performs antimicrobial functions:
  - Antibacterial
  - Antifungal
  - Anthelmintic (kills worms)

Table 5.3 Effects of Garlic and Onion Consumption on Serum Lipids Under Carefully Matched Diets

Garlic/Onion Consumption Level	*Cholesterol Level*	*Triglyceride Level*
Garlic 50 g/week onion 600 g/week	159 mg/dL	52 mg/dL
Garlic 10 g/week onion 200 g/week	172 mg/dL	75 mg/dL
No garlic or onions	208 mg/dL	109 mg/dL

devoted to garlic, and my book *The Healing Power of Herbs* gives much attention to garlic.

Much of the therapeutic effect of garlic is thought to be due to volatile factors of garlic that are composed of sulfur-containing compounds: allicin, diallyl disulfide, diallyl trisulfide, and others. Other constituents of garlic include additional sulfur-containing compounds, high concentrations of trace minerals (particularly selenium and germanium), glucosinolates, and enzymes. The compound allicin is mainly responsible for the pungent odor of garlic.[16]

Garlic appears to be an important protective factor against atherosclerosis and heart disease. Many studies have found that garlic decreases total serum cholesterol levels while increasing serum HDL-cholesterol levels. HDL-cholesterol, often termed the "good" cholesterol, is a protective factor against heart disease. Garlic has also demonstrated blood-pressure-lowering action in many studies. Garlic has been shown to decrease systolic pressure by 20 to 30 mm Hg and diastolic pressure by 10 to 20 mm Hg in patients with high blood pressure.[17]

In a 1979 population study, researchers studied three populations of vegetarians in the Jain community in India who consumed differing amounts of garlic and onions.[18] Numerous favorable effects on blood lipids, as shown in Table 5.3, were observed in the group that consumed the largest amount. The study is quite significant because the subjects had nearly identical diets, except with respect to garlic and onion ingestion.

The therapeutic uses of garlic are quite extensive. Its use as a food should be encouraged, despite its odor, especially in individuals with elevated cholesterol levels, heart disease, high blood pressure, diabetes, candida infections, asthma, infections (particularly respiratory tract infections), and gastrointestinal complaints. As many of the therapeutic compounds in garlic have not been found in cooked, processed, and proprietary forms, the broad range of beneficial effects attributed to garlic can best be obtained from fresh, raw garlic—although limited, specific effects can be obtained from the other forms. For medicinal purposes, at least three cloves of garlic per day is recommended; for protective measures, at least three cloves per week is a good idea.

Selection and Preparation

Buy fresh garlic. Do not buy garlic that is soft, shows evidence of decay such as mildew or darkening, or is beginning to sprout. When juicing garlic, it is best to remove the garlic clove from the bulb and wrap it in a green vegetable like parsley. This accomplishes two things: it prevents the garlic from popping out of the juicer, and the chlorophyll helps bind some of the odor. It is a good idea to juice the garlic first, so the other vegetables will remove the odor from the machine. Garlic, whether chopped, sliced, or crushed, is a valuable addition to many foods, improving not only their nutritional benefits but also their flavor. Garlic is used liberally in many recipes in *The Healing Power of Foods Cookbook.*

Jerusalem Artichoke

The Jerusalem artichoke is native to North America and is often referred to as a "sun-choke." Jerusalem artichokes are not part of the artichoke family; in fact, they are members of daisy family (Compositae) and are closely related to the sunflower. The name *Jerusalem* is thought to be an English corruption of Ter Neusen, the place in the Netherlands from which the plant was introduced into England. The plants were originally cultivated by the Native Americans.

Key Benefits

Jerusalem artichokes, like the globe artichoke, are a rich source of inulin, a polysaccharide or starch that the body handles differently from other sugars. In fact, inulin is not utilized by the body for energy metabolism at all. This makes Jerusalem artichokes extremely beneficial to diabetics. Jerusalem artichoke polysaccharides have actually been shown to improve blood-sugar control.[19] Since the body does not utilize the primary carbohydrate in Jerusalem artichokes, the calorie content is virtually nil, only 7 calories per 100 g (roughly 3½ ounces).

Although inulin is not utilized by the human body, it does provide nutrition to health-promoting bacteria in the intestinal tract. Specifically, inulin promotes the growth of bifidobacteria, a cousin of *Lactobacillus acidophilus,* the primary organism in live yogurt cultures.[20] Bifidobacteria are the primary organisms found in mother's milk, and they are thought to be critical to maintaining a healthy balance of intestinal microflora throughout an individual's lifetime. Bifidobacteria are effective inhibitors of many disease-causing organisms; exhibit antitumor activity; help reduce serum cholesterol levels; and may provide some B-vitamins. Bifidobacteria dairy products and supplements are available in the marketplace. However, Jerusalem artichokes and flour have been shown to be effective in promoting bifidobacteria growth in the intestinal tract.[21]

Jerusalem artichokes may also have some immune-enhancing activity, since inulin enhances a component of our immune system known as complement. Complement is responsible for increasing such host defense mechanisms as neutralization of viruses, destruction of bacteria, and speeding the movement of white blood cells (neutrophils, monocytes, eosinophils, and lymphocytes) to areas of infection. Many medicinal plants, including echinacea and burdock, owe much of their immune-enhancing effects to inulin. Jerusalem artichoke is one of the richest sources of inulin available.

Selection and Preparation

Fresh Jerusalem artichokes should be firm, with fresh-looking skin. They make excellent additions to vegetable juices and salads (grated or thinly sliced), or they can be cooked like potatoes. Jerusalem artichoke flour can be used in quantities of up to 10 percent of the total flour content in breads, pastas, and other baked goods.

Jicama

Jicama, pronounced "HEE-ka-ma," is a turnip-shaped root vegetable native to Mexico and Central America.

Key Benefits

Jicama's high water content makes it a fantastic vegetable to juice. Like most root vegetables, it is especially high in potassium. Its flavor is very similar to that of a water chestnut. In fact, many Oriental restaurants substitute jicama for the more expensive water chestnut.

Selection and Preparation

High-quality jicama should be firm and heavy for its size. Jicama that is shriveled, soft, or unusually large is likely to be tough and woody and to contain less water. Jicama can be added to vegetable juices, served raw in relish trays and salads, or used in Asian dishes such as stir-fries as a replacement for water chestnuts. The Jicama Salad recipe in *The Healing Power of Foods Cookbook* utilizes jicama and Jerusalem artichokes.

Kale and Other Greens

Kale is a member of the cabbage or cruciferous family. Kale is probably the closest relative of wild cabbage in the whole cabbage family. Kale and collards are essentially the same vegetable, except that kale has leaves with curly edges and is less tolerant to heat. Collards and kale are native to Europe, where they have been cultivated for many centuries as food for people and livestock. In the United States, kale and collards are grown primarily on the east coast, from Delaware to Florida. Other greens of the cabbage family, such as mustard greens, turnip greens, kohlrabi, and watercress, offer similar benefits to kale and collards and can be used similarly.

Key Benefits

Kale and collards are rich in essential vitamins and minerals. They are especially rich in calcium, potassium, and iron. A cup of kale or collards actually has more calcium than a cup of milk. Furthermore, they contain almost three times as much calcium as they do phosphorus. High phosphorus consumption has been linked to osteoporosis, because excessive phosphorus reduces the utilization and promotes the excretion of calcium.

As members of the cabbage family, kale and collards exhibit the same anticancer properties (see page 108). Kale and collards are also excellent sources of many anutrients, especially pigments like carotenes and chlorophyll. Kale and collards are among the most nutritious of all vegetables.

Selection and Preparation

High-quality kale, collards, and other greens are fresh, tender, and dark green. Avoid greens that show dry or yellowing leaves, evidence of insect injury, or decay. Greens make excellent additions to fresh vegetable juices; typically one-third of the volume should be composed of the greens juice, since its flavor can be quite strong. A salad spinner is a great way to dry the leaves and prepare them for juicing. Usually the leaves can be fed into the juicer intact; large leaves may need to be cut. Greens can be utilized in salads, although kale can be quite tough. Greens can also be steamed or used in soups. Here are some of the recipes from *The Healing Power of Foods Cookbook* that utilize kale and other greens: Greens, Walnuts, and Raisins; Steamed Kale; and Swiss Chard and Garlic with Pasta.

Leeks

Leeks are related to onions and garlic. While the bulbs of garlic and onions are typically the edible portion, with leeks the leaves and stems are eaten, rather than the long narrow bulb.

Key Benefits

Leeks share many of the same healthful qualities as onions and garlic, only they are less dense. Consequently, larger quantities of leeks must be consumed to produce similar effects to those of onions and garlic. Presumably, leeks can lower cholesterol levels, improve the immune system, and fight cancer just as onions and garlic do.

Selection and Preparation

Leeks should have broad, dark, solid leaves and a thick white neck, with a base about 1 inch in diameter. Leeks with yellowing, wilted, or discolored leaves should be avoided. Leeks can be utilized in ways similar to onions. The following recipes in *The Healing Power of Foods Cookbook* utilize leeks: Leek and Tomato Casserole and Spicy Hot Leeks.

Lettuce and Similar Greens

Lettuce is native to the Mediterranean region and is a member of the daisy and sunflower family (Compositae). The ancient Greeks and Romans hailed lettuce as a medicinal plant. Augustus Caesar went so far as to erect a statue in honor of lettuce, believing that it had aided his recovery from illness. Lettuce is a major salad crop in the United States. Among the numerous types of lettuce are Iceberg, Romaine, Butterhead, and Looseleaf varieties. Other green leafy vegetables that do not belong to the cabbage family, such as endive, have benefits similar to lettuce's.

Key Benefits

In general, the darker the lettuce, the greater the nutrient content: Romaine > Looseleaf > Butterhead > Iceberg. Lettuce is a good source of chlorophyll and vitamin K.

Selection and Preparation

Good-quality lettuce looks fresh, crisp, and free from any evidence of decay. Avoid lettuce that has a rusty appearance and signs of decay. A salad spinner is a great way to dry the leaves and prepare them for use in salads or for juicing.

Onions

Onions, like garlic, are members of the lily family. Onions originated in the central part of Asia, from Iran to Pakistan and northward into the southern part of Russia. There are numerous forms and varieties of onion, as it is cultivated worldwide. Common varieties are white globe, yellow globe, red globe, and green (shallots). With globe onions, the part used is the fleshy bulb; with green onions, both the long slender bulb and the green leaves are used. Chives, another member of the onion family, are used as a culinary herb. Chives complement the flavor of onions, potatoes, carrots, spinach, and most other vegetables.

Key Benefits

Onions, like garlic, contain various organic sulfur compounds. Onions also have the enzyme alliinase, which is released when an onion is cut or crushed, causing conversion of trans-S-(1-propenyl)cysteine sulfoxide into the so-called lacrimatory or crying factor (propanethial S-oxide). Other constituents include flavonoids (primarily quercetin), phenolic acids (for example, ellagic, caffeic, sinapic, and p-coumaric acids), sterols, saponins, pectin, and volatile oils.[22]

Although not nearly as valued a medicinal agent as garlic, onions have been used almost as widely. Onions produce many of the same healthful effects as garlic. There are, however, some subtle differences that make one more advantageous than the other under certain conditions.

Like garlic, onions and onion extracts have been shown in several clinical studies to decrease blood lipid levels, prevent clot formation, and lower blood pressure. Onions have been shown to exert significant blood-sugar-lowering action, comparable to that of prescription drugs (tolbutamide and phenformin) often given to diabetics. The active blood-sugar-lowering principle in onions is believed to be allyl propyl disulphide (APDS), although other constituents such as flavonoids may play a significant role as well. Experimental and clinical evidence suggests that APDS lowers glucose by competing with insulin (also a disulfide molecule) for breakdown sites in the liver, thereby increasing the insulin's lifespan. Other mechanisms, such as increased liver metabolism of glucose or increased insulin secretion, have also been proposed.[23]

Onion has been used historically for asthma. Its action in asthma is due to its ability to inhibit the production of compounds which cause the bronchial muscle to spasm along with its ability to relax the bronchial muscle.[24]

An onion extract was found to destroy tumor cells in test tubes and to arrest tumor growth when tumor cells were implanted in rats. The onion extract was shown to be unusually nontoxic: a dose 40 times higher than the dose required to kill the tumor cells had no adverse effect on the host. In addition, green onions (scallions) have been shown to exhibit significant therapeutic activity against leukemia in mice.[25]

Again, liberal use of *Allium* species (garlic, onions, leeks, and others) appears particularly indicated, considering the major disease processes (such as atherosclerosis, diabetes, and cancer) of the twentieth century.

Selection and Preparation

Globe onions should be clean and hard, and should have dry smooth skins. Avoid onions with developed seedstems, misshapen bulbs, or evidence of decay. Green onions should have fresh-looking green tops and a white neck; ones with yellowing, wilted, or discolored tips should be avoided. Cooked onions can be eaten on their own, either steamed or boiled. I have actually seen my mother eat raw Walla Walla sweet onions as if they were apples, but onions are usually used to flavor and enhance other vegetables and recipes. Onions are utilized in many recipes in *The Healing Power of Foods Cookbook.* If you are a real onion lover, you may want to try the recipe for Stuffed Onions.

Parsley

Parsley, like carrots and celery, is a member of the umbelliferous family. Native to the Mediterranean, unfortunately most parsley is now used most often as a garnish instead of in foods.

Key Benefits

Parsley is extremely rich in numerous nutrients, in chlorophyll, and in carotenes. The high cholorphyll content of parsley can help mask the odor and taste of many other foods, including garlic. Ingesting parsley has been shown to inhibit the increase in humans of urinary mutagenicity following ingestion of fried foods. This is most likely due to the chlorophyll, but other compounds in parsley such as vitamin C, flavonoids, and carotenes have also been shown to inhibit the cancer-causing properties of fried foods.

Parsley has benefits that extend well beyond its chlorophyll content. It has long been used for medicinal purposes and is regarded as an excellent "nerve stimulant." Empirical evidence seems to support this and probably explains why so many juice enthusiasts label parsley-containing juices "energy drinks."

Selection and Preparation

Parsley can be grown at home or purchased fresh from the grocery store. It should be bright, fresh, green, and free of yellowed leaves and dirt. Slightly wilted parsley can be revived to freshness in cold water. Fresh parsley is used in vegetable juices, salads, and as a flavoring agent and garnish. Numerous recipes in *The Healing Power of Foods Cookbook* utilize parsley for its nutritional and flavorful effects.

Parsnip

The parsnip (*Pastinaca sativa*), like parsley, carrots, and celery, is a member of the umbelliferous family. The parsnip's carrotlike root is the edible portion of the plant. Native to the Mediterranean, parsnip is not very popular in the United States, not only because few people really enjoy the taste, but also because it grows slowly and therefore is not very profitable for farmers to grow.

Key Benefits

Parsnip provides similar nutritional value to potatoes, although parsnips contain only about 80 percent of the protein and vitamin C content of potatoes.

Selection and Preparation

Smooth, firm, well-shaped parsnips are preferred. Avoid soft, flabby, or shriveled roots. Parsnips are most often puréed, mashed, whipped, or added to soups and stews. The following recipes in *The Healing Power of Foods Cookbook* utilize parsnips: Carrot and Parsnip Soup with Vegetables; Spinach and Parsnip Soup; and Gingered Tempeh and Vegetables.

Potatoes

Potatoes are members of the Solanaceae or nightshade family and are native to the Andes Mountains of Bolivia and Peru, where they have been cultivated for over 7,000 years. Sometime during the early part of the sixteenth century, potatoes were brought to Europe by Spanish explorers. Potatoes are a hearty crop and became a favorite food in Ireland in the 1800s largely as a result of the tremendous rise in population coupled with a declining economy. Because 1½ acres of land could produce enough potatoes to feed a family of five for a year, most Irish families came to depend on potatoes for food. Several hundred varieties of potatoes are grown worldwide.

Key Benefits

Potatoes are excellent sources of many nutrients, including potassium and vitamin C. Potatoes themselves are low in calories: a medium-sized potato contains only 115 calories. Unfortunately, however, most Americans eat the potato in the form of french fries, hash browns, potato chips, or baked potatoes smothered in butter or sour cream. The protein quality in potatoes is also quite high. Although they have about the same protein content as corn or rice, potatoes also contain lysine, an essential amino acid often lacking in grains. Potatoes, like other foods of the nightshade family, may aggravate arthritis in some individuals.

As an interesting side note, boiled potato-peel dressings may offer effective treatment for skin wounds in some Third World countries where modern skin graft procedures are not available. Preliminary studies conducted at a children's hospital in Bombay, India, where a dressing prepared from boiled potato peelings attached to standard gauze bandages was used, found that the dressings demonstrated good therapeutic effect in promoting healing and keeping the burn from becoming infected.[26] Patients noted pain relief, while physicians noted reduced levels of bacterial contamination and faster healing as a result of the boiled potato-peel dressings.

Selection and Preparation

Use only high-quality potatoes that are firm and display the characteristic features of its variety. Avoid wilted, leathery, or discolored potatoes—especially those with a greenish tint. Potatoes can be boiled, baked, mashed, or fried. The following recipes in *The Healing Power of Foods Cookbook* feature potatoes: Curried Potatoes; Mashed Potatoes with Onion Gravy; and Indonesian Curried Vegetable Stew with Coconut Milk.

Radish

The radish is a member of the cabbage family that is believed to have originated in the eastern part of the Mediterranean and in western Asia. There are numerous varieties of radish. The most popular variety in the United States is the small, round, red radish; while in Asian cultures, the daikon may weigh up to 5 pounds.

Key Benefits

In addition to being an excellent source of vitamin C and potassium, the radish, like the beet, has been used as a medicinal food for liver disorders.

Selection and Preparation

Good-quality red radishes should have their greens intact. The greens should look fresh, with no signs of spoilage. Slightly flabby greens can be restored to freshness if stored in the refrigerator in water; if it is too late, simply cut off the greens. The radish root should be firm, smooth, and vibrant red versus soft, wrinkled, and dull-colored. Fresh radishes with the greens attached can be stored for 3 to 5 days in the refrigerator, but radishes with the greens removed can be stored in the refrigerator for 2 to 4 weeks. Radishes are best utilized in salads.

Spinach

Spinach is believed to have originated in southwestern Asia or Persia. It has been cultivated in many areas of the world for hundreds of years, not only as a food, but also as an important medicinal plant in many traditional systems of medicine.

Key Benefits

There is much lore regarding spinach. It was regarded historically as a plant with remarkable abilities to restore energy, increase vitality, and improve the quality of the blood. There are sound scientific reasons why spinach would produce such results—primarily the fact that spinach contains twice as much iron as most other greens. Spinach, like other chlorophyll- and carotene-containing vegetables, is a strong protector against cancer.

Selection and Preparation

Fresh spinach should be dark green, fresh-looking, and free of any evidence of decay. Slightly wilted spinach can be revived to freshness in cold water. Raw spinach can be used in fresh vegetable juices and salads. Spinach is best cooked by gently steaming it until leaves are tender. Spinach is used in a wide range of recipes. The following recipes in *The Healing Power of Foods Cookbook* feature spinach: Spinach and Parsnip Soup; Spinach Salad; Spinach Dip; and Winter Pesto.

Squash, Pumpkins, and Gourds

Squash belong to the gourd or melon family (Cucurbitaceae). Native to Central America, squash spread throughout North and South America in pre-Columbian times. Shortly after the discovery of America, squash were brought back to Europe and Asia, where production eventually surpassed that in America. The leading producers of squash are China, Egypt, Turkey, and Romania.

The many types of squash generally fall into two major categories: summer and winter. Summer squash include yellow, white bush scallop, and zucchini. Winter squash include pumpkins, butternut, acorn, and spaghetti.

Key Benefits

Squash are an excellent food, providing edible flesh and seeds. Summer squash, due to their higher water content (95 percent, compared to 81 percent), are not as nutrient-dense as the winter varieties. Summer squash are excellent diet foods because they are very low in calories (14 calories per 3½ ounces). Summer squash do provide fair amounts of potassium, carotenes, and vitamin C. Winter squash—especially the darker-flesh varieties such as pumpkin and acorn—provide exceptional amounts of carotenes, complex carbohydrates, potassium, and many B-vitamins. Like other carotene-rich vegetables, squash have been shown to exert a protective effect against many cancers, particularly lung cancer. The nutritional benefits of the seeds are discussed in Chapter 9.

Selection and Preparation

When selecting squash, make sure that they exhibit the proper color, firmness, and other qualities or characteristics that the variety selected should have. Summer squash are usually left unpeeled and are cooked whole, sliced, or cubed. Delicious steamed, stir-fried, or sauteed, summer squash can also be used in mixed vegetable dishes and casseroles. Winter squash are usually prepared by first removing the fibrous matter and seeds from the center and then baking, broiling, or steaming them. Spaghetti squash is often prepared as a substitute for spaghetti by baking or steaming it until the rind softens; then it is cut in half lengthwise, and the spaghetti strands are removed. Pumpkin and other varieties are often mashed like potatoes and either eaten as such or used in breads, cakes, muffins, and pies.

Sweet Potatoes and Yams

Sweet potatoes are not members of the potato (Solanaceae) family; rather, they are members of the Convolvulaceae family. The sweet potato is native to Mexico and Central and South America. In the United States, we tend to call the darker, sweeter sweet potato a yam. In actuality, however, it is not a yam but another variety of sweet potato. True yams are native to Southeast Asia and Africa and differ slightly from the sweet potato. True yams have very little carotene.

Key Benefits

Unlike yams, sweet potatoes are very rich in carotenes. The darker the variety, the higher the concentration. Sweet potatoes are also rich in vitamin C, calcium, and potassium. Sweet potatoes are far more nutritious than Irish potatoes.

Selection and Preparation

Use only high-quality sweet potatoes that are firm and display the characteristic features of the variety being selected. Remember: the darker the variety, the higher the carotene content. As a bonus, American "yams" are sweeter and taste better. Avoid wilted, leathery, or discolored sweet potatoes, especially those with a greenish tint. Sweet potatoes are great on their own, or they can be prepared in ways similar to Irish potatoes. The following recipes in *The Healing Power of Foods Cookbook* utilize sweet potatoes: Sweet Potato Pumpkin Soup and Spiced Yams.

Tomatoes

At one time tomatoes were believed to be poisonous; now they are one of the world's leading vegetable crops. The tomato, like many other members of the Solanaceae or nightshade family, originated in Central and South America.

Key Benefits

The tomato is packed with nutrition, especially when fully ripe; red tomatoes have up to four times more beta-carotene than green tomatoes. Tomatoes supply good amounts of vitamin C, carotenes, and potassium. Tomatoes, like other members of the nightshade family, may aggravate arthritis in some individuals.

Selection and Preparation

Good-quality tomatoes are well-formed, plump, fully red, firm, and free from bruise marks. Avoid tomatoes that are soft or show signs of bruising or decay. Raw tomatoes can be juiced or used in salads. Tomatoes are used in sauces, stir-fries, and many other dishes. Numerous recipes in *The Healing Power of Foods Cookbook* utilize tomatoes or tomato sauce.

Turnip

The turnip is a member of the cabbage family. Rutabagas, which are similar to turnips, are actually a cross between turnips and kale. Once a popular food in Europe, turnips lost popularity as the potato rose to prominence. Both the root and the greens (see page 119) are edible.

Key Benefits

Although turnips are considered a "starch" vegetable, they provide only one-third the calories of an equal amount of potatoes. Turnip greens supply many times the nutrient content of the turnip root. As a cabbage-family vegetable, turnips provide numerous health benefits (see page 108). Turnips and rutabagas contain especially high amounts of compounds (goitrogens) that interfere with thyroid function. Their use by individuals with low thyroid function should be limited. If turnips and rutabagas are eaten on a regular basis, high-iodine-containing foods (such as kelp) or iodine supplements must also be consumed.

Selection and Preparation

Turnip roots should be firm and smooth, with no visible signs of mold or decay. Avoid soft, shriveled or large turnips, since they are less nutritious and less tasty. Turnips are most often prepared by boiling the diced turnip in water and then mashing them. Mashed turnips can be served alone or mixed with an equal amount of potato. Turnips are also used in soups, stews, and vegetable casseroles.

6

The Healing Power of Fruits

When most people think of fruit, they think of sweet, soft, succulent, refreshing, and delicious natural foods like apples, oranges, berries, and melons. However, by strict definition, a fruit is the ripened ovary of a female flower. This scientific definition thus covers what we commonly call fruit, as well as nuts and some vegetables, including squash, pumpkins, and tomatoes. Although most fruits are seasonal, modern transportation methods make a wide variety of fresh fruits available to most people year-round.

In general, fruits are excellent sources of many vital antioxidant nutrients and anutrients such as vitamin C, carotenes, flavonoids, and polyphenols like ellagic acid. Regular fruit consumption, like regular vegetable consumption, has been shown to offer significant protection against many chronic degenerative diseases including cancer, heart disease, cataracts, and strokes.

Since fruits contain a fair amount of natural fruit sugar (fructose), people are generally recommended to limit their intake to no more than four servings or two 8-ounce glasses of fresh fruit juice per day. People who suffer from hypoglycemia, diabetes, candidiasis, or gout are probably best advised to eat the fruit in its whole form or to drink the fresh juice with food or dilute it with an equal amount of pure water.

Although fructose is 1½ times sweeter than sucrose (white sugar), it is handled differently by the body. To be utilized, fructose must be changed into glucose in the liver; consequently blood-sugar (glucose) levels do not rise as rapidly after fructose consumption as they do after consumption of sugars. Sucrose, which is composed of one molecule of glucose and one molecule of fructose, causes an immediate elevation in blood-sugar level. While most diabetics cannot tolerate sucrose, most can tolerate moderate amounts of fruits and fructose without loss of blood-sugar control. In fact, they tolerate fruits much better than they do white bread and other refined carbohydrates.[1]

Regular fruit consumption may also help control the appetite and promote weight loss. While aspartame (NutraSweet), glucose, and sucrose may increase the appetite, several studies have found that fructose actually decreases the quantities of calories and fat consumed. Typically, the studies gave the subjects food or drink containing an equivalent amount of fructose or other sweetener 30 minutes to 2½ hours before allowing them to consume as much food as they desired at a dinner buffet. The studies were designed in "double-blind" fashion, so that neither the observers nor the participants knew who had been given what. Consistently, subjects receiving the fructose-sweetened food or drink ate substantially fewer calories and less fat than did those in the groups receiving aspartame, sucrose, or glucose.[2]

Since fruits contain fructose in a natural form, consuming a serving of fruit or fruit juice at least 30 minutes before dinner may significantly suppress the appetite, resulting in fewer calories' being consumed. And when fewer calories are consumed, weight loss is much easier to achieve. Fruits make excellent between-meal snacks.

Figure 6.1 shows the geographical origins of various fruits. Table A.2 in the Appendix identifies the nutritive value of edible parts of selected fruits.

Apple

The apple originated in the Caucasus Mountains of western Asia and eastern Europe. The apple is often referred to as the king of fruits. In the United States, more than 25 varieties of apple are available. The most popular variety is the Delicious. Good apples for juicing are the Delicious (both red and golden yellow), Granny Smith, and Winesap varieties.

Key Benefits

Apples are a good (but not great) source of many vitamins and minerals, particularly if they are unpeeled. Unpeeled apples are especially high in non-pro-vitamin-A carotenes and pectin. Pectin is a remarkable type of fiber that has been shown to exert a number of beneficial effects. Because it is a gel-forming fiber, pectin can improve the intestinal muscle's ability to push waste through the gastrointestinal tract. Pectin also binds to and

Figure 6.1 The origins of our modern fruits.

Europe	Africa	Middle East	India	China	Central Asia	South Pacific	North America	Central America	South America
Apple	Akee	Apple	Cantaloupe	Apricot	Cranberry	Banana	Blueberry	Acerola	Cherimoya
Blackberry	Cantaloupe	Cantaloupe	Citron	Citron	Currant	Breadfruit	Cranberry	Avocado	Guava
Cranberry	Tamarind	Cherry	Lemon	Jujube	Elderberry	Durian	Currant	Grapefruit	Passionfruit
Currant	Watermelon	Date	Lime	Kiwi fruit	Gooseberry	Jackfruit	Elderberry	Papaya	Pineapple
Elderberry		Fig	Mango	Kumquat	Medlar	Mangosteen	Pawpaw	Sapodilla	Soursop
Gooseberry		Grape		Lemon		Plantain	Plum	Sapote	Strawberry
Medlar		Mulberry		Litchi nut		Rambutan	Raspberry		
Plum		Pear		Loquat			Strawberry		
Raspberry		Pomegranate		Nectarine					
Strawberry		Quince		Orange					
		Raspberry		Peach					
				Persimmon					
				Plum					
				Tangerine					

eliminates toxins in the gut, as well as helping lower cholesterol levels and promote weight loss.[3]

Apples contain many compounds that possess significant anticancer actions. Research demonstrates that many of these compounds are found in much higher concentrations in fresh apples. Fresh whole apples and fresh apple juice contain approximately 100 to 130 mg per 100 g (roughly 3½ ounces) of ellagic, chlorogenic, and caffeic acids, however, the content of these compounds in cooked or commercial apple products is at or near zero—another strong case for eating your fruits and vegetables fresh.

Selection and Preparation

You should definitely buy organic apples if they are available. The recent publicity about the dangerous chemical known as alar (applied to apples to make them ripen uniformly) led producers to curtail its use to an extent, but many other chemicals are still sprayed on apples. In addition, apples are often waxed to keep them fresh longer. Be aware that even organic apples may appear "waxy" because apples have a natural coating of a wax-like substance.

Fresh apples should be firm, crisp, and well-colored. If an apple lacks color, it is likely to have been picked before it was fully mature and then artificially ripened. Apples picked when mature have more color, better flavor, and a longer storage life than apples picked too early. Check out the hardness of the apple—a fresh apple will produce a characteristic snap when you apply pressure to the skin with a finger. Overripe apples will not give you a crisp snap, and they will feel softer.

For maximum nutritional benefit, apples should be consumed in their fresh form—either whole or as juice. In juicing, one key use of apples is as a component in mixes with other fruits and vegetables because of its sweet but not overpowering flavor. Since very small amounts of cyanide are contained in the seeds of apples, many people recommend that you core the apples to remove the seeds before juicing. This is probably a good idea, but I rarely do it, because the amount of cyanide in the apple seeds is extremely minute and—since there is very little liquid in the seed—the seed generally gets shot out the back of the juicer anyway.

Apricot

The apricot is technically classified as a "drupe" or fleshy, one-seeded fruit containing a seed enclosed in a stony pit. The apricot is in the same family as the almond, the cherry, the peach, and the plum. Apricots originated in China. Alexander the Great is believed to have brought the apricot to Greece and ultimately to Western civilization.

Key Benefits

Apricots are good sources of potassium, magnesium, iron, and carotenes. Dried apricots are quite popular, but most contain high levels of sulfur dioxide, which is added to the fruit during the drying process to inactivate enzymes that would otherwise cause the fruit to spoil. Alternative preservation methods (such as blanching) are available that do not necessitate the use of sulfur.

Selection and Preparation

Fresh, ripe apricots should be a uniform golden-orange color, round, and about 2 inches in diameter. Ripe apricots yield to a gentle pressure on the skin. If the fruit is quite hard or relatively yellow in appearance, it is unripe; if it is quite soft or mushy, it is overmature. Fresh apricots are usually best when in season, June through August. Eat them plain or in fruit salads, or juice them.

Apricots should be washed if organic, and soaked or sprayed with a biodegradable wash and then rinsed if nonorganic. Slice them in half and remove the pit.

Since apricots are drier (85 percent water) than most other fleshy fruits, they do not lend themselves to being the sole component of a juice. Fortunately, apricots mix quite deliciously in a base of other fruits, especially apples, oranges, and peaches. Here are a couple of my favorite apricot juice recipes:

Apricot–Orange Juice

4 apricots

2 oranges

Apricot–Pear Juice

4 apricots

1 pear

Avocado

The fruit of the avocado tree (*Persea americana*) is typically used as a vegetable. Native to Central America, avocados are now grown in most tropical and subtropical countries. California produces about 80 percent of the U.S. avocado crop.

Key Benefits

The fat content of an avocado is around 20 percent, or roughly 20 times that of other fruits. The oils provided by an avocado are primarily unsaturated fatty acids, including oleic acid and linoleic acid. Avocados are an excellent source of vitamin E, many B-vitamins, and potassium. In fact, one avocado has the potassium content of two or three bananas. Of course, an avocado also has about three times as many calories as a banana. The total calorie content of an average-size avocado is 300 calories. Again, this is much higher than the calorie count of other fruits.

Selection and Preparation

Ripe avocados should yield slightly to gentle pressure. Hard avocados can be ripened by storing them at room temperature. Refrigeration will slow down ripening. Avoid overripe, rancid avocados with brown meats. Avocados mix deliciously in salads and in guacamole dip.

Banana

Although it looks like a tree, the banana plant is actually a very large barkless plant. The difference between a tree and a plant is that a tree has wood in the stem above the ground. Bananas are thought to have originated in Malaysia and spread to India, the Philippines, and New Guinea. The most popular type of banana is the large yellow, smooth-skinned variety familiar to most Americans. This banana is known as the Manqué or Gros Michel (Big Mike). Other varieties familiar to many are the smaller red-skinned variety known as the Red Jamaican and the larger green bananas known as plantains. Plantains are used similarly to a vegetable, in that they are usually fried or cooked. Bananas are the second leading fruit crop in the world.

Key Benefits

Bananas are full of nutrition, especially potassium. An average-size banana contains a whopping 440 mg of potassium and only 1 mg of sodium. Plantain bananas show some promise in the treatment of peptic ulcers.[4]

Selection and Preparation

Fresh bananas are best when they are yellow (with no green showing) and speckled with brown. Bananas with green tips are not quite ripe, but they will continue to ripen if stored at room temperature. After ripening, bananas may be stored in the refrigerator; and while the skin will turn dark brown, they will remain fresh for 3 to 5 days. Bananas that are bruised, discolored, or soft have deteriorated and should not be used.

Bananas do not lend themselves to juicing, but you can make fresh juice and mix it with a banana in a blender. In the summer, try freezing a banana and mixing it with fresh apple–strawberry juice in the blender to make a delicious "smoothie."

Berries

Blackberries, blueberries, raspberries, strawberries, currants, and other berries are discussed here as an aggregate. Berries are native to many parts of the world, especially in the Northern Hemisphere. Hundreds of varieties of berries now exist as a result of accidental and intentional crossbreeding (hybridization).

Key Benefits

Berries are rich in vital nutrients, yet low in calories. Hence, berries are excellent foods for individuals with a "sweet tooth" who want to improve the quality of nutrition without increasing the caloric content of their diet. Juices prepared from fresh berries typically contains fewer than 100 calories per 8 ounces and provide a rich source of potassium, pure water, water-soluble fibers, and flavonoids. The flavonoids—and mainly a group of flavonoids known as anthocyanidins—are responsible for the colors of the berries. For example, the purplish-black color of blackberries is due to the anthocyanidin known as cyanidin, while the red color of strawberries is due to the anthocyanidin known as pelargonidin. The beneficial effects of flavonoids are discussed in Chapter 4.

Berries have long been used for a wide range of medicinal effects. Today, more and more research supports many of the folk uses of berries. For example, during World War II, British Royal Air Force pilots consumed bilberry (a variety of blueberry) preserves before their night missions. The pilots believed, based on folk medicine, that the bilberries would improve their ability to see at night. After the war, numerous studies demonstrated that blueberry extracts do in fact improve nighttime visual acuity and lead to quicker adjustment to darkness and faster restoration of visual acuity after exposure to glare.[5]

Bilberry extracts have been used by physicians for medicinal purposes in Europe since 1945. Most of the therapeutic applications have involved eye complaints. Results have been most impressive in individuals with retinitis pigmentosa, sensitivity to bright lights, diabetic retinopathy, and macular degeneration. Additional research suggests that bilberries may protect against the development of cataracts and glaucoma, and may be quite therapeutic in the treatment of varicose veins, hemorrhoids, and peptic ulcers.[6]

Most clinical studies have utilized various berry extracts—primarily bilberry and black currants—concentrated for anthocyanoside content. To achieve a similar concentration using fresh fruit, a daily intake of at least 16 ounces (1 pint) of fresh juice would be required.

Berries, especially strawberries, are good sources of the anticancer compound ellagic acid. In one study, strawberries topped a list of eight foods most closely linked to lower rates of cancer death among a group of 1,271 elderly people in New Jersey. Those who ate the most strawberries were three times less likely to develop cancer than those who ate few or no strawberries.[7]

Selection and Preparation

Buy the freshest berries possible. Eat them whole or in fruit salads, or juice them. If berries are not in season, purchase unsweetened frozen berries, and use them to make smoothies in the blender with fresh juice. The berries should be washed if organic, and soaked or sprayed with a biodegradable wash and then rinsed if nonorganic.

Cantaloupe or Muskmelon

In the United States, what we commonly refer to as a cantaloupe is actually a muskmelon. True cantaloupes are seldom grown in the United States.

Cantaloupes are thought to have originated in either Africa or the Middle East. The cantaloupe is now grown all over the world.

Key Benefits

Cantaloupes are extremely nutrient-dense, as defined by quality of nutrition per calorie. An entire 1-pound cantaloupe seldom contains more than 150 calories, yet it provides excellent levels of carotenes, potassium, and other valuable nutrients—especially if the skin is also juiced. Cantaloupe has been shown to contain the compound adenosine, which is currently being used in patients with heart disease to keep the blood thin and to relieve angina attacks.[8]

Selection and Preparation

There are three major signs of a ripe cantaloupe: (1) no stem, but a smooth, shallow basin where the stem was once attached; (2) thick, coarse, and corky netting or veining over the surface; and (3) a yellowish-buff skin color under the netting. Overripeness is characterized by pronounced yellowing of the skin and a soft, watery, and insipid flesh. Small bruises do no harm, but large bruised areas should be cut away. Examine the stem scar to make sure that no mold is growing in it. Keep cantaloupes at room temperature if they are still a little hard, or in the refrigerator if fully ripe. Eat them plain or in fruit salads, or juice them.

Cherries

Cherries are grown in every state and in most parts of the world, but where the cherry comes from is not known. There are basically two types of cherries: sweet and sour. More than 500 varieties of sweet cherries exist, including Bing, black, Windsor, and Napoleon. There are also more than 270 varieties of sour cherries. Sometimes sour cherries are referred to as tart, pie, or red cherries. The sweet cherries are best for juicing. In general, the darker the cherry, the better it is for you.

Key Benefits

Consuming the equivalent of ½ pound of fresh cherries per day has been shown to be very effective in lowering uric acid levels and preventing attacks of gout. Cherries, like berries, are rich sources of flavonoids. Specifically, anthocyanidins and proanthocyanidins are the flavonoid molecules that give these fruits their deep red-blue color; they are remarkable in their ability to prevent collagen destruction (see pages 89, 91).

Selection and Preparation

Good cherries have bright, glossy, plump-looking surfaces and fresh-looking stems. They should be firm, but not hard. Overmature cherries are usually easy to spot. Soft, leaking flesh, brown discoloration, and mold growth are all indications of decay. After removing the stone, eat cherries plain or in fruit salads, or juice them.

Cranberries

Cranberries grow wild in Europe, North America, and Asia. However, almost all of the world's cranberry crop is produced in the United States. Most Americans associate cranberries with Thanksgiving and Christmas dinner, but more and more individuals are eating or drinking these berries throughout the year.

Key Benefits

Cranberries are quite bitter and have been used by many more people for their medicinal than for their nutritional benefits. Cranberries and cranberry juice have been used to treat bladder infections and have proved to be quite effective in several clinical studies. In one study of patients with active urinary tract infections, drinking 16 ounces of cranberry juice per day was shown to produce beneficial effects in 73 percent of the subjects (44 females and 16 males). Furthermore, withdrawal of the supplemental cranberry juice from the diets of those who had benefited resulted in recurrence of bladder infection in 61 percent.[9]

Many people believe that the action of cranberry juice is due to its acidification of the urine and to the antibacterial effects of a cranberry component, hippuric acid. But these are probably not the major mechanisms of action. To acidify the urine, at least 1 quart of cranberry juice would have to be consumed. In addition, the concentration of hippuric acid in the urine as a result of drinking cranberry juice is insufficient to inhibit bacteria. Nonetheless, a positive effect of cranberry juice in the treatment of bladder infection has been noted at a consumption level of only 16 ounces of cranberry juice per day.[10] These data indicate that another mechanism is more likely.

Recent studies have shown that components in cranberry juice reduce the ability of *E. coli* to adhere to the lining of the bladder and urethra.[11] In order to infect, bacteria must first adhere to the mucosa. By interfering with such adherence, cranberry juice greatly reduces the likelihood of infection and helps the body fight off infection. This is the most likely explanation for cranberry juice's positive effects in bladder infections.

Of seven juices studied (cranberry, blueberry, grapefruit, guava, mango, orange, and pineapple), only cranberry and blueberry contained this inhibitor.[12] Blueberry juice is a suitable alternative to cranberry juice in the treatment of bladder infections.

Most cranberry juice drinks on the market contain only one-third cranberry juice, mixed with water and sugar. Fresh cranberry juice naturally sweetened with fresh apple, pear, or grape juice is preferable.

Selection and Preparation

Ripe cranberries are plump, red, shiny, and firm. Poor quality is indicated by shriveling, dull appearance, and softness. Fresh cranberries can be stored in a refrigerator for several months with only minimal loss of moisture or nutritional value. If you have grown accustomed to cranberry juice, here is a healthful alternative to the sugar-filled cranberry drinks sold in cans or bottles. This is a great drink around the holidays. Juice the cranberries first, followed by the lemon, grapes, and apple wedges.

Zesty Cran–Apple Juice

2 apples
1 handful of grapes
½ cup cranberries
½ lemon

Dates

The date palm is considered to be the first tree cultivated by human beings. Mature trees can achieve a height of up to 100 feet. The fruits grow in clusters that can contain up to 200 dates and can weigh up to 25 pounds. Native to the Middle East and North Africa, dates remain an important food in these areas.

Key Benefits

Dates primarily provide sugars. The sugar content consists of varying amounts of simple sugars. The total sugar content can range from 60 to 70 percent.

Selection and Preparation

Most dates are left on the tree to sun-dry. Avoid dates that show any visible signs of microbial growth. Dates can be eaten on their own or used in baked goods, salads, and other dishes.

Figs

The fig tree is native to the Middle East and to the Mediterranean and is among the world's first cultivated trees. Figs are grown in moderate climates all over the world. The five leading world producers are Turkey, Greece, the United States, Portugal, and Spain. Approximately 99 percent of the U.S. crop is grown in California.

Key Benefits

Figs are high in natural simple sugars, minerals, and fiber. They are fairly rich in potassium, calcium, magnesium, iron, copper, and manganese. Figs are often recommended for nourishing and toning the intestines.

Selection and Preparation

Although raw figs are available, dried figs are the most popular form. Typically, dried figs are preserved with potassium sorbate to help keep them moist without spoiling. Dried figs can be consumed on their own or can be utilized in baked goods (fig bars), in jams, and in fruit dishes.

Grapefruit

The grapefruit was first noticed on Barbados in 1750; by 1880 it had become an important commercial crop in Florida. The best grapefruits are grown in Florida and Texas. For juicing purposes, it is best to utilize grapefruits with a red-pink meat, such as the Ruby Red or Star Ruby.

Key Benefits

Fresh grapefruit is low in calories, but is a good source of flavonoids, water-soluble fibers, potassium, vitamin C, and folic acid. Grapefruit, like other citrus fruits, has been shown to exert some anticancer effects in human population studies and in animal studies. Grapefruit pectin has been extensively studied by researchers at the University of Florida led by Dr. James Cerda since 1973. Grapefruit pectin has been shown to possess similar cholesterol-lowering action to other fruit pectins.[13] The whole fruit contains more pectin than the juice. The edible portion of the whole fruit contains approximately 3.9 percent pectin. Since most of the cholesterol-lowering studies used 15 grams of grapefruit pectin to produce a 10 percent drop in cholesterol levels, this would mean that eating approximately two grapefruit per day would lower a person's risk of heart disease by 20 percent. Of course, eating other foods rich in pectin and other soluble fibers would have similar effects.

Recently, grapefruit consumption has been shown to normalize hematocrit levels.[14] The word *hematocrit* refers to the percentage of red blood cells per volume of blood. The normal hematocrit level is 40 to 54 percent for men and 37 to 47 percent for women. Low hematocrit levels usually reflect anemia. High hematocrit levels may reflect severe dehydration or an increased number of red blood cells. A high hematocrit reading is associated with an increased risk for heart disease, because it means that the blood is too viscous (thick).

Naringin, a flavonoid isolated from grapefruit, has been shown to promote the elimination of old red blood cells from the body. This evidence prompted researchers to evaluate the effect on hematocrit levels of eating a half to one whole grapefruit per day. As expected, the grapefruit lowered high hematocrit levels. However, researchers were surprised to find that it had no effect on normal hematocrit levels and that it actually increased low hematocrit levels.[15]

This balancing action is totally baffling to most drug scientists, but not to experienced herbalists who have used terms such as alterative, amphiteric, adaptogenic, or tonic to describe this effect. It appears that, in addition to possessing currently understood actions, many foods and herbs possess actions that are not yet fully understood. For example, many natural compounds in herbs and foods appear to aid body control mechanisms in normalizing many of the body's processes. When a certain body function is elevated, the herb or food will have a lowering effect; and when a certain body function decreases, it will have a heightening effect. Grapefruit appears to have this effect on hematocrit levels.

Selection and Preparation

Fresh grapefruits of good quality are firm but springy to the touch, well-shaped, and heavy for their size. If the grapefruit is soft, wilted, flabby, or has green on the skin, it should not be consumed. Eat grapefruits by themselves or in fruit salads, or juice them.

Some people are allergic to citrus peels. When such allergies are suspected, caution must be exercised, and the grapefruit peel should not be eaten. Citrus peels contain some beneficial oils; but these oils can interfere with some body functions, so they must not be consumed in any significant quantity. For example, citrus peels contain a compound known as citral that is antagonistic to some of the effects of vitamin A.

Grapes

Grapes have been eaten since prehistoric times and were cultivated as far back as 5000 B.C. Grapes are the leading fruit crop in the world. There are three basic types of grapes: Old World, North American, and Hybrids. Old World grapes account for over 95 percent of the grapes grown worldwide. Old World grapes are versatile and may be used as table grapes, raisins, and wine. North American grapes, including the Concord and the Niagara, are available in seedless varieties and are good for juice and as table grapes, but not for raisins. Hybrids are crosses between Old World and North American grapes and are used primarily in wine production.

Key Benefits

Grapes provide similar nutritional benefits to other berries. Nutritional quality can be enhanced by juicing whole grapes that contain seeds. In Europe, a grapeseed extract rich in flavonoids that are known as procyanolic oligomers or leukocyanidins is widely used in treating varicose veins and other venous disorders. These flavonoids are extremely powerful antioxidants and have also been shown to reverse atherosclerosis.[16]

Selection and Preparation

Grapes do not ripen after harvesting, so look for grapes that are well colored, firmly attached to the stem, firm, and wrinkle-free. Green grapes are usually the sweetest. After purchase, grapes should be stored in the refrigerator, where they will maintain their freshness for several days. Eat them whole or in fruit salads, or juice them.

Kiwifruit

The kiwifruit was developed in New Zealand from a smaller, less tasty fruit, the Chinese gooseberry. Since kiwifruits are now grown in California, more and more Americans are discovering this deliciously nutritious fruit. The kiwifruit is a small oval fruit that is brown and fuzzy on the outside. Inside, it contains a sherbet-green meat surrounding small jet-black edible seeds.

Key Benefits

Kiwifruits are rich in enzymes if juiced unpeeled and with the seeds. Kiwifruit are also rich in vitamin C and potassium.

Selection and Preparation

Kiwifruits should feel firm, but not rock-hard. They should give slightly when pressed. Eat them plain or in fruit salads, or juice them. Kiwifruit mixes deliciously with most other fruits, especially grapes, apples, and oranges.

Lemon

The lemon originated somewhere in Southeast Asia. Since lemon trees are more sensitive to freezing temperatures than are other citrus trees, lemons have been the most difficult citrus fruit to cultivate. But unlike other citrus trees, the lemon tree bears fruit continuously. California and Florida lead the United States in the production of lemons.

Key Benefits

Lemons are rich in vitamin C and potassium. The vitamin C content and storage capacity of lemons made them useful for sailors in the battle against scurvy during long voyages. Lemons also contain a substance known as limonene, which is used to dissolve gallstones and shows extreme promise as an anticancer agent.[17] The highest content of limonene is found in the white spongy inner parts of the fruit.

Selection and Preparation

A ripe lemon should have a fine-textured, deep-yellow skin and should be firm to the touch. Deep-yellow-colored lemons are usually less acidic than the paler or greenish-yellow varieties. They are also usually thinner-skinned and yield a larger proportion of juice. Avoid dried out, shriveled, or hard-skinned fruit.

Lemons are most often consumed as "lemonade." Jay Kordich, the Juiceman, has an outstanding recipe for lemonade: juice four apples and one-quarter of a lemon (with the skin), and serve over crushed ice.

Lime

The lime is similar to the lemon, only smaller and greener. Like the lemon, the lime originated somewhere in Southeast Asia; and like lemons, limes were used by sailors in the battle against scurvy during long voyages—especially by British sailors. Hence the term *limeys.*

Key Benefits

Limes do not differ much in nutritional value from lemons.

Selection and Preparation

Limes should be green in color and heavy for their size. If limes show purple- to brown-colored spots, this is a sign that they are decaying. Limes can be used in place of lemons in most dishes.

Mango

Mangoes originated in India, but they are now grown in many tropical locations including California, Hawaii, and Florida. Mangoes are one of the leading fruit crops in the world. In fact, more mangoes are consumed by more people in the world on a regular basis than are apples.

Key Benefits

Mangoes are a good source of potassium, vitamin C, carotenes, and flavonoids. Mangoes provide a rich assortment of antioxidants, and they are delicious when ripe.

Selection and Preparation

A ripe mango will yield to pressure much as an avocado will. Mangoes should be yellowish-green, with a smooth skin and a sweet fragrance. Avoid fruit that is too hard or soft, bruised, or smells of fermentation. Eat them plain or in fruit salads, or juice them. Mangoes yield a relatively thick juice, so you'll want to juice it with higher-water-content fruits such as apples, pears, and oranges.

Orange

The modern-day orange evolved from varieties native to southern China and Southeast Asia. Oranges are by far the leading fruit crop of the United States. Personally I prefer the California orange (the Valencia) to the Florida variety, although the latter typically generates more juice. Mandarin oranges, tangerines, tangelos, and citrons provide benefits similar to those of the orange.

Key Benefits

Everyone knows that oranges are an excellent source of vitamin C. Equally important to the nutritional value of oranges is its supply of flavonoids. The combination of vitamin C and flavonoids makes oranges a very valuable aid in strengthening the immune system, supporting connective tissues of the body (including the joints, gums, and ground substance), and promoting overall good health.

Consuming oranges and orange juice has been shown to protect against cancer, to support the immune system, and to help fight viral infections.[18] In addition to having vitamin C and flavonoids, oranges contain good amounts of carotenes, pectin, potassium, and folic acid. The pectin in oranges possesses similar properties to grapefruit pectin in lowering cholesterol levels.

Selection and Preparation

Fresh oranges are of the best quality when they are well-colored, heavy, and firm, with fine-textured skin. Look out for molds and severely bruised or soft-puffy oranges. Oranges keep well in the refrigerator for more than a week. Eat them plain or in fruit salads, or juice them.

Papaya

The papaya originated in Central America. The green unripe papaya is the source of papain, a protein-digesting enzyme similar to bromelain. Papain is used commercially in many meat tenderizers.

Key Benefits

Papayas are rich in antioxidant nutrients such as carotenes, vitamin C, and flavonoids. Papayas also contain good amounts of many minerals, especially potassium and magnesium. Although the ripe fruit does not contain as much papain as the unripe fruit, it does contain some. In addition to its commercial uses, papain has a number of medicinal applications, including use in such conditions as indigestion, chronic diarrhea, hay fever, sports injuries and other causes of trauma, and allergies. Basically, papain is used in a similar manner as bromelain.[19]

Selection and Preparation

Papayas should be yellow-green in color and firm (but not rock-hard) to the touch. Overmature papayas are soft and usually show signs of decay. Papayas contain small black seeds that are edible but quite bitter. Eat papayas plain or in fruit salads, or juice them.

Peaches and Nectarines

The peach, like many other fruits, is native to China. The numerous varieties of peaches fall into two basic categories: freestone and clingstone. This refers to how easily the pit can be removed from the fruit. Popular freestone varieties include Elberta, Hale, and Golden Jubilee. Popular clingstone varieties are Fortuna, Johnson, and Sims. Nectarines are essentially peaches without the fuzz.

Key Benefits

Two peaches or nectarines or 8 ounces of pure juice contains fewer than 100 calories but provides some important nutrients like potassium, carotenes, flavonoids, and natural sugars.

Selection and Preparation

Fresh peaches and nectarines should be fairly firm. Fruits purchased before they are fully ripe will ripen at home if kept at room temperature. The color indicates the variety of the peach more than ripeness; hence it should not be used as a gauge of ripeness. Be on the lookout for bruises and signs of spoilage. Once ripe, peaches should be stored in the refrigerator. Eat them plain or in fruit salads, or juice them. Peaches yield a relatively thick juice, so you'll want to juice them with apples or pears.

Pear

The pear originated in western Asia, but it is now cultivated throughout much of the world. There are numerous varieties of pears. The best varieties for juicing include Bosc, Anjou, Bartlett, and Comice.

Key Benefits

Pears are an excellent source of water-soluble fibers, including pectin. In fact, pears are actually higher in pectin than apples. This makes them quite useful in helping to lower cholesterol levels and in toning the intestines.

Selection and Preparation

As pears ripen, their skin color changes from green to the color characteristic of the variety. Bosc pears turn brown; Anjou and Bartlett pears turn yellow; and Comice pears have a green mottled skin. Fresh pears are best when they yield to pressure much as a ripe avocado does. Unripe pears will ripen at home if stored at room temperature. Once ripe, they should be refrigerated. Eat them plain or in fruit salads, or juice them. Firm pears are much easier to juice than soft pears. Pears, like apples, can be added to vegetable-based juices to improve the juices' flavor.

Pineapple

The pineapple is native to South America. The United States ranks as one of the world's leading suppliers of pineapples, although all of its pineapples are produced in Hawaii. The edible flesh of the pineapple has a characteristic flavor often described as a mixture of apple, strawberry, and peach.

Key Benefits

The virtues of bromelain, the protein-digesting enzyme complex of pineapple, have already been discussed in Chapter 4. Briefly, bromelain has proved to be useful in treating a number of health conditions, including angina, arthritis, indigestion, upper respiratory tract infections, athletic injuries, and trauma.

In a study conducted at the Cancer Research Center of Hawaii at the University of Hawaii, an extract of pineapple significantly inhibited the growth of tumor cells in cell cultures.[20] In this study another enzyme, known as peroxidase, was indicated to be the major antitumor component. This would indicate that fresh pineapple may have effects beyond its bromelain content. Fresh pineapple is rich in enzymes, vitamin C, and potassium, and low in calories.

Selection and Preparation

The main thing to be concerned about is the presence of decayed or moldy spots; check the bottom stem scar. Ripe pineapples have a fruity, fragrant aroma, are more yellow than green in color, and are heavy for their size. Eat them (peeled and cut up) on their own or in fruit salads, or juice them. Pineapple makes a fantastic base for low-calorie fruit drinks, especially when mixed with berries.

Plums and Prunes

Like peaches and apricots, plums are classified as a drupe because of their hard pit or stone surrounded by soft, pulpy flesh and a thin skin. Plums originated in Europe and Asia. There are five main types of plums: European, Japanese, American, Damson, and Ornamental. A prune is a dried plum, just as a raisin is a dried grape.

Key Benefits

Plums and prunes are often eaten for their laxative effects. Prunes are more effective than plums in this capacity. Plums are good sources of carotenes, flavonoids, potassium, and iron.

Selection and Preparation

Plums vary in color and size. They may be as small as a cherry or as large as a peach; and their skin may be green, yellow, blue, or purple. Select fresh plums based on the color characteristic of the variety. Ripe plums are firm to slightly soft. Avoid plums that have skin breaks, brownish discoloration, or excessive softness. Eat them plain or in fruit salads, or juice them. Plums are fairly harsh if juiced alone, but they mix very well with pears.

Watermelon

Watermelons originated in Africa, but have been cultivated since ancient times in Europe and Asia. Today watermelons are grown worldwide in tropical, semitropical, and temperate climates. The most common watermelon consumed in the United States is light to dark green with stripes or mottling on the outside, covering bright red flesh peppered with dark brown or black seeds. The flesh may also be pink, orange, yellow, or white.

Key Benefits

Watermelon, as its name would imply, is an excellent source of pure water. It is very low in calories. Watermelon is also an excellent diuretic.

Selection and Preparation

People tap on watermelons to determine whether they sound hollow and are therefore ripe; however, this practice does not guarantee success. Look for watermelons that have a smooth surface and a cream-colored underbelly. Despite the best precautions, it is difficult to judge the quality of a watermelon without cutting it in half. Once it is cut, indicators of a good watermelon include firm, juicy red flesh and dark brown to black seeds. The presence of white streaks in the flesh or white seeds usually indicates immaturity. Watermelon can be eaten on its own, used in fruit salads, or juiced.

7

The Healing Power of Grains

Grains are without question the most important food crop in the world, providing the "staff of life" for most people on this planet. Grains have fueled the growth of civilization; and as the earth's population continues to grow, people's reliance on grains is greater than ever.

A grain is most often the seed of a member of the grass family; members of this family are commonly referred to as "cereal" grains. The word *cereal* is derived from Ceres, the Roman goddess of agriculture. Grains were among the first cultivated crops, and archaeological evidence shows that wheat and barley were used over 10,000 years ago by people living in the so-called "Fertile Crescent"—a broad crescent-shaped area that curved northward and eastward from what is now the eastern border of Egypt, to the Taurus Mountains of southern Turkey, across to the Zagros Mountains of western Iran, and down to the Persian Gulf (see Figure 7.1). By about 5000 B.C., grain farming was well established along the Nile in Egypt.

Other areas of the world began grain farming a bit later. By 4000 B.C., millet farming was well established along the upper Yellow River in China. About the same time, rice was being cultivated in Southeast Asia. Since dried grains store well, it is not surprising that their cultivation spread as people traveled to new lands.

The cultivation of grains and the development of grain foods like bread contributed greatly to the spread of civilization. Without grains, civilization probably would not have developed as it has. Several factors promoted the spread of grain cultivation: (1) an increase in population; (2) changes in climate; (3) the domestication of animals; and (4) the development of commerce.

The creation of a consistent food supply through agriculture led quantitatively to increased reproduction and qualitatively to healthier people who were better equipped to deal with the environment. As the population

Figure 7.1 The Fertile Crescent, where cultivation of grains began.

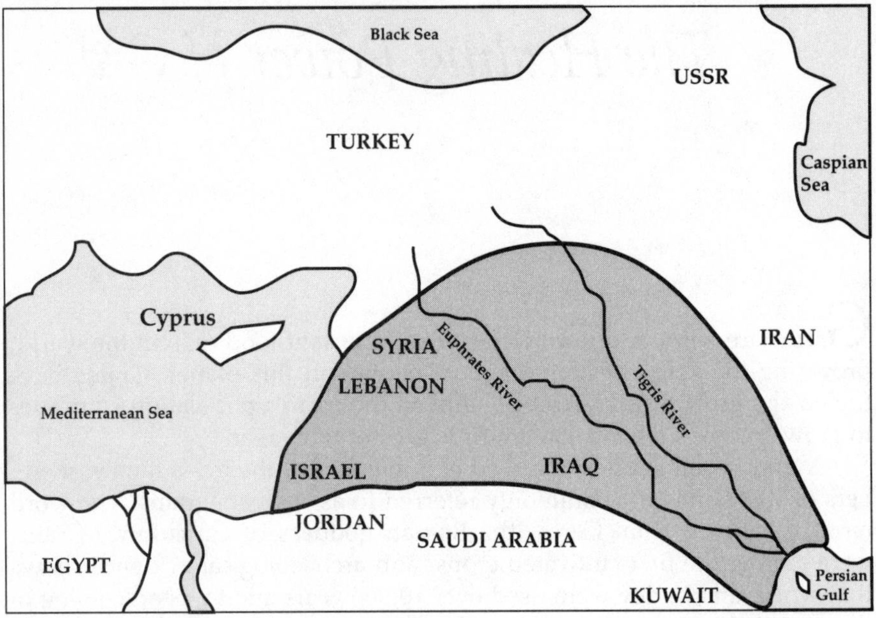

of early villages increased, more land had to be cultivated in order to sustain them. Eventually people were forced to relocate to new areas, anyway. As the land changed, so did the natural habitat and culture. This increased people's dependence on farming, which in turn required inhabitants of villages to work together cooperatively. Every major densely populated ancient civilization in the world developed because it was largely composed of grain farmers.

Climatic events obviously played a major role in the development of agriculture. Of particular significance was the global warming trend between 5500 and 3000 B.C. that resulted in the melting of much of the world's polar ice caps and mountain glaciers. The rising sea level forced many farmers in low-lying areas to migrate to places of higher elevation. Concurrently, the melting of mountain glaciers allowed some grain farmers to migrate northward into Central Europe.

Also important to the spread of grain and civilization was the domestication of animals. Animals such as the ox, the donkey, and the camel were used to help till the soil and to carry the harvested grain. This led, in turn, to increased commerce.

The Green Revolution

In ancient times, as the population of a village grew, so did the villagers' dependence upon grains. Today, as our global population multiplies, we depend on grains for food more than ever. In addition to their numerous health benefits, grains and other plant foods offer a solution to world hunger.

Throughout history, improvements in farming techniques and the development of improved hybrids (crossbreeds) of specific grains have led to better crop yields. However, since not much farmland remains uncultivated, there is an ever growing need for even better utilization of existing land to feed the world's population. The so-called Green Revolution refers to recent breakthroughs in agriculture that have the potential to double or triple the supply of grains and other foods for the world's expanding population and, more immediate, for the developing countries of the world. We are in the midst of this Green Revolution.

The "father" of the Green Revolution is Norman Borlaug, an American agricultural scientist who in 1970 was awarded the Nobel Peace Prize for his breeding of higher-yielding varieties of wheat at the International Maize and Wheat Improvement Center in Mexico. Borlaug's wheat, a hybrid of wheat varieties from the United States, Russia, Japan, and Mexico has numerous favorable traits: (1) short stature of the wheat stalk, which prevents the wheat from growing too tall and falling or breaking; (2) an increased number of grains per plant; (3) strong resistance to disease; and (4) improved tolerance to the environment (climate, day length, and so on).

Similar improvements have been made in rice, most notably by the International Rice Research Institute in the Philippines, which in 1968 released the IR-8 rice strain. This "miracle" rice is a cross between a Chinese semidwarf strain and a tall Indonesian strain; it yields three times as much grain as the older types. Originally the IR-8 strain was a bit chalky, with a strange taste; however, these defects have been overcome and other improvements have been introduced through further breeding.

The Green Revolution is not limited to grains. Improvements are continually being made in the production of all crops. In terms of satisfying the world's food requirements, however, grains and legumes are viewed as being the most important prospective answers. The two foods work well together in many respects. The amino acid patterns complement each other in such a way that the shortcomings of one are compensated for by the other. Specifically, the low lysine content of grains is compensated by the high lysine content of legumes, while the low methionine and cysteine content of many legumes is compensated for by the higher methionine and cysteine content of grains. Furthermore, certain legumes, like peanuts and

Figure 7.2 Wheat anatomy.

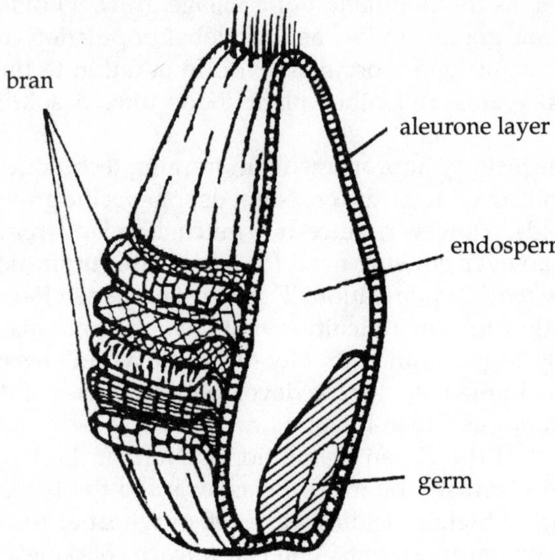

soybeans, convert nitrogen gas from the air into soil ("fixed") nitrogen. The soil is then suitable for grain cultivation. After the grains have depleted the nitrogen, the legumes can once again be planted to renourish the soil with nitrogen. Eventually, grains and legumes may be produced that yield higher-quality protein.

Whole vs. Refined Grains

The anatomy of structure of a grain is basically the same for all grains. The illustration and description of a grain of wheat in Figure 7.2 is representative. The bran is composed of tissues between the outer seed coat and the aleurone layer of the endosperm. The endosperm is the storage compartment of the grain and is composed primarily of protein and carbohydrate. The germ contains the embryo or sprouting section of grain.

Typically in the production of flour, the bran, the aleurone layer, and the germ are removed, leaving only the endosperm. This has a good point and a bad point. The bad point is that removing the bran and the germ results in the loss of many key nutrients (see Table 7.1). The good point is

Table 7.1 Nutrient Losses Due to Removing Bran and Germ from Wheat

Nutrient	*Percentage Loss*
Thiamine	97%
Vitamin B_6	94%
Niacin	88%
Chromium	87%
Magnesium	80%
Potassium	77%
Zinc	72%
Fiber	70%
Essential fatty acids	70%
Riboflavin	68%
Calcium	60%
Pantothenic acid	57%
Protein	25%

that the flour's shelf life is increased. While this may be an important advantage in many parts of the world, it is not so in the United States. To compensate for the loss of nutrients, the flour is "enriched" with specific nutrients, including iron, thiamine, riboflavin, and niacin. The levels of these nutrients in enriched flour are slightly higher than they are in whole-wheat flour. The addition of other nutrients is optional.

This same sort of refining is done with whole grains as well. For example, the overwhelming amount of rice consumed in the world is eaten as white rice. White rice is produced in several stages. First, the rice is milled, to separate the outer portions of the grain (husk, bran, and aleurone), as well as the germ, from the endosperm. At this point, the rice may be sold as "brown rice" or milled (polished) at least three more times to produce white rice. The secondary polishing results in significant nutrient loss. Of particular importance is the loss of thiamine (vitamin B_1).

A severe deficiency of thiamine results in a condition known as beriberi, which is characterized by extreme loss of appetite, congestive heart failure, water retention, psychosis (disorientation, hallucinations, loss of memory, and so on), muscle pain, and other symptoms of disturbed nerve function. In past centuries, beriberi was relatively common in Asia, among sailors, and in prisons. Prior to the late 1890s, the cause of beriberi was not known. The first clue was discovered in 1873, when a Dutch naval doctor observed that European sailors had significantly fewer cases of beriberi than did sailors recruited from the East Indies. By decreasing the amount of white rice in the sailor's diets, crews were able to decrease the rate of beriberi. Still, medical experts thought that beriberi was caused by some toxin or infectious agent in the white rice. Takaki, a Japanese naval doctor, was the first to report that beriberi seemed to be a nutritional deficiency. He based his conclusion on the success he had in reducing the amount of beriberi among Japanese sailors by giving them additional meat, dry milk, and vegetables. The Dutch physician Eijkman's classic experiments in the 1890s began to clarify the role of diet in beriberi.[1]

Eijkman noticed that feeding fowl polished white rice caused them to develop symptoms similar to beriberi. By adding rice polishings (the material removed from whole rice to produce white rice) to the feed, Eijkman was able to cure the fowl of their form of beriberi. His associate later demonstrated that adding green peas, green beans, and meat to the diet of fowl that were otherwise subsisting on polished rice could likewise prevent beriberi in fowl. From this, they deduced correctly that something in natural foodstuffs prevented beriberi. In 1911, Funk, working at the Lister Institute of London, isolated from rice polishings what he thought was the substance that could cure/prevent beriberi. Funk termed his discovery a "vitamine." What Funk had actually isolated, however, turned out to be the antipellagra vitamin, niacin (vitamin B_3). In 1926, pure thiamine, the true antiberiberi vitamin, was isolated by two Dutch scientists, Jansen and Donath, working in Java. Today, white rice is often enriched with thiamine and other nutrients lost during milling. Beriberi is still prevalent in many parts of Asia, however, where polished, unenriched rice supplies up to 80 percent of the total calories. Beriberi and many other nutrient deficiencies in Third World countries could be prevented if the people simply ate whole grains.

The story of beriberi and the discovery of thiamine highlights the value of whole grains over polished grains. In addition to supplying many known nutrients, whole grains provide substantially more anutrients and possibly many unknown compounds with health-promoting properties as well. Instead of removing natural nutrients from the grains and then adding back a limited number of these in the form of synthetic replacements, wouldn't it make more sense to eat whole grains?

Whole grains are a major source of complex carbohydrates, dietary fiber, minerals, and B-vitamins. The protein content and quality of whole grains is greater than that of refined grains. Diets rich in whole grains have been shown to protect against the development of chronic degenerative diseases, especially cancer, heart disease, diabetes, varicose veins, and diseases of the colon including colon cancer, inflammatory bowel disease, hemorrhoids, and diverticulitis.

Preparation and Uses of Whole Grains

Grains are used in various foods—breakfast cereals, pasta, bread, casseroles, and so on. Perhaps the most healthful way to enjoy the nutritional benefits of whole grains is simply by boiling or steaming them. This can be done with the help of a double-boiler or grain steamer. The most common method, however, is to bring the appropriate amount of water (see Table 7.2) to a boil in a pot, add the appropriate amount of whole grain, bring to another boil, reduce heat, cover, and simmer for the appropriate amount of time.

Whole grains are great diet foods: low in calories, high in fiber, and high in complex carbohydrates. Since cooking grains in water tremendously increases their water content, this (along with the high fiber content of whole grains) provides incredible bulking action. In other words, whole grains are quite satisfying due to their high bulk. Whole grains can be used as breakfast cereals, side dishes, casseroles, or part of the main entrée. *The Healing Power of Foods Cookbook* contains many whole-grain recipes. Table 7.2 presents a guide to yields in cooking grains.

Over 8,000 different species of plants supply grains, but only a handful of these play a significant role in the human diet. The major food grains—wheat, rice, corn, and oats—will be discussed next, followed by a brief description of some of the more popular minor food grains. Table A.3 in the Appendix identifies the nutritive value of edible plants of selected grains as well as of selected grain products.

Table 7.2 Guide for Cooking Grains

Grain (1 cup dry)	*Cups of Water*	*Cooking Time*	*Yield*
Barley	3	1–4 hours	3½ cups
Brown rice	2	45 minutes	3 cups
Buckwheat (kasha)	2	15 minutes	2½ cups
Millet	3	45 minutes	3½ cups
Oats	2	30 minutes	3 cups
Quinoa	2¼	20 minutes	2 cups
Whole wheat			
Berries	3	2 hours	2⅔ cups
Bulgur	2	15–20 minutes	2½ cups
Cracked	2	25 minutes	2⅓ cups
Wild rice	3	1 hour	4 cups

The Major Food Grains

Wheat

Wheat provides more nourishment for more people throughout the world than does any other food. More than one-third of the world's population utilizes wheat as a main dietary staple. Wheat also accounts for the largest cropland area of any food, as more than 22 percent of all available cropland is devoted to growing wheat. The major wheat-producing countries in the world are Russia, the United States, China, and India. The leading wheat-producing states in the United States are Kansas, North Dakota, Oklahoma, Texas, Washington, and Montana.[2]

First cultivated in the Fertile Crescent and later in Egypt, wheat has been an extremely important grain throughout history. Indeed, the development of Western civilization can be linked to the history of wheat. The reverential place wheat held in almost every major culture is noted in various ways. In Western culture, the Lord's Prayer alludes to the importance of wheat and bread: "Give us this day our daily bread."

Wheat is used in various products, but primarily as flour for bread and baked goods. One key reason why wheat is better suited for bread making than is any other grain is its high gluten content. Gluten is composed of two proteins (gliadin and glutenin) that are found in many grains but are found in their highest quantities in wheat, followed by rye (a distant second), oats, and barley. Gluten gives flour elasticity and strength, and allows breads to "rise." After kneading, gluten traps the carbon dioxide produced by yeast or a chemical leavening agent, resulting in the expansion or "rising" of the dough.

Some people cannot tolerate gluten: either they are allergic to it or they lack the ability to digest it. Celiac disease, also known as nontropical sprue, is an intestinal disorder caused by the inability to utilize gluten. It is characterized by diarrhea, malabsorption of nutrients, and an abnormal small intestine structure that reverts to normal when dietary gluten is removed and avoided thereafter. Celiac disease is discussed further in Chapter 14.

Wheat bran is a popular bulk laxative. A third of a cup per day is sufficient for this purpose. In addition to fiber, wheat bran also contains most of the B-vitamins and about 20 percent of the total protein content of whole wheat. Wheat bran contains fiber compounds known as phytates that can impair the absorption and utilization of several minerals, including calcium, zinc, iron, and copper. Anyone taking large amounts (more than ⅓ cup per day) of wheat bran regularly for its laxative effect would be wise to supplement the diet with additional minerals.

Whole-grain wheat and wheat germ are good sources of vitamin E and octacosanol, two very important antioxidants.

Rice

Rice is by far the most important grain in Eastern Asia, where 94 percent of the world's rice crop is grown and consumed. In China, Japan, Thailand, and Indonesia, the annual per capita rice consumption is 200 to 400 pounds. In comparison, the United States contributes little more than 1 percent of the total rice crop, with a yearly per capita consumption of less than 8 pounds.

Contrary to most people's perception, rice does not have to grow in water. The rice fields or paddies are flooded as an efficient method of weed and insect control and to produce higher yields.

Brown rice is quite nutritious and is comparable in caloric, vitamin, and mineral content to whole wheat. Rice bran, like oat bran, can help lower serum cholesterol levels. In addition to its fiber components, rice bran contains gamma-oryzanol, a compound with profound beneficial effects. Gamma-oryzanol not only lowers cholesterol, it exerts growth-promoting powers as well.[3] Presumably, since whole-grain brown rice contains rice bran and gamma-oryzanol, it has cholesterol-lowering effects, too. Although wheat has a higher protein content than brown rice (8 percent), the protein quality of brown rice is better.[4] Unfortunately, most of the rice consumed is white rice, not brown rice.

In the process of polishing white rice, essential oils are lost; fiber content, protein content, and quality decrease; minerals are lost; and significant reductions occur in B-vitamins such as thiamine (80 percent), riboflavin (50 percent), niacin (65 percent) and vitamin B_6 (50 percent). Because rice is such a major component in Eastern Asian diets—accounting for 60 to 80 percent of the calories—stripping away these key nutrients causes nutritional deficiencies that would not exist if the people simply ate brown rice.

For nearly 100 years, efforts have been made in many parts of Asia to improve the nutritional quality of the diet by encouraging people to eat more unmilled rice and by introducing other dietary changes. However, these efforts have largely failed, because people have resisted changing their dietary practices. They simply prefer the white rice to the more natural brown rice. The result? General malnutrition and beriberi remain common in many areas of Asia.

Enriched rice has been suggested as a way to reduce the rate of beriberi among rice-eating populations. This process involves spraying selected vitamins and minerals on the polished white rice and then sealing them in place with an edible film. This treated rice is then mixed in with ordinary white rice in a proportion of 1 part enriched rice to 200 parts ordinary white rice. The result is a white rice that has the same levels of thiamine, iron, and niacin as brown rice. Although enrichment has been shown to be effective on a limited scale, major obstacles (including the cost of the vitamins and the enrichment process) must be overcome before it can be utilized worldwide. Obviously, it would not be necessary at all if people would simply eat brown rice instead of white rice.

Wild rice is native to the Great Lakes Region of North America. Wild rice is higher in protein content and lower in fat than other grains. It can be cooked in the same ways as brown rice.

Corn

Many people are surprised that corn is considered a grain. Internationally, corn is referred to as *maize* because the term *corn* is often used to indicate whatever happens to be the leading cereal grain in an area. In the United States this is, appropriately, corn. In England, *corn* refers to wheat; and in Scotland and Ireland, *corn* refers to oats. So, to avoid confusion, the word maize is used. In this book, however, *corn* will refer to what Americans know as corn.

Corn is another contribution from America, where corn has been cultivated for over 3,000 years. Just as wheat was the "staff of life" in European culture, corn was similarly viewed by Native Americans and early European settlers. The cultivation of corn was deeply embedded in religion, ceremonies, and customs of the Native Americans.

While yellow corn predominates today, the Native Americans prized corn with colorful kernels—blue, red, pink, and black—or with bands, spots, or stripes. The difference in color is due primarily to concentrations of different pigments (such as carotenes and flavonoids) contained in the aleurone (the outer layer of the endosperm).

While corn is an important food crop in the United States, more than 75 percent of it is grown specifically for use as animal feed.[5] Corn provides complex carbohydrates, essential fatty acids, and vitamin E. The protein content of corn (8 to 11 percent) is lower than that of many other grains. The protein quality is also lower than most other grains, due to low levels of both lysine and tryptophan. Corn is also a poor source of niacin: 50 to 80 percent of its niacin content is bound in such a way that it cannot be utilized by the body. People relying primarily on corn run the risk of developing pellagra, a disease caused by a deficiency of niacin. An exception to this involves people who consume cornmeal in the form of tortillas. During the process of mixing cornmeal with lime (calcium carbonate) and water, the niacin is unbound and made available to the human body.

Corn and corn by-products (corn syrup, cornmeal, corn oil, and so on) are used in various products. Two special preparations of corn that deserve comment are grits and polenta. Grits are made from coarsely ground grain (in this case, corn) from which the bran and the germ has been removed. Therefore, grits provide less nutrition than does whole corn. Grits are often enriched with vitamins and minerals to replace those lost during processing. Grits are a popular breakfast grain. Polenta is simply cooked cornmeal (whole or degerminated). Polenta can be eaten on its own or substituted for pasta in recipes.

Oats

Oats are a relatively newly cultivated grain. They have been cultivated for only about 2,000 years. Although substantially less oats are produced than wheat, rice, or corn, I include oats as a major grain due to their well-known health benefits and their popularity in the United States. Oats are the fourth-leading grain produced in the United States (after corn, wheat, and sorghum), in number of bushels produced.

Thanks to an explosion of marketing information, most Americans are now aware of the cholesterol-lowering effects of oats. Since 1963, more than 20 clinical studies have examined the effect of oat bran on serum cholesterol levels.[6] Various oat preparations containing either oat bran or oatmeal have been used, including cereals, muffins, breads, and entrées. The overwhelming majority of these studies have demonstrated a very favorable effect of oats on cholesterol levels. In individuals with high cholesterol levels (above 220 mg/dl), consuming the equivalent of 3 grams of soluble oat fiber typically lowers total cholesterol by 8 to 23 percent. This is highly significant, given that, with each 1 percent drop in serum cholesterol level, there is a 2 percent decrease in the risk of developing heart disease. The 3 grams of fiber specified would be provided by approximately one bowl of ready-to-eat oat bran cereal or oatmeal. Although oatmeal's fiber content (7 percent) is less than that of oat bran (15 to 26 percent), the polyunsaturated fatty acids appear to contribute as much to the cholesterol-lowering effects of oats as does the fiber content. Although oat bran has a higher fiber content, oatmeal is higher in polyunsaturated fatty acids. This makes oatbran and oatmeal quite similar in effectiveness. Although individuals with high cholesterol levels will see significant reductions in these levels as a result of frequent oats consumption, individuals with normal or low cholesterol levels will see little change.

The Minor Food Grains

Amaranth

Amaranth is an ancient food of the Aztecs and Mayans of Central America that is now being "rediscovered." Due to its recent introduction into the modern food supply, amaranth tends to be less allergenic than many other grains. Although more expensive than many other common grains, its cost may be justified in allergic individuals. Amaranth is available as whole grains, as flour, and in breakfast cereals. It can be used similarly to wheat.

Barley

Barley is one of the oldest cultivated grains in the world. Although used as a food crop, barley is probably most valued as an ingredient in alcoholic beverages such as beer and barley-wine. Barley is the fourth-ranking cereal crop in the world, behind wheat, rice, and corn. Russia is by far the leading barley producer in the world, followed by France, China, Great Britain, Canada, and Germany. North Dakota and Idaho are the leading U.S. producers. Most of the barley produced (80 percent) is used in the manufacture of alcoholic beverages (beer and whiskey) or as livestock feed.[7]

Nutritionally, barley provides similar benefits to corn. Like oats and rye, barley grains are covered with hulls or husks that are best removed before using the remainder for food purposes. Different machines are used to scour or pearl the indigestible husk and all or part of the bran layer. Barley groats are the least processed, but their use is limited to porridge. Pot barley is the next-least-processed pearled whole-grain barley; it is used primarily in mushroom and barley soups. Pearl barley is more processed than pot barley and is used much as rice is. The flavor of barley blends well in vegetable soups, legume dishes, casseroles, and many other recipes. Barley flour can be used in place of wheat flour in recipes for bread and other baked goods.

Buckwheat

Native to Asia, buckwheat comes from a plant that is not a grass. The plant produces a fragrant flower, followed by the development of buckwheat groats—little triangular grains covered by a fibrous shell. Most of the world's buckwheat supply is grown in Russia, Poland, and Eastern Europe, where it is an important food item.

Buckwheat lacks the bran and germ, but still provides a good fiber content. Unlike the other grains, buckwheat is high in lysine, which makes buckwheat complementary to other grains in providing a higher-quality protein when combined.

In Russia, kasha—a cooked, mashed buckwheat dish—is a popular breakfast cereal. In Japan, buckwheat flour is combined with wheat flour to make Soba noodles; and whole buckwheats are soaked, steamed, dried, and then milled to remove the hulls to make a product (known as Soba-mai) that is used much as rice is. In the United States, buckwheat flour is used most often to make buckwheat pancakes.

Millet

Millet is a major part of the diet for many people living in India, Africa, China, and Russia. At one time millet was an important crop in Europe as well, but it was largely replaced by corn and the potato. More than 94 percent of the entire world's millet production occurs in Asia and Africa. Although the protein content of millet can vary between 5 and 20 percent, with an average of 10 to 12 percent, millet is generally superior to wheat, corn, and rice in protein content.

Quinoa

Quinoa, like amaranth, is a rediscovered grain. Native to Central America, quinoa is a quick-cooking (20 minutes) whole grain. It can be used as a main dish or as a side dish. Quinoa is available at most health-food stores. It is probably the least allergenic of the grains.

Rye

Rye appears to have originated in central Asia before spreading westward into Eastern Europe. It is used primarily as a bread grain and is second only to wheat in this application. Interestingly, as living standards rise, the consumption of rye bread falls. Russia is by far the leading producer of rye, followed by Poland, Germany, and Turkey. Most of the rye grown in the United States is used as livestock feed.[8]

Rye fiber supplies a rich source of noncellulose polysaccharides, with a high water-binding capacity. By binding water in the intestinal tract, rye breads give the sensation of fullness. Dry rye breads or crackers rich in fiber may be the most useful for this purpose; look for products without unnecessary oils and salt.

Because rye grows well in poor soil and in moist climates, it is a fertile growing medium for the ergot fungus. Ergot grows out of the flowering stalk as a hornlike dark fruiting body that resembles a deformed grain.

During the Middle Ages, ergot was responsible for frequent epidemics of what was called Holy Fire or Saint Anthony's Fire—a condition characterized by loss of blood flow to the extremities, resulting in intense pain and eventually gangrene along with mental derangement. The compounds responsible for these symptoms are chiefly alkaloids, of which LSD (lysergic acid diethylamide) is a variant. Today, small amounts of ergot compounds are used in the medical treatment of migraines, Parkinson's disease, and shock.[9]

Sorghum

Sorghum has been cultivated in Africa and Asia for over 4,000 years. Sorghum is known as chicken corn, guinea corn, and kafficorn. It is usually grown in hot, dry regions where corn cannot be grown successfully. Although sorghum is the fifth leading grain crop in the world (after wheat, rice, corn, and barley), less than 2 percent of the sorghum grown in the United States, which is the world's leading producer, is used in foods, in alcohol production, or for seed. The rest, 98 percent, is used as livestock feed. Nutritionally, sorghum is comparable to corn.[10]

Triticale

Triticale is a hybrid of wheat and rye. It is attracting considerable interest because its protein content is higher than wheat's. However, it requires fertile, well-watered soil for best growth; it yields less grain per acre than does wheat; and it is susceptible to ergot.

8

The Healing Power of Legumes

Legumes (beans) are among the earliest of cultivated plants. Fossil records demonstrate that even prehistoric people domesticated and cultivated them for food. Today, legumes are a mainstay in most diets of the world. This extremely large category of plants contains over 13,000 species and is second only to grains in supplying calories and protein to the world's population. Compared to grains, legumes supply about the same number of total calories, but they usually provide two to four times more protein. Legumes combine with grains to form complete proteins.

Legumes are often called "the poor person's meat." However, they might better be known as the "healthy person's meat." Many legumes, especially soybeans, demonstrate impressive health benefits. Diets rich in legumes are used to lower cholesterol levels, improve blood glucose control in diabetics, and reduce the risk of many cancers. Legumes contain many important nutrients and anutrients. Many of these are detailed in Table A.4 in the Appendix.

Legumes are all very similar in shape and structure. The cotyledon, like the endosperm in grains, determines the nutritional content of the seed; it functions in providing the nutrition required to get the sprout established.

Legumes and Flatulence

One problem with legumes is increased intestinal flatulence (gas) or intestinal discomfort. Most humans pass gas a total of 14 times per day, with a total volume of 1 pint. About half of the gas is swallowed air, and another 40 percent is carbon dioxide released by the bacteria in the intestines. The remaining 10 percent is a mixture of hydrogen, methane, sulfur compounds, and by-products of bacteria such as indoles, skatoles, ammonia, and hydrogen sulfide. This last fraction is responsible for the offensive odors.

The flatulence-causing compounds in legumes are primarily oligosaccharides, which are composed of three- to five-sugar molecules linked together in such a way that the body cannot digest or absorb them. Because the body cannot absorb or digest these oligosaccharides, they pass into the intestines, where bacteria break them down. Gas is produced by the bacteria as they digest the oligosaccharides. Navy and lima beans generally produce the most offensive gases, while peanuts produce the least, because of their respective levels of these compounds.[1]

The quantity of oligosaccharides in a legume (and hence the amount of flatulence produced by it) can be significantly reduced by properly cooking or sprouting it. A commercial enzyme preparation (Beano) is also available to help reduce flatulence.

Cooking Dried Legumes

Although most legumes can be purchased precooked in cans, cooking your own offers significant economic and health benefits. Cooking your own legumes will produce three times the amount for the same money as canned products.

Dried legumes are best prepared by first soaking overnight in an appropriate amount of water (see Table 8.1). This is best done in the refrigerator, to prevent fermentation. Soaking usually reduces the required cooking time dramatically. If soaking overnight is not possible, here is an alternate method: place the dried legumes in an appropriate amount of water in a pot; for each cup of dried legumes, add ¼ teaspoon of baking soda; bring to boil for at least 2 minutes; and then set aside to soak for at least an hour. The baking soda will soften the legumes and help break down the troublesome oligosaccharides. The baking soda will also help reduce the amount of cooking time. After soaking, beans should be simmered with a minimum of stirring, to keep them firm and unbroken. A pressure cooker or crock pot can also be used.

Sprouting Legumes

Since legumes are actually seeds, they contain all the essential factors to enable the plant to sprout and develop. Sprouting is thought not only to increase the nutritional value for many of these foods, but to improve their

Table 8.1 Guide for Cooking Legumes

(1 Legume cup dry)	*Water*	*Cooking Time (if presoaked)*	*Yield*
Black beans	4 cups	1½ hours	2 cups
Blackeye peas	3 cups	1 hour	2 cups
Chick peas	4 cups	2½–3 hours	2–3 cups
Kidney beans	3 cups	1½ hours	2 cups
Lentil or split peas	3 cups	½–1 hour	2 cups
Lima beans	2 cups	1½ hours	2 cups
Navy beans	3 cups	1–1½ hours	2 cups
Pinto beans	3 cups	2–2½ hours	2–3 cups
Soybeans	4 cups	3 hours	2 cups

digestibility as well. Many sprouts, such as alfalfa, mung bean, garbanzos (chick-peas), and lentils are available at grocery stores. Alfalfa sprouts are by far the most popular.

Sprouting at home is quite easy for most nuts, seeds, grains, and legumes. All you need is a large glass jar; or better yet, invest in a sprouting jar equipped with different types of lids. After rinsing, place the item to be sprouted in the jar, and cover it with water for 24 hours. You may need to rinse the item once or twice and re-cover it with water. After the initial 24 hours, pour out the water, rinse, and allow the moist sprouts to sit in an area without direct sunlight. Rinse the sprouts twice daily. Once the item has sprouted (usually one to three days), it can be placed in more direct sunlight if desired. Most sprouts will be ready to eat in a day or two after they have sprouted.

Soybean

The soybean is preeminent among legumes both in dietary importance and in the quantity of information that has been gathered about its health benefits—much of which applies to other legumes as well.

The soybean plant (*Glycine max*) is native to China, where it has been cultivated for food for well over 13,000 years. The ancient Chinese considered the soybean their most important crop and a necessity for life. Thanks largely to the United States, which accounts for over 50 percent of the world's production, the soybean is now the most widely grown and utilized legume, accounting for well over 50 percent of the world's total legume production. In terms of dollar value, the soybean is the United

States' most important crop, ranking above corn, wheat, and cotton. Unfortunately, in the United States, despite its use in a variety of food products, the soybean is still used primarily for animal feed (protein meal) and for its oils. Since the 1970s, however, Americans have markedly increased their consumption of traditional soyfoods (such as tofu, tempeh, and miso) and of so-called "second-generation" soyfoods that simulate traditional meat and dairy products. Consumers can now find soy milk, soy hotdogs, soy sausage, soy cheese, and soy frozen desserts at their grocery stores.

The increase in soyfood consumption is attributed to several factors, including economics, health benefits, and environmental concerns. Soybeans provide a great amount of nutrition per acre. In fact, 1 acre of soybeans can provide nearly 20 times the amount protein that the same area of land could produce if used for raising beef. Human use of and reliance on soybeans will grow as the world's population continues to grow and as its food supply continues to shrink.

Key Benefits

A review of the benefits of soy could fill a large book. It is one of the world's most important foods, especially as a protein source (soybeans contain 38 percent protein). Compared to other legumes, soybeans are higher in essential fatty acids (the total fat content is 18 percent) and much lower in carbohydrates (31 percent). Other nutrients supplied by soybeans in good amounts include vitamin E, calcium, phosphorus, and iron.

The key benefits of soy relate to its excellent protein content, its essential fatty acid and lecithin levels, its fiber constituents, its anticancer components, and its estrogenic activity. Each of these will be discussed separately, but the topics are intricately interrelated.

Protein Content Although the amino acid profile of soy is not perfect, as it is somewhat low in methionine and tryptophan, it is still regarded as equal in protein quality to animal foods. When soy is combined with grains high in methionine (like corn), an extremely high-quality protein is made. Soybased infant formulas are a universally accepted staple for babies who cannot tolerate milk-based formulas. Soy protein–based products provide the same order of growth and development in infants and of protein nutrition in adults as do milk-based formulas.[2] However, the human body appears to handle plant proteins and animal proteins differently. For example, experimental studies in animals and humans have shown that isolates of soy protein tend to lower cholesterol levels, while protein from animal sources (particularly casein from milk) tend to raise them.[3] Researchers have yet to determine exactly how vegetable proteins like soy protein lower cholesterol levels; several factors have been observed that might account for the reduction. The cholesterol-lowering effect of soy protein formulations is more apparent when serum cholesterol levels are high. Human studies have shown that total cholesterol and LDL (the bad) cholesterol are both reduced, as are elevated triglyceride levels.[4] From a practical perspective, consumers should be wary of casein-containing (that is, milk-based) meal replacement formulas such as Ultra SlimFast. Casein has been shown to increase cholesterol levels and the risk of developing gallstones.[5]

Essential Fatty Acids, Phytosterols, and Lecithin Soybeans have a total fat content of approximately 18 percent, of which 85 percent is unsaturated and 15 percent is saturated. The unsaturated portion is composed of linolenic (9 percent of total oil content), linoleic (50 percent), and oleic (26 percent) acids. The essential fatty acid content of soybeans supports their cholesterol-lowering and anticancer effects.

Soybeans are the primary commercial source of lecithin (phosphatidylcholine). Unrefined soy oil contains approximately 3 percent lecithin. During refining, the lecithin is removed as an "impurity" and then sold for use in baked goods, prepared foods, and pharmaceutical preparation. Lecithin is an excellent emulsifier for helping oils and water mix. Lecithin also has been shown to produce numerous beneficial health effects. A commercial lecithin preparation containing up to 90 percent phosphatidylcholine (a major component of the cellular membranes in humans) has demonstrated positive effects in lowering cholesterol levels, improving liver and gallbladder function, and repairing various neurological disorders.[6] Phosphatidylcholine plays an important part in maintaining the myelin sheath that surrounds nerve cells, and it acts as a precursor to the neurotransmitter acetylcholine. Phosphatidylcholine has been investigated in the treatment of Alzheimer's disease, Parkinson's disease, Tourette syndrome, and Huntington's disease.[7] The results have sometimes shown a positive effect and sometimes no effect. It is not known to what degree the lecithin or choline content of soybeans contributes to the beneficial effects.

Soybeans, like most other seeds, nuts, and legumes, contain compounds known as phytosterols. These plant compounds are structurally similar to cholesterol and steroid hormones. Phytosterols function to inhibit the absorption of cholesterol by blocking absorption sites. The cholesterol-lowering effects of phytosterols are well documented.[8] Phytosterols have also been shown to enhance immune functions, inhibit the Epstein-Barr virus, prevent chemically induced cancers in animals, and exhibit numerous anticancer effects.[9] Soybeans are especially rich in phytosterols, especially beta-sitosterol. A 100-gram (3½-ounce) serving of soybeans provides approximately 90 mg of beta-sitosterol, while unrefined soybean oil provides 315 mg per 100 mg. Refined soybean oil provides much less—132 mg per 100 mg.

Fiber Components Soybeans contain a mixture of fiber components. Approximately 94 percent of the total fiber content is composed of insoluble fiber, and 6 percent is soluble. Of the insoluble fiber, approximately 90 percent consists of hemicelluloses. Numerous health effects of soy fiber have been demonstrated in clinical studies. Its effectiveness is largely due to its ability to perform the following actions:

Increase fecal bulk
Increase fecal water content
Decrease intestinal transit time
Reduce blood cholesterol and triglyceride levels
Improve glucose tolerance
Increase insulin sensitivity

These effects of soy fiber make soybeans and other soy fiber–containing foods useful in cases of constipation, diarrhea, high cholesterol level, or diabetes.

Anticancer Compounds In June 1990, the National Cancer Institute held a workshop to examine the relationship between soybean consumption and cancer.[10] Soybean consumption is thought to be one of the major reasons for the relatively low rates of breast and colon cancers in Japan and China. Studies in animals have demonstrated that diets composed of as little as 5 percent soybeans can significantly inhibit chemically induced cancers. Soybeans contain many known and proposed anticancer compounds. In addition to containing fiber and other well-recognized anticancer nutrients and anutrients, soybeans bear several other potent anticancer agents in relatively high concentrations. The most interesting of these are isoflavones, phytosterols, and protease inhibitors.

Protease Inhibitors Soybeans, like other legumes, nuts, and seeds, contain compounds that inhibit the action of the protein-digesting enzymes (proteases). These compounds, referred to as *protease inhibitors,* are part of the seed's defense against destruction. For example, because of protease inhibitors, many seeds are indigestible when eaten by birds and are excreted intact so that they can still sprout new plants. Does this mean that humans cannot digest these foods either? Not necessarily. In humans, compensatory mechanisms, such as increased pancreatic enzyme output, can counteract some of the protease inhibition. In addition, most (but not all) protease inhibitor activity is destroyed by cooking or sprouting.

Consumption of raw soybeans, which contain considerable quantities of protease inhibitors, was one of the first dietary factors shown to inhibit the growth of experimental cancers in animals. Numerous studies in animals have confirmed a possible anticancer effect when they are fed soyfoods containing protease inhibitors.[11] However, although this anticancer effect may be due in part to protease inhibition, the same degree of inhibition has been produced by feeding animals soyfoods without the protease inhibitors. Furthermore, the anticancer effects of the protease inhibitors may not be direct. Pancreatic enzyme preparations containing proteases—and other proteases, like bromelain—have long been used in Europe and by alternative healthcare practitioners in the United States to treat cancer. Some clinical evidence suggests that this is quite beneficial.[12] The use of proteases in treating cancer appears to contradict the animal studies demonstrating that protease inhibition inhibits cancers. But on closer examination, it appears that feeding animals (and humans) protease inhibitors actually stimulates output of more pancreatic proteases. Although the proteases may be inhibited from digesting the protease inhibitors, their other functions may not be affected. Such functions include activating certain immune functions.[13]

As a side note, one possible effect of consuming protease inhibitors in the form of raw nuts, seeds, grains, and legumes is an increase in the output of the hormone cholecystokinin by the intestines. Increased cholecystokinin levels in the blood result in feelings of satiety and a significant reduction in appetite.[14]

Isoflavones Isoflavones are also known as *phytoestrogens,* signifying their mild estrogenic activity. The isoflavonoids in soybeans possess about 0.2 percent of the estrogen activity of estradiol, the principal human estrogen. Isoflavones actually bind to estrogen receptors. Their weak estrogenic action is actually an antiestrogenic effect, preventing the binding of the body's own estrogen to the receptor. This effect does not disrupt the normal reproductive and fertility functions of estrogen, but it may counteract some of the hormone's cancer-causing potential.[15]

Many tumors, especially breast cancers, are sensitive to estrogen, meaning that many tumors grow in response to estrogen binding to cell receptors and stimulating tumor growth. Tamoxifen, a drug used to block estrogen in the treatment of breast cancer, is similar to isoflavones in structure and action. Experimental studies in animals have demonstrated that soy isoflavonoids are extremely effective in inhibiting mammary tumors. The isoflavonoids work not only by occupying estrogen receptors, but also by triggering other, unrelated mechanisms. Researchers have concluded that the anticancer activity of soy isoflavones may not be limited to estrogen-dependent tumors.[16]

Estrogenic Activity The isoflavones and phytosterols of soybeans produce a mild estrogenic effect. This effect may be very important in menopausal and postmenopausal women. Consuming 1 cup of soybeans per day would provide approximately 300 mg of isoflavone, the equivalent of about 0.45 mg of conjugated estrogens or one tablet of Premarin, a popular estrogen used for menopausal symptoms.

In a study of postmenopausal women, those who consumed enough soyfoods to provide about 200 mg of isoflavone per day demonstrated signs of estrogenic activity when compared to a control group.[17] Specifically, the women consuming the soyfoods demonstrated an increase in the number of superficial cells that line the vagina. Presumably, soyfood consumption may offset some of the vaginal drying and irritation frequently experienced by postmenopausal women.

Estrogens are widely prescribed for postmenopausal women in an attempt to prevent osteoporosis. This may not be necessary if proper diet and lifestyle measures are followed (see pages 327–30). Furthermore, a diet rich in isoflavonoids may be a suitable alternative. In addition to their estrogenic activities, isoflavonoids demonstrate other beneficial effects in preventing bone loss.

Phytoestrogens may exert a balancing effect when estrogen levels are high, as is commonly seen in the premenstrual syndrome (PMS).[18] Consuming soyfoods is the most economical (and possibly the most beneficial) way to increase the intake of phytoestrogens.

Preparations and Uses

Soybeans can be utilized in their whole cooked or sprouted form—on their own or in recipes. Soybeans can be substituted for other beans in soups, stews, casseroles, and other dishes. From a nutritional standpoint, combining one part soy to three parts grain, especially corn, produces a high-quality protein source.

Miso Miso is a fermented soy paste that is made by inoculating trays of rice with a mold, *Aspergillus oryzae,* and leaving it to mold abundantly. A ground preparation of cooked soybeans and salt is then mixed in, and the mass is allowed to ferment for several days before being ground into a paste that has the consistency of peanut butter. The entire process may take 10 to 40 days, depending on the temperature. Miso is used primarily as a flavoring material in soups and on vegetables. Miso may provide some vitamin B_{12} to vegetarians.

Soy Flour, Protein Concentrates, and Protein Isolates Excluding soybeans used for oil, more than 90 percent of the soybeans consumed by people in the United States are eaten in the form of soy protein products. These may range from soy flour to soy protein concentrates to soy protein isolates. All are made from defatted soybean flakes, and they range in protein content from 40 to 90 percent.

Soy flour is extremely rich in protein; typically it contains 40 to 50 percent protein. Soy flour and soy protein concentrates (typically 70 percent protein) can be added to baked goods, such as breads, rolls, buns, bagels, pancakes, and waffles, to improve their protein quality. Soy protein concentrates are also used to produce meat analogues and to act as an extender of ground beef.

Soy protein isolates (90 to 95 percent protein) are used in various products, including infant formulas, meal replacement formulas, meat products, dairy-type whipped toppings, frozen desserts, and milk alternatives. The benefits of soy protein isolates over casein-based meal replacement formulas have already been discussed.

Soy Milk Soy milk is increasing in popularity due to improvements in its commercial production. Classically, soy milk is produced by soaking the beans in water, grinding the soaked beans, and filtering the liquid. Commercially available soy milks may be produced in this manner, or they may be produced from soy protein concentrates and isolates. On its own, soy milk is not especially palatable. To enhance the flavor, makers add various natural flavors such as vanilla, chocolate, and carob. Consumers can even find soy milk frozen desserts that offer a delicious and healthful alternative to ice cream.

Soy Sauce Soy sauce is a salty brown sauce made, like miso, by fermenting soy with *Aspergillus oryzae* and wheat. Soy sauce originated in China over 2,500 years ago. It was introduced into Japan in the seventh century A.D. The average annual per capita intake of soy sauce in Japan is about 3 gallons. High-quality soy sauce supplies good amounts of free amino acids, but its popularity is primarily due to the flavor that it imparts to other foods. Reduced-sodium soy sauce is a more healthful choice.

Tempeh Tempeh, an Indonesian specialty, is a chunky-textured cake of cooked soybeans fermented by the addition of *Rhizopus oligosporus*. Since this organism produces vitamin B_{12}, tempeh may provide this vitamin to vegetarians. However, we should not assume that fermented foods like tempeh and miso are excellent sources of vitamin B_{12}. In addition to the tremendous variation in B_{12} content of these foods, some evidence indicates that the form of B_{12} in the foods is not exactly suited to body requirements. Vegetarians should supplement their diets with vitamin B_{12}.

Tofu Tofu or bean curd is now a well-known food. After soy sauce, it is the biggest seller among soyfoods in the United States. Tofu is made from soy milk by coagulating the soy proteins with calcium or magnesium salts (nigari). The remaining liquid (whey) is then discarded, and the curds are pressed to form a cohesive bond. The degree of pressing produces soft, regular, or firm tofu.

Tofu is an excellent food from a nutritional and health perspective. Substituting tofu for cheese has demonstrated impressive results in lowering blood cholesterol levels, both in men and in women. Although tofu is rather bland on its own, it is quite good at taking on the flavor of other ingredients that it is cooked with, making it extremely versatile. Tofu serves as the major component of many "second-generation" soy products.

Common Dried Beans

Included in this category are dried French, kidney, navy, snap, stringless, and green beans. These are all different varieties of the common bean (*Phaseolus vulgaris*). The ancestors to the modern varieties were cultivated over 7,000 years ago by predecessors of the Incas, Aztecs, and Mayans. Its cultivation was spread by migrating bands of Native Americans throughout the Americas. Early European explorers and settlers of the fifteenth, sixteenth, and seventeenth centuries were introduced to the bean by these natives. In fact, the basic recipes for Boston baked beans and succotash were derived from dishes made by the native Americans.

The key nutritional benefits of common beans are quite similar to those of soybeans except that the former are much lower in fat content (usually only 1 to 2 percent). Their protein content and quality are quite similar. Beans also offer an excellent source of complex carbohydrates and fiber. Beans are quite versatile and can be prepared in a variety of ways.

Adzuki Bean

The adzuki bean (*Phaseolus angularis*) has been cultivated in Japan and China for hundreds of years and ranks second to soybeans in popularity there. Dried adzuki beans provide about the same nutritional value as common dried beans. They have a particularly favorable calcium-to-phosphorus ratio (4:1) for helping prevent osteoporosis. Adzuki beans form an important part of the Zen macrobiotic diet. They can be cooked and utilized in the same manner as other legumes.

Alfalfa

Most people are surprised to learn that alfalfa (*Medicago sativa*) is a member of the pea family and, therefore, is a legume. Alfalfa is primarily grown as forage for lifestock. Alfalfa-leaf tablets are available at health-food stores as a dietary supplement, and most Americans are familiar with alfalfa sprouts. Alfalfa sprouts provide numerous nutritional benefits; they are a good source of vitamin C, carotenes, chlorophyll, vitamin K, and many other nutrients. Alfalfa sprouts are now widely available and can be found in most grocery stores, or you can sprout your own. The sprouts can be used in salads and in sandwiches.

Carob

Most consumers are familiar with carob as an alternative to chocolate as a flavoring agent, but they may not know exactly what carob is. Carob is the fruit pod of the carob tree (*Ceratonia siliqua*), originally native to the Middle East and cultivated in the Mediterranean. Carob is also known as St. John's bread, locust bean, and locust pod. These names derive from the belief that carob pods were the food referred to in the Bible (Matthew 3:4) as the "locusts" that St. John ate with honey while traveling in the desert.

Interest in carob as an alternative to chocolate began in the 1920s. Carob, which is naturally sweeter than chocolate, can be used in some recipes without a sweetener and does not contain the stimulant properties of chocolate. Is carob a more healthful choice than chocolate? It all depends on what else accompanies them. Both chocolate and carob products tend to be high-calorie foods rich in fats and sugar.

Chick-pea

Chick-peas or garbanzos (*Cicer arietinum*) are thought to have originated in what is now Turkey. Although the chick-pea is now grown in all semidry and subtropical areas of the world, India and Pakistan grow over 80 percent of the world's chick-pea crop. The chick-pea has become a major crop in Pakistan and India because it is extremely drought-tolerant and provides excellent protein (when combined with grains) for the large vegetarian populations of these countries. Most of the chick-peas are utilized in "dahls," hummous, falafel, and other dishes of India and the Middle East.

Fava Bean

Native to North Africa and the Mediterranean region, the fava or broad bean (*Vicia faba*) was the major bean grown throughout the Old World prior to the introduction of the common bean. Fava beans resemble lima beans but are larger. The fava bean has a very interesting history. According to legend, the Greek philosopher and mathematician Pythagorus could have avoided his death at the hands of an angry mob if he had escaped through a field of fava beans. Why didn't Pythagorus run? Historians believe he suffered from favism—a painful blood condition brought on by eating fava beans or by inhaling the pollen from the flowering plant. Evidently, Pythagorus chose the lesser of two evils. Favism is caused by an inborn error of metabolism, a genetic defect, that cause the red blood cells to rupture after the individual consumes fava beans or inhales the plant's pollen. There is no known way to remove or inactivate the responsible substances. Favism is thought to affect up to 35 percent of some Mediterranean populations and 10 percent of American Blacks. Symptoms of favism include dizziness, nausea, and vomiting, followed by severe anemia. People susceptible to favism should definitely avoid fava beans.

Fava beans provide similar nutritional benefits to common beans, and they are used in various Mediterranean and Chinese dishes.

Lentil

Lentils (*Lens esculenta*) are among the oldest cultivated plants in the world. Archaeologists have found lentil seed at the sites of Middle and Near Eastern farming villages that existed over 8,000 years ago. Lentils do not significantly differ in nutritional content from other common legumes. Lentils are of particular benefit in the dietary management of blood-sugar disorders, because they prevent the level of blood glucose from rising rapidly after a meal.[19] Lentils can be prepared in various ways, but they are usually used in soups, casseroles, and stews.

Lima Bean

The lima bean is thought to be named after Lima, Peru, the area where it was first cultivated. Archaeological evidence shows that large-seeded limas were first cultivated in Peru more than 7,000 years ago. Lima beans are now grown in many parts of the world. The leading producers in the United States are California, Delaware, Wisconsin, and Maryland. The nutritional content of lima beans does not differ substantially from that of other common beans. Lima beans are available dried or as fresh green limas. Obviously, beans fresh in their pods are preferable. Green and dried limas are typically prepared and served on their own, in salads, in soups, and in stews.

Mung Bean

The mung bean (*Phaesolus aureus*) was native to India, but it has long been cultivated in China and Southeast Asia. Most mung beans are consumed as bean sprouts. Most grocery stores now have a ready supply of fresh mung bean sprouts, or you can sprout your own. Mung bean sprouts are most often used in salads, stir-fried vegetables, and Asian dishes.

Peas

The garden pea (*Pisum sativum*) appears to have been derived from the field pea (*Pisum arvense*) through centuries of cultivation and selection for certain desired characteristics. This occurred in both Europe and Asia. Today, almost 80 percent of the world's crop is utilized as dried peas rather than as fresh peas. In the United States, however, this is reversed, with 90 percent of the peas being eaten as green peas. Wisconsin, Washington, and Minnesota are the biggest producers of green peas; Russia and China are by far the leading producers of dried peas.

Peas are lower in calcium and phosphorus than beans are, but they provide similar levels of protein, carbohydrate, and fat. Green peas are a good source of vitamin C and carotenes, whereas dried peas contain very little of these nutrients. Since dried peas lack water, they are denser in calories than fresh peas are.

Peas are available fresh in pods, canned, frozen, or dried. Although fresh peas are almost always available, most people find it too much of a hassle to shell the peas (although the entire pod is edible). Frozen peas are the leading frozen vegetable sold. Dried peas are most often utilized in soups, while fresh peas are usually eaten steamed on their own or with other vegetables.

String Beans

The string or snap bean is a member of the common bean family (*Phaseolus vulgaris*). In addition to their use as a dried bean, string beans are available fresh in the pod. Whole string beans (with pods) are excellent foods for weight-loss: they contain very few calories per serving, while providing excellent nutrition and dietary fiber. Popular methods of preparing string beans are steaming, stir-frying, and baking in casseroles.

9

The Healing Power of Nuts, Seeds, and Oils

Nuts and seeds are the vehicle for plant reproduction. Locked inside them is the potential for an entire plant. It is truly amazing to think that a giant oak tree began its life as an acorn. Nuts and seeds provide excellent human nutrition; they are especially good sources of essential fatty acids, vitamin E, protein, and minerals. Because of their high oil content, nuts and seeds are often used as sources of oils for use in salad dressings, cooking, and cosmetic preparations. This chapter discusses some of the common nuts, seeds, and vegetable oils.

Nuts, Seeds, and Vegetable Oils: An Overview

The term *nut* commonly refers to the shell-encased seed of a tree. However, many foods we consider nuts, such as peanuts, do not fit the strict definition of a nut. Peanuts are actually legumes. There are over 300 types of nuts, and every plant has a seed, but relatively few are important as food crops.

In terms of worldwide production, the coconut is by far the most widely grown and utilized nut crop, followed by the peanut. In fact, coconuts and peanuts account for roughly 94 percent of the world's nut production.[1] One main reason for this is that coconuts and peanuts provide oils that are among the leading ingredients of cooking oils, margarines, and shortening.

In the United States, peanuts are easily the leading nut crop, accounting for more than 70 percent of the country's yearly nut production.[2] The next most common nut crops in the United States are almonds, walnuts, and pecans. Unfortunately, most nuts are consumed after they have been fried in fat and salted, or as ingredients in cookies, candies, and confections.

As more Americans are seeking more healthful food choices, nut and seed consumption is on the rise. Nuts and seeds, like the plant foods discussed in previous chapters, are rich in both nutrients and anutrients. In addition to fiber components, important anutrients in nuts and seeds include protease inhibitors, ellagic acid, and other polyphenols. Table A.5 in the Appendix identifies many of the nutritive values of these foods.

Because of the high oil content of nuts and seeds, you might suspect that frequent consumption of nuts would increase the rate of obesity. But a large population study of 26,473 Americans found that obesity was less common among people who consumed the most nuts than in other groups. A possible explanation is that the nuts produced satiety, a feeling of appetite satisfaction. This same study also demonstrated that higher nut consumption was associated with some protection against heart attacks (both fatal and nonfatal).[3]

Oils

Nuts and seeds have long been used as a source of vegetable oils for culinary, medicinal, and cosmetic purposes. For food purposes, oils can be used in salad dressings and sauces, in baking, and for cooking foods. Certain oils offer advantages over others for certain applications. For example, olive, sesame, soy, and canola oil are more stable than other vegetable oils, so they are preferred for use when exposing foods to heat. Canola oil is made from rapeseeds from which a toxic oil, erucic acid, has been removed. It has gained incredible popularity in a short period of time because it is being promoted for its high level (7 percent) of omega-3 oils. Although soy oil has a slightly higher omega-3 oil content (9 percent) and flax oil is even higher (58 percent), these highly polyunsaturated oils are less stable than canola oil. Highly polyunsaturated oils such as flax, safflower, and sunflower are not recommended for exposure to heat because the heat changes the chemical structures of the fatty acids and forms free radicals. These oils are best suited for salad dressings.

Certain oils are best avoided. In addition to margarine and shortening, cottonseed, coconut, and palm oil should not be used. Coconut and palm oils consist primarily of saturated fat, while cottonseed oil may contain toxic residues because cotton plants are so heavily sprayed during cultivation and because the oil contains gossypol, a substance known to inhibit sperm function. In fact, gossypol is being investigated as the "male birth control pill." Its use as an antifertility agent began after studies demonstrated that men who had used crude cottonseed oil as their cooking oil had low sperm counts followed by total testicular failure.[4]

For medicinal purposes, flaxseed, evening primrose, and black currant oils are the most popular vegetable oils. Black currant and evening primrose oils are used because they contain gamma-linolenic acid, an omega-6 fatty acid that eventually acts as a precursor to the favorable prostaglandins of the 1 series (see page 42 for a description of prostaglandin metabolism). However, flaxseed oil is not only less expensive, it may provide greater benefits due to its high concentration of linolenic acid, an omega-3 fatty acid. Flaxseed oil also contains linoleic acid, which is easily converted to gamma-linolenic acid in most people. Marine lipids rich in eicosapentaenoic (EPA) and other omega-3 oils are also quite popular.

Table 9.1 lists the fat content and fatty acid composition of selected nuts, seeds, and vegetable oils.

Table 9.1 Fat Content and Fatty Acid Composition of Selected Nuts, Seeds, and Vegetable Oils, in Percentages

Food	*Fat Content (%)*	*Fatty Acid Composition (% of total fats)*			
		18:3ω3	*18:2ω6*	*18:1ω9*	*Saturated Fats*
Almond	54	0	17	78	5
Brazil nut	67	0	24	48	24
Canola	30	7	30	54	7
Cashew	42	0	6	70	18
Corn	4	0	59	24	17
Coconut	35	0	3	6	91
Filbert	62	0	16	54	5
Flaxseed	35	58	14	19	9
Macadamia nut	72	0	10	71	12
Olive	20	0	8	76	16
Peanut	48	0	29	47	18
Pecan	71	0	20	63	7
Pistachio	54	0	19	65	9
Pumpkin seed	47	15	42	34	9
Rice bran	10	0	35	48	17
Sesame seed	49	0	45	42	13
Soy	18	9	50	26	15
Sunflower	47	0	65	23	12
Walnut	60	5	51	28	16

18:3ω3 = Linolenic acid
18:2ω6 = Linoleic acid
18:1ω9 = Oleic acid

How Oils Are Produced

In a modern oil-pressing factory, the starting material (seed, nut, grain, or legume) is first mechanically cleaned to prepare it for either chemical or mechanical extraction. With chemical extraction, the material is typically rolled into meal (for example, seed meal or cornmeal) and then mixed with a chemical solvent such as hexane. Once the solvent has separated the oil from the meal, the mixture is exposed to high heat to distill the solvent. Although most of the solvent is removed by this means, traces can still be found. The oil to be produced is usually further processed (degummed, bleached, deodorized, and so on) to produce a "refined" oil. A refined oil is one that has had some of its "impurities"—vitamin E, lecithin, chlorophyll, carotenes, aromatic oils, and free fatty acids—removed. Many of these impurities have important health-promoting properties. In the process of refining, the oil is exposed not only to extremely high heat, but also to caustic substances such as phosphoric acid and sodium hydroxide. Because the refined oil has been stripped of most of its natural protection against damage, synthetic antioxidants like BHT are then added.

The mechanical method usually differs only in how the oil is initially extracted. The seeds are typically cooked at high temperatures for up to two hours and then mechanically pressed through an expeller. The pressure can be as high as several tons per square inch. This results in the generation of heat, usually around 200°F. The higher the heat, the better the oil yield. Oil pressed in this manner can be filtered and sold as "cold-pressed" (no external heat was added during the extraction) or as natural, crude, or unrefined oil. Or it can be processed further to produce a refined oil. Even oil that has undergone refinement can still be labeled cold-pressed as long as no external heat was applied during the extraction.

Although far from ideal, the best oils commonly available in the United States are the cold-pressed unrefined oils. Do not expect these oils to taste as "clean" as the highly processed commercial varieties you may have grown accustomed to. Cold-pressed unrefined oils still retain much of their original flavor.

Selecting and Storing Nuts and Seeds

In general, nuts and seeds, due to their high oil content, are best purchased and stored in their shells. The shell is a natural protector against free-radical damage caused by light and air. Make sure that the shells are free from splits, cracks, stains, holes, or other surface imperfections. Do not eat or use moldy nuts or seeds, since these may not be safe. Also avoid limp, rubbery, dark, or shriveled nut meats. Store nuts and seeds in their shells in a cool, dry environment. If whole nuts and seeds in their shells are not available, make sure that the ones you obtain are stored in airtight containers in the refrigerator or freezer. Packages of crushed, slivered, and broken nut pieces are usually rancid. Prepare your own from the whole nut if a recipe calls for these.

Nut and Seed Preparations

Besides simply eating nuts and seeds as snacks, you can add them to many foods for their unique flavor. With the aid of a food processor, nut and seed butters can be prepared. Most nuts and seeds have enough natural oils, but occasionally you may need to add some additional oil. Keep nut butters in airtight containers in the refrigerator.

Since nuts and seeds, like grains and legumes, contain the essential factors needed for the plant to grow and develop, they can also be sprouted. Sprouting is thought to increase the item's nutritional value and its digestibility (see page 167 for instructions on sprouting at home).

Almond

The almond (*Prunus amygdalus*) is a small deciduous tree closely related to the peach, apricot, and cherry. Unlike in these other drupes, however, in the almond the outer fleshy layer is quite tough and becomes the hull at maturity. This hull must be cracked to free the sweet-tasting nut.

The almond is thought to have originated in western Asia and North Africa. California is the major almond producing area in the world, because almonds grow best where summers are long and hot and winters are mild. In fact, almond growing is second only to the grape growing in terms of crop acreage in California.

Almonds are packed with nutrition. Their high fat content (up to 60 percent) translates into a high calorie content. Just 100 grams (3½ ounces) of almonds provide nearly 600 calories. Almonds are rich in polyunsaturated oils, protein (20 percent), potassium, calcium, iron, zinc, and vitamin E. Almonds also contain some amygdalin, which is better known as "laetrile." This has resulted in almonds' gaining a reputation as an anticancer food. However, unlike apricot kernels, almonds are safe to consume, even in large amounts. Since almonds have a high ratio of arginine to lysine, they should be avoided by individuals susceptible to cold sores or herpes infections; arginine promotes (and lysine prevents) the activation of the virus.[5]

Almonds can be eaten on their own. The almond should be sweet tasting. If it has a bitter taste, this is usually a sign that prussic acid levels are too high. Bitter or rancid-testing almonds should not be eaten. Almonds can also be added to fruit and vegetable salads, baked goods, and breads.

Brazil Nut

Brazil nut trees (*Bertholletia excelsia*) are native to the Amazon valley in Bolivia and Brazil. It is still the only area where the tree grows. The Brazil nut tree can grow to a height of 100 feet. The nuts fall to the ground when they are ripe. This can be lethal, because the nuts are housed in woody pods containing up to 20 nuts and weighing up to 5 pounds. Harvesters have to protect themselves from the falling pods by wearing hard hats and shields. Approximately 40,000 metric tons of Brazil nuts are exported annually to the United States and Europe.[6]

Brazil nuts are similar in nutritive value to almonds, but they have a higher fat content. Brazil nuts are good sources of methionine and cysteine, making them a good complementary protein source for vegetarians.

Because of their high fat content, brazil nuts can turn rancid quite rapidly if they are not kept in the shell in a cool, dry area. Shelled nuts, even if stored in the refrigerator, easily turn rancid. Brazil nuts are best eaten fresh from the shell as a snack food.

Cashew Nut

The cashew tree (*Anacardium occidentale*) is native to coastal areas of northeastern Brazil, but it is now cultivated in India and Africa as well. Cashew nuts are seeds that adhere to the bottom of the cashew apple.

Cashews have a lower fat content than do most other nuts. Approximately 65 percent of the fat content is derived from unsaturated fatty acids; however, oleic acid, a monounsaturated oil, accounts for roughly 90 percent of this unsaturated fatty acid content, while linoleic acid accounts for only 10 percent. Cashew nuts are lower in vitamin E and calcium than most nuts, but they are a good source of magnesium, potassium, iron, and zinc.

Have you ever noticed that cashews are always sold without shells? That is because the outer shell contains a caustic oil that can damage the skin when touched. The shell must therefore be removed. Due to their high content of oleic acid (versus polyunsaturated oils), cashews are more stable than most other nuts. Still, they should be stored in an airtight container in the refrigerator to protect them from getting rancid. Cashews can be eaten on their own in either raw or roasted form. Cashews can also be added to many fruit and vegetable salads for a "nutty" taste.

Chestnut

The chestnut tree (*Castanea crenata*) is native to southern Europe and the Middle East, but it is now grown in many areas throughout the world. China, Italy, Japan, and Spain are the principal growers of chestnuts. The chestnut is enclosed in a rough envelope known as a burr. After the burrs fall to the ground, they are gathered and the chestnuts are removed.

Chestnuts are considerably higher in carbohydrate and much lower in calories, protein, and fat than are other nuts. Typically a chestnut contains three to four times more carbohydrate, one-half the calories, one-third the protein, and about one-fifteenth the amount of fat that other nuts have. Actually, the overall nutrient composition of chestnuts is quite close to that of dry cereal products made from corn or rice. Chestnuts, although they contain lower amounts than other nuts, are still good sources of potassium, magnesium, iron, and manganese.

Due to their low fat content, properly dried chestnuts store quite well. Chestnuts are most often consumed after being roasted in the fireplace during the winter holidays. The roasted chestnuts are often ground into flour for baking cookies and candies.

Coconut

The coconut is the fruit of the coconut palm tree (*Cocus nucifera*). Coconuts are native to the tropical and subtropical parts of the world, where they are used extensively as food. In fact, coconuts are by far the most widely grown and used nut crop in the world. Coconuts yield milk, oil, meat, and meal. Because coconut oil contains predominantly saturated fats, it is extremely stable, making it a popular ingredient in candies, baked goods, shortening, margarines, and deep-fat frying. The oil is also used in soaps, lotions, shampoos, and detergents.

Coconuts, like most nuts, contain significant amounts of fat. The fresh mature nut meat contains over 50 percent water and approximately 35 percent coconut oil, 10 percent carbohydrates, and 3.5 percent protein. One cup of the meat provides approximately 500 calories. The fresh milk provides about 600 calories per cup and is composed of 25 percent coconut oil, 5 percent carbohydrates, and 3 percent protein. Dried coconut meat provides nearly 900 calories per cup and is composed of 65 percent fat, 23 percent carbohydrate, and 7 percent protein. The protein content of coconut is of lower quality than that of other nuts, because it is deficient in the essential amino acids lysine and methionine.

Mature coconuts are available in most grocery stores. They should be stored in a dry, cool area. Coconut meat is also available in cans or packages as shredded coconut. Shredded coconut is often sweetened with sugar and preserved with propylene glycol (antifreeze). It may be best to buy whole coconuts and prepare your own shredded coconut with the aid of a food processor.

Whole green coconuts are harvested when the meat is soft and rubbery. After cutting or sawing the husk and shell, you can easily scoop out the meat with a spoon. It can then be eaten on its own or added to baked goods for flavor.

Mature coconuts are harvested after the shell has become quite hard and the meat is firm. To prepare mature coconuts, first punch out the "eyes" and drain off the coconut milk. The milk can be used as a beverage or flavoring agent, or it can be added back to the meat later on. After removing the milk, break the shell by striking it with a hammer; then remove the meat and peel it. The meat can be consumed on its own, ground in a food processor for use in fruit salads or baked goods, or combined with the milk for any of these uses.

Filbert (Hazel Nut)

The filbert is the seed of the filbert or hazel tree (*Corylus maxima*). They are called filberts because they ripen at about the time of St. Philibert's Day, August 20. The filbert tree grows to a height of 6 to 12 feet and is native to Europe, Asia, and North America. It does best in moist, temperate climates. The principal growing areas are Turkey, Italy, and Spain. Oregon is the major filbert supplier in the United States. The nuts are allowed to fall to the ground where they are gathered by hand or by mechanical devices. In addition to their use as a food, filberts are used to make liqueurs (such as Frangelico), and the oil is used in cosmetics and perfumes.

Filberts provide similar nutritional benefits to almonds, although they are higher in fat and a little lower in protein. A 100-gram (3½-ounce) portion supplies 634 calories. Filberts can be eaten fresh from the shell as a snack food, or they can be added to baked goods and desserts.

Flax (Linseed)

Flax (*Linum usitatissimum*) is native to the Mediterranean. It has been used not only as a food, but also for its fibers, which can be woven into linen cloth. Although whole flaxseeds contain a toxic glucoside, their oil is detoxified by heating. Flax has been used as a food item for well over 5,000 years.

Flaxseed flour and defatted flaxseed meal, because of their high content of lignans (see page 83), are being used for investigations into the association between high lignan consumption and lowered risk for sex-hormone-dependent cancers such as breast cancer. Plant lignans are converted into enterolactone and enterodiol by intestinal bacteria. These hormonelike substances produce a number of protective effects against breast cancer and are thought to be one of many protective factors against breast cancer in a vegetarian diet. This is supported by studies showing that women with breast cancer and omnivores typically excrete much lower levels of lignans in their urine than do vegetarian women.[7] To substantiate this protective effect, many researchers have constructed animal studies. In one, supplementing a high-fat diet with flaxseed flour at a level of 5 percent of total calories reduced the early markers for mammary cancer in rats by over 55 percent.[8] Lignans are found in many other seeds, grains, and legumes.

Although whole flaxseeds are quite nutritious and may offer anticancer benefits, the oil is more highly prized. Flaxseed oil is rich in linolenic acid, an omega-3 oil. The majority of scientific studies on omega-3 oils have utilized fish oils (EPA and docosahexanoic acids), but linolenic acid is a precursor to EPA and exerts many of the same effects as EPA, as well as several on its own. Omega-3 oils are recommended for treating or preventing high cholesterol levels; high blood pressure and other cardiovascular diseases; cancer; auto-immune diseases such as multiple sclerosis and rheumatoid arthritis; allergies and inflammation; many skin diseases, including eczema and psoriasis; and many others.[9]

Flaxseed oil may indeed be the most advantageous oil for medical use. One tablespoon per day provides an amount sufficient for most of these indications as well as for a good dietary supplement. Flaxseed oil should definitely be cold-processed.

Macadamia Nut

Most people assume the macadamia tree (*Macadamia ternafolia*) is native to Hawaii; however, it is actually native to Australia. It was brought to Hawaii in the 1890s, where it has flourished. It grows best in well-drained soils and moist semitropical climates.

One reason macadamia nuts have such a wonderful flavor is that they have a high fat content (72 percent). Their protein content is low (8 percent) compared to that of other nuts. From a nutritional standpoint, macadamia nuts offer very little other than calories.

Macadamia nuts are most often available in packages or cans as fried, salted snacks or as candies. Unshelled nuts store quite well in a dry environment. Macadamia nuts can be eaten on their own as a snack or used to enhance the flavor of baked goods and confections.

Olive

Technically speaking, the olive is a fruit. Olives are discussed in this chapter, however, because of their high oil content. First cultivated in Greece, the olive does best in warm, dry climates and in various types of soil. Italy and Spain produce over 50 percent of the world's olives and olive oil. California is by far the leading olive producer in the United States.

The total fat content of olives (15 to 35 percent) makes them a fine candidate for oil production. Olive oil contains 75 percent oleic acid, a monounsaturated fatty acid. Like other unsaturated fatty acids, oleic acid has been shown to lower blood cholesterol levels.

Raw olives are quite bitter and must be processed to remove the bitterness before they are edible. Processing involves soaking the olives in strong salt solutions; hence olives have a high salt content. Olives are available green or ripe (black), canned or bottled.

Olive oil is available in different grades. Extra virgin olive oil is the initial unrefined oil from the first pressing of the fruit, virgin olive oil refers to all oil produced from the first pressing, and pure olive oil usually means a lower-quality oil produced from subsequent pressings. Chemically the difference between an extra virgin oil and a virgin oil involves the amount of free oleic acid. "Virgin" is allowed to contain up to 4 percent free oleic acid; "fine virgin," "superfine virgin," and "extra virgin," respectively, are allowed 3, 1.5, and 1 percent free oleic acid levels.

Peanut

The most popular nut, the peanut, is not a nut at all; it is a legume. The peanut begins as an aboveground flower that eventually forms a stalklike stem that pushes into the ground, swells, and grows into a peanut. The peanut plant (*Arachis hypogaea*), a small bush, is native to South America. It was spread by Portuguese explorers to East Africa and by Spanish explorers to the Philippines. Later, it came to North America via Africa and the slave trade. The plant grows best in tropical or subtropical climates.

The world's largest producers are India, China, and the United States. Georgia is by far the leading peanut-producing state in the United States. Peanuts are the largest nut crop in the United States, accounting for more than 70 percent of the country's entire nut production.[10]

Peanuts contain roughly 50 percent fat, 26 percent protein, and 19 percent carbohydrates. The fat consists of predominantly (75 percent) unsaturated fatty acids. The protein content is the highest among the common nuts. Peanuts are also an excellent source of B-vitamins and minerals, especially potassium, magnesium, calcium, zinc, and iron.

Peanuts are available whole (either raw or roasted) in unshelled or shelled form, as peanut butter, and as ingredients in snack foods and candies. In the United States, approximately 50 percent of all peanuts are eaten as peanut butter; 25 percent are consumed as roasted peanuts, either shelled or unshelled; and another 25 percent are consumed in candies.[11] Peanut butter was first prepared in 1890 by a St. Louis physician who prescribed it to his patients as a nutritious, easily digested food. Commercially available peanut butter is made by grinding dry-roasted peanuts and (usually) adding hydrogenated oils to help stabilize it—that is, to keep the oil from separating out. Obviously, given the detrimental health effects of hydrogenated oils, commercial peanut butters containing hydrogenated oils should not be used. Several peanut butter suppliers use only peanuts in their peanut butter; for an even better product, grind your own fresh peanut butter. Most health-food stores and many grocery stores now have nut grinders on their premises for making fresh peanut butter. Store fresh or opened peanut butter in the refrigerator.

Peanuts are susceptible to molds and fungal invasions. Aflatoxin, a poison produced by a fungus (*Aspergillus flavus*), is of particular concern. This toxin is a known carcinogen. In fact, aflatoxin is twenty times more toxic than DDT and is one of the most potent cancer-causing compounds known. Aflatoxin has also been linked to mental retardation and lowered intelligence. [12] A rural region of Georgia, where people eat a diet high in homegrown peanuts, has twice the national average rate of mental retardation; even trace amounts of aflatoxin in the diet of pregnant women can lead to mental retardation in their infants.

To help prevent aflatoxin ingestion, the FDA enforces an administrative guideline of 20 parts per billion as the maximum of aflatoxin permitted in all foods and animal foods, including peanut butter and other peanut products. To protect yourself further from aflatoxin ingestion, make sure that raw peanuts have been stored in a dry, cool environment. The fungus grows when the temperature is between 86° and 96°F and when the ambient humidity is high. Roasted peanuts offer more protection against aflatoxin than do raw peanuts. And although roasting results in loss of some nutrients, it is thought to improve the digestibility of peanuts. Unsalted, dry-roasted peanuts are more healthful choices than salted or oil-roasted peanuts.

Peanuts make an excellent snack and are also used extensively in Asian dishes. Around the world, peanuts and peanut products are an important food, especially in areas where high-quality nutrition may otherwise be lacking.

Pecan

The pecan tree (*Carya illinoensis*) is a type of hickory that is native to North America—specifically, to the valleys of the Mississippi River and its tributaries. The pecan tree can grow to a height of 180 feet, although most mature trees are 75 to 90 feet high. The United States is by far the leading producer of pecans; very few pecans are produced outside the United States. Most of the pecans are grown in the South, with Georgia producing about 40 percent of the U.S. crop.

Pecans are another delicious nut that owes much of its flavor to its high fat content (71 percent). Pecans are similar to macadamia nuts in this respect, but they contain slightly higher amounts of protein, minerals, and B-vitamins.

Because of their high oil content, pecans should definitely be purchased in shells. Pecans may be eaten on their own or added to various baked goods, salads, desserts, cereals, and other foods; the sweet flavor of pecans is compatible with a wide range of foods.

Pine Nuts

Pine nuts are the seeds of certain species of pine trees. The nuts are locked within the pine cone. Pine nuts are similar to almonds in nutritional content. They are extremely susceptible to rancidity and should be kept in airtight containers in the refrigerator. Pine nuts are used in pesto sauces and other vegetarian dishes.

Pistachios

The pistachio tree (*Pistacia vera*) is a small tree native to the Middle East and western Asia. Pistachios have become quite popular in Mediterranean and Middle Eastern cuisines. The introduction of the pistachio tree to California has resulted in increased popularity of pistachios in the United States as well.

Pistachios are quite similar in nutritional content to almonds, except that they are richer in iron and thiamine, and lower in calcium and niacin. Pistachios are 55 percent fat and 20 percent protein, and they are excellent sources of most B-vitamins, potassium, iron, magnesium, and calcium.

Pistachios are most often available roasted in the shell. Avoid salted pistachios and ones that have been dyed red. Pistachios are most commonly eaten as snacks, but they can also be added to confections, desserts, and baked goods.

Pumpkin Seeds

The pumpkin as a vegetable is described in Chapter 5. Pumpkin seeds, like other squash seeds, are packed with nutrition and are excellent sources of essential fatty acids, protein (29 percent), and minerals. Pumpkin seeds have long been used by naturopathic physicians in treating prostate disorders, due to their high content of essential fatty acids and zinc. Deficiencies of or an increased requirement for these nutrients has been linked to the high rate of benign enlargement of the prostate. Some evidence indicates that supplying these key elements to the prostate may improve the symptoms of prostate enlargement.[13] Pumpkin seeds have also been used to help expel intestinal parasites, especially helminths or worms.[14]

Pumpkin seeds are best obtained in their natural state from pumpkins. After being removed from the pumpkin, the seeds need to dry. This usually takes a few days. After the seeds have dried, the tough adhering shell can be removed. Pumpkin seeds are excellent raw, but they can also be roasted.

Sesame Seeds

Sesame (*Sesamum indicum*) was one of the very first food crops and definitely the first crop grown for its edible oil. Thought to have originated in India, the sesame plant grows to a height of 2 to 4 feet. It produces tiny pink or white flowers and small pods that encase flat seeds ranging in color from white to dark brown. Currently, sesame seeds must be harvested by hand to prevent damage; thus, production is limited to countries where labor is inexpensive and plentiful. In addition to its use as a food or oil, sesame oil is used in cosmetic and pharmaceutical preparations.

Sesame seeds have an average oil content of 50 percent, along with a protein content of 25 percent. The protein is composed of a very favorable amino acid profile (high methionine and cysteine content) that complements many other vegetarian protein sources, such as soy, peanuts, and other legumes, to form a more complete protein. Sesame seeds are also an excellent source of calcium and other minerals. Since the sesame seed hull contains 2 to 3 percent oxalic acid—a compound that can interfere with calcium utilization—and has a bitter flavor, the hull is often removed.

Like most nuts and seeds, sesame contains lignans. Sesamin, a lignan that exists exclusively and abundantly in sesame, has demonstrated remarkable antioxidant effects.[15] This action is put to good use in stabilizing sesame products. However, sesamin demonstrates additional benefits. In particular, sesamin has been shown to inhibit the absorption of cholesterol from the diet and to inhibit the manufacture of cholesterol in the liver in rats. This preliminary research suggests that sesame seeds and oil, as rich sources of sesamin, may be able to lower blood cholesterol levels significantly.[16]

Sesame seeds are available in many forms: dry, cleaned, and with hulls; white and without hulls; toasted; as defatted sesame flour; and as sesame butter (tahini). Hulled sesame seeds offer the greatest nutritional benefits. In addition to their use as a snack and as a food, sesame seeds are often added as a decorative and flavoring agent to breads, buns, and rolls.

Sunflower Seeds

The sunflower (*Helianthus annuus*) is a tall, strong, bright yellow flower that is native to the Americas. The sunflower plant can grow to a height of 20 feet, and the flower can be as large as 30 inches in diameter. Most sunflower seeds are used to make oil. The leading producers of sunflower oil are Russia, the United States, Argentina, and Romania. North Dakota, Minnesota, and California are the leading producers in the United States.

Sunflower seeds are excellent sources of the essential fatty acid linoleic acid, making them particularly useful whenever the benefits of linoleic acid are desired, such as for lowering blood cholesterol levels and for preventing heart disease. Sunflower seeds also provide an excellent protein content and a very good amino acid profile. Sunflower seeds provide good levels of vitamin E and B-vitamins, along with many minerals, including iron. In fact, a serving of sunflower seeds contains more than 30 percent more iron than a serving of raisins, a popular source of iron.

Whole sunflower seeds are available, raw or roasted, with or without hulls. Fresh raw sunflower seeds with hulls provide the greatest nutritional benefit. They are usually dehulled with the fingernails or teeth to liberate the whole seed. Roasted seeds, even with the hull on, have a relatively short shelf life. Roast your own by spreading seeds in a baking tray and setting it in the oven for 15 minutes at 350°F. Salted sunflower seeds should be avoided.

Sunflower seeds are a good snack food, and they make a delicious and highly nutritious addition to breads, rolls, and salads.

Walnut

Walnut trees are native to Asia, Europe, and North America. They are large, long-living trees and can grow to a height of 150 feet. The two walnut species of greatest commercial importance are the English walnut (*Juglans regia*) and the black walnut (*Juglans nigra*). The English walnut is preferred because its nuts are easier to shell. A walnut is usually 1½ to 2½ inches in diameter and oblong to round in shape. The nut is surrounded by an outer, leathery husk and an inner wrinkled shell that houses the meat. The United States provides more than half of the world's production of walnuts, despite the fact that they are grown for commercial purposes exclusively in California. Besides providing nuts, walnut trees are also a popular shade and ornamental tree, and a source of hardwood used in furniture.

Walnuts are among the most nutritious of nuts, since their water content is low (3 to 4 percent). Walnuts provide good levels of oils (60 percent), protein (20 percent), vitamin E, calcium, iron, and zinc. Walnuts are often regarded as a "brain food." This conception probably stems from the wrinkled, brainlike, appearance of its shell, as well as from its excellent nutritional profile.

Walnuts are best purchased as whole, uncracked nuts. Whole walnuts stored in a cool, dry environment can be stored for up to one year. Walnuts can be eaten alone as a snack food, or they can be used in baked goods, salads, and other dishes.

10

The Healing Power of Common Herbs and Spices

Technically, herbs are plants that do not have a woody stem; if a plant has a woody stem, it is referred to as a shrub, bush, or tree. However, the term *herb* is also used to describe a plant or plant part that is used for medicinal purposes. A spice technically describes a plant product that has aromatic properties and is used to season or flavor foods. Most spices are derived from bark (for example, cinnamon), fruit (for example, red and black pepper), seed (for example, nutmeg), or other part of a tree or shrub or herb, while herbs used in cooking are typically composed of leaves and stem. This makes for an easy way of distinguishing herbs from spices. But can herbs be spices, and can spices be herbs? Yes, of course. Many herbs are used to flavor foods, thus meeting definition of a spice; and most spices can be used for medicinal purposes, thus meeting the second definition of an herb.

Plants as Medicine

Before we discuss the use herbs and spices in foods, let's consider their use as medicines. Specifically, let's answer the following question: Are herbs effective medicinal agents, or is their use merely a reflection of folklore, outdated theories, and myth? To the uninformed, herbs are generally thought of as ineffective medicines used prior to the advent of more effective synthetic drugs. To others herbs are simply sources of compounds to isolate and then market as drugs. But to some, herbs and crude plant extracts are effective medicines to be respected and appreciated.

For many of the people of the world, herbal medicines are the only therapeutic agents available. It is difficult to assess the extent to which plants are used as medicines throughout the world, but the World Health Organization has estimated that perhaps 80 percent of the more than 4 billion people in the world rely on traditional medicines for their primary health care needs. Since botanical medicine accounts for the major part of traditional therapies, it can be safely stated that the majority of the people of the world rely directly on plants as medicines. Unfortunately, most people in the United States have little idea of the tremendous value of plants as medicine.

Although botanical medicine has existed since the dawn of time, the ways in which plants actually affect human physiology remain largely unknown. Many plants clearly do contain compounds that exert a high degree of pharmacological (druglike) activity. Indeed, for the past 30 years, about 25 percent of all prescription drugs in the United States have contained active constituents obtained from plants. One of the great fallacies promoted by the U.S. medical establishment has been that many natural therapies (including herbal medicine) lack any firm scientific basis. This assertion is simply untrue. In fact, during the last 10 to 20 years, there has been an explosion of scientific information concerning plants, crude plant extracts, and nutritional substances from plants as medicinal agents.

People often ask, "What advantages do herbal medicines possess over synthetic drugs?" As a general rule, herbs are less toxic than their synthetic counterparts and offer less risk of side effects. Obviously, there are exceptions to this rule. In addition, an herb's mechanism of action is often specifically to correct the underlying physiological imbalance or other cause. In contrast, a synthetic drug is often designed to alleviate a symptom or effect without addressing the underlying cause. Moreover, with many plants, the whole plant or crude extract is much more effective than are isolated constituents.

Herbal medicine will certainly continue to play a major role in the medicine of the future. There is a growing appreciation of the harmonious healing properties that herbs possess, particularly in Europe and Asia. People in the United States are beginning to become more aware of the tremendous medicinal value of herbs as well. Without a doubt, the medicine of the future will make good use of herbal medicine: the medicine of the past will be the medicine of the future.

The difference between past and future uses will be due to the growing sophistication of herbal medicine. With the continuing advancement of science and technology, the quality of herbal medicines available has greatly improved. Improvements in cultivation techniques, coupled with improvements in quality control and standardization of potency, will continue to increase the effectiveness of herbal medicines.

One major development in herbal medicine involves improvements in extraction and concentration processes. An extract is a concentrated form of the herb, obtained by mixing the crude herb with an appropriate solvent and then partly or completely removing the solvent. When an herbal tea bag is steeped in hot water, the resulting fluid is actually a type of herbal extract known as an infusion. The water serves as a solvent, removing some of the medicinal properties from the herb. Teas are often better sources of bio-available compounds than are powdered herbs, but they are relatively weak in action compared to tinctures, fluid extracts, and solid extracts.

In terms of potency, there is usually no real comparison between an extract and the ground dried herb. The extract is more effective, has a higher concentration of active ingredients, has a longer shelf-life, and has a greater degree of standardization. The term *standardization* refers to guaranteeing the potency of an herb by stating the level of active compounds per dose. This would be like guaranteeing that each cup of coffee contained the same amount of caffeine. Standardization of this sort allows for accurate dosage recommendations and consistent clinical responses.

Many herbs have profound medicinal effects but do not lend themselves to being used in foods. If you are interested in herbal medicine and would like to learn more, please get a copy of my book *The Healing Power of Herbs*.

Cooking with Herbs and Spices

Have you ever heard the expression "Add a little spice to your life"? This little message reflects the belief that herbs and spices add a great deal to foods. Without herbs and spices, many foods taste dull and bland. It is amazing what herbs and spices can do to some of the most simple foods. Consider the potato. On its own, the potato is fairly mild and simple in taste; but add a little tarragon, dill, or ground red pepper and you have a whole new experience.

It is best to use herbs in their fresh form. To prepare most fresh herbs for use, first remove the stems; then put the leaves into a measuring cup, and (with your kitchen shears upright) mince them to the desired size. If using a recipe that calls for a dried herb, simply multiply the amount specified by four. Since dried herbs are more concentrated than fresh, you will have to use more of the fresh.

To season enough vegetables to serve four people, start with 1 teaspoon of fresh or ¼ teaspoon of crushed dried herb. Taste, and then add a little more if needed.

Table 10.1 Complementary Foods and Seasonings

Food	*Seasoning*
Asparagus	chives, lemon balm, sage, tarragon, thyme
Beans, rice, and other legumes and grains	cumin, garlic, mint, onions, oregano, parsley, saffron, sage, thyme
Broccoli	basil, dill, garlic, oregano, tarragon, thyme
Cabbage	basil, cayenne pepper, cumin, dill, marjoram, sage
Carrots	anise, basil, chives, cinnamon, clove, cumin, dill, ginger, marjoram, mint, parsley, sage, tarragon, thyme
Corn	chives, lemon balm, saffron, sage, thyme
Eggplant	basil, cinnamon, dill, garlic, marjoram, mint, onion, oregano, parsley, sage, thyme
Peas	chives, rosemary, tarragon, thyme
Potatoes	basil, chives, coriander, dill, oregano, parsley, rosemary, sage, tarragon, thyme
Pumpkin and winter squash	basil, cardamom, cinnamon, clove, ginger, marjoram, rosemary, sage
Spinach	anise, basil, chives, cinnamon, dill, rosemary, thyme
Tomatoes	basil, chives, coriander, dill, garlic, marjoram, oregano, parsley, rosemary, sage, tarragon, thyme

Matching Vegetables with Herbs and Spices

Some combinations of foods and seasonings are more appealing than others. Table 10.1 lists some complementary pairings that can be used as a starting point.

Thousands of herbs and spices are in use around the world. The discussions that follow cover some of the more commonly used herbs and spices.

Anise

Anise (*Pimpinella anisum*) is a member of the same plant family as celery, fennel, dill, and carrots—the Umbelliferae. The seed (called aniseed) is most often used, for its strong licorice flavor.

Key Health Benefits

Like fennel, anise is a rich source of coumarin compounds. Anise also contains a relatively high concentration of volatile oils. Together, the compounds in anise exert a broad range of health benefits, but primarily they help expel gas (carminative effect), relax intestinal spasms (antispasmodic effect), and relieve cough.

Selection

Aniseed is available whole or ground. Whole is preferable, since many of the volatile oils quickly become lost after grinding.

Uses

The strong licorice flavor of anise makes it very popular in cakes, cookies, and breads. It also mixes well with spinach and carrots.

Basil

There are many species of basil, but the most common is sweet basil (*Ocimum basilicum*). This annual plant has green leafy stems that give it a bushy appearance. Although basil can achieve a height of 2 feet, it rarely is allowed to do so. Native to India, Africa, and Asia, basil is now cultivated extensively throughout the world. In addition to the plant's use as an aromatic herb, the aromatic oil of sweet basil is used in cordials (such as Chartreuse), cosmetics, perfumes, and soaps.

Key Health Benefits

As basil is a member of the mint family, it possesses many of the same medicinal effects. Its historical uses mirror that of many of the mints, including use as a digestive aid, as a mild sedative, and as a palliative for headaches. In China, the medicinal use of basil can be traced back 3,000 years. Basil is still used in China to treat spasms of the intestinal tract, kidney ailments, and poor circulation. The volatile oil of one variety of sweet basil has been shown to possess antibacterial, as well as anthelminthic (antiworm), activities.

Selection

Basil can often be found fresh in grocery stores. This is the best way to buy it, as it is the most aromatic form of the herb. Look for crisp, vibrant green basil with no signs of decay. Dried basil can be used if fresh basil is not available.

Uses

Basil adds a clovelike taste to foods. It can be used alone, but it also mixes well with other herbs and spices, including garlic, thyme, and oregano. Basil is often added to tomato sauces and pestos. It can substitute for oregano in most recipes. Perhaps the most well-known use of basil is as an ingredient in pesto. Pesto is great over pasta or potatoes. Most pestos contain a lot of parmesan cheese, which means extra saturated fat and sodium. The Healthy Pesto recipe in *The Healing Power of Foods Cookbook* is a more healthful version.

Cardamom

True cardamom (*Elettaria cardamomum*) is a perennial plant with simple erect stems (or canes) that can reach a height of 10 to 12 feet. The fruit contains up to 18 seeds, and these seeds are used whole or ground as a spice. Cardamom is native to southern India, Ceylon, and Malaysia. Not surprisingly, it found its way into curry powder. Cardamom is also used in many desserts, especially pastries, and as a fragrance in soaps, detergents, lotions, and perfumes.

Key Health Benefits

Cardamom has been used as a medicine in India and China since the beginning of recorded history. Its prime uses are similar to those of cinnamon and ginger: as a carminative, a digestant, and a stimulant.

Selection

Cardamom can be purchased as whole or ground seeds. It is best to buy them whole and grind them yourself.

Uses

Cardamom tastes like an airy, gentle ginger, with a touch of pine. Although rarely used alone, cardamom enhances the flavor of pumpkins and other squash, sweet potatoes, pastries, and many other foods. Cardamom is often combined with cumin, coriander seed, and other ingredients of curry.

Cayenne Pepper and Paprika

Cayenne or red pepper is the fruit of *Capsicum annuum*, a shrubby, tropical plant that can grow to a height of 3 feet. The fruit is technically a berry. Paprika is a milder and sweeter-tasting fruit produced from a different variety of capsicum. Although cayenne pepper is native to tropical America, it is now cultivated in tropical locations throughout the world and has found its way into the cuisine of many parts of the world, particularly Southeast Asia, China, Southern Italy, and Mexico.

Key Health Benefits

The folk use of cayenne pepper is quite extensive. It has been used for asthma, fevers, sore throats and other respiratory tract infections, digestive disturbances, and cancers, and it has been used as an ingredient in various poultices. From a nutritional standpoint, cayenne peppers are full of nutrients, particularly vitamin C and carotenes. However, most of the beneficial effects of cayenne pepper are thought to be due to the compound capsaicin. Capsaicin is responsible for the irritating (hot) effect of red pepper when it is applied to the skin or ingested. This effect is mediated by a compound known as "substance P." (The P stands for pain.) Capsaicin causes the release of substance P from nerve cells, which results in irritation and pain; once substance P is released, however, capsaicin works to block the re-uptake of substance P. The net result is that capsaicin depletes substance P, thereby blocking the pain sensation. Capsaicin-containing formulas have shown impressive results when applied to the skin in cases of psoriasis, rheumatoid arthritis, and post-herpes pain (postherpetic neuralgia).

Cayenne pepper exerts beneficial effects internally, too. Perhaps most important are its effects on stimulating and enhancing digestion. Much of this effect occurs through stimulation of gastric acid secretion. Although people with active peptic ulcers may be bothered by "spicy" foods containing cayenne pepper, spicy foods in normal individuals do not cause ulcers. In fact, some evidence supports the idea that spicy foods containing cayenne and turmeric may actually help heal peptic ulcers.

Cayenne pepper also exerts a number of beneficial effects on the cardiovascular system. Specifically, it reduces a person's likelihood of developing atherosclerosis, by reducing blood cholesterol and triglyceride levels, reducing platelet aggregation, and increasing fibrinolytic activity. "Fibrinolytic activity" refers to the body's ability to prevent the formation of bloodclots, which might otherwise induce a heart attack, stroke, or pulmonary embolism. Cultures in which large amounts of cayenne pepper are consumed are associated with a much lower rate of these diseases.

Interestingly, capsaicin, although hot to the taste, has actually been shown to lower body temperature by stimulating the cooling center of the hypothalamus in the brain. The ingestion of cayenne peppers by people in cultures native to the tropics appears to offer them a way to cope with high temperatures.

Selection

Cayenne peppers are available in various forms: whole fresh, whole dried, crushed dried, or ground. Select according to recipe specifications.

Uses

Cayenne pepper adds a hot flash to foods. Cayenne pepper can be added to many different foods and is used frequently in Cajun, Creole, Spanish, Mexican, Szechuan, Thai, and East Indian recipes.

Although cayenne is a component of chili powder (which can have a similar appearance), chili power is actually a combination of several spices, usually including cayenne, cumin, turmeric, ginger, and oregano.

Super Chili Powder Recipe

2 tablespoons paprika

½ teaspoon ground cayenne

1 tablespoon turmeric

½ teaspoon oregano

⅛ teaspoon cumin

⅛ teaspoon coriander

1 pressed clove garlic

¼-inch slice of ginger, finely minced

Cinnamon

Cinnamon comes from the inner bark of an evergreen tree native to Sri Lanka, southwestern India, and southern Asia. After it is peeled away from the tree, it curls up into "sticks" as it dries. In addition to its usefulness as a spice, cinnamon or its oil can be used as flavoring agents in pharmaceutical, personal health, and cosmetic products. Cinnamon is also frequently used in incense.

Key Health Benefits

Cinnamon has its own distinct flavor. It also has a long history of use in both Eastern and Western cultures as a medicine. Some of its reported uses include treatments in cases of arthritis, asthma, cancer, diarrhea, fever, heart problems, insomnia, menstrual problems, peptic ulcers, psoriasis, and spastic muscles. Scientific studies support some of these uses. Some of the confirmed effects of cinnamon are as a sedative, an anticonvulsant, a diaphoretic, a diuretic, an antibiotic, and an antiulcerative.

Cinnamon is often used in multicomponent Chinese herbal formulas, some of which have been studied for their clinical effects. For example, cinnamon combined with Chinese thoroughwax (*Bupleuri falcatum*) and Chinese peony (*Paeonia lactiflora*) has been shown to produce satisfactory results in the treatment of epilepsy. Out of 433 treated cases (most of whom were unresponsive to anticonvulsant drugs), 115 were cured and another 79 improved greatly. Improvements were noted not only in the form of clinical symptoms but also by improvements in the form of brain-wave patterns. Other clinical studies have shown cinnamon-containing formulas to be useful in cases of the common cold, influenza, and frostbite.

Here is a great tea to drink when you feel a cold coming on:

Cinnamon–Ginger Tea

1-inch slice of fresh ginger
¼ teaspoon cinnamon
¼ lemon
1 cup hot water

If you own a juice extractor, juice the ginger and lemon and then add the juice to a cup of water. If not, grind the ginger and squeeze the juice from ½ lemon and add these to the water.

This is a diaphoretic tea, meaning that it will warm you from the inside and promote perspiration. Both ginger and cinnamon have confirmed diaphoretic activity. This drink is good for you even when you don't have a cold—if you just want to warm up and feel good.

Selection

Cinnamon is available as dried "sticks" or ground.

Uses

Cinnamon is a vital ingredient in Indian, Moroccan, Indonesian, Middle Eastern, Greek, Chinese, and other cuisines. It is an extremely versatile spice that complements a wide variety of foods and other spices.

Cloves

Cloves are the unopened flower bud of the clove tree (*Syzygium aromaticum*). Native to the Spice Islands of Indonesia, cloves are now cultivated in Tanzania, Madagascar, India, Brazil, the Philippines, and other warm regions. In addition to the bud's use as a spice, clove oil is used in toothache remedies, dental cements, and other materials and as a fragrance in toothpastes, soaps, lotions, and perfumes. A major portion of the world's clove production goes to Indonesia for use in kretak cigarettes, which contain a mixture of two parts tobacco to one part cloves. When smoked, these cigarettes produce a crackling noise.

Key Health Benefits

The pain-relieving properties of cloves and clove oil have been known for centuries, especially in the treatment of toothaches. A home remedy for a toothache is to apply a few crushed cloves to the tooth or hold them in the mouth. Cloves taken primarily as a tea have been administered for abdominal problems, particularly in cases of indigestion, nausea, and parasitic infections. Clove oil is a potent antibiotic.

Selection

Cloves are available whole, ground, or as clove oil. Select the form based on the intended use.

Uses

Cloves possess a distinctive flavor that is often used to spice up dishes, especially in the cuisines of Russia, Scandinavia, Greece, India, and China. Cloves have also been used to make an "old-time" air freshener known as a pomander. To make this, simply place whole cloves in a medium-size orange. You may want to wear a thimble to protect your finger as you push in the cloves, or use an ice pick to puncture the orange's skin before inserting the cloves. About 2 ounces of whole cloves should suffice. Scatter the cloves all over the orange, filling in the spaces as you go. When you are finished, the entire orange should be covered with cloves. To prevent the evaporation of volatile clove oils, use a fixative such as orris root powder. Simply dust the pomander with the fixative, and then place it in a dark, airy spot to allow it to age for four weeks. Once dry, the pomander can be decorated with a ribbon and placed anywhere you wish—in a dresser drawer, in a closet, hanging in a room, or in a decorative bowl.

Coriander/Cilantro

Coriander (*Coriandrum sativum*) is a bright green annual with slender, erect, hollow stems. The parts of the plant used include the leaves (commonly sold as cilantro or Chinese parsley) and the dried ripe fruits (commonly called coriander seeds).

Key Health Benefits

Coriander has been used as a medicine for thousands of years in India and China. Even Hippocrates is said to have used coriander in medicines. Its prime uses are similar to those of other aromatic spices such as cardamom, cinnamon, and ginger: as a carminative, a digestant, and a stimulant. Poultices made from coriander have been recommended for joint pain.

Selection

Coriander is available as a whole seed or ground. Whole is preferable. If the recipe calls for ground coriander, simply grind the whole seed yourself. Coriander leaves (cilantro) and roots can also be used, if they can be found.

Uses

The flavor of coriander seeds and cilantro has been described as a "bold sage flavor and tangy citrus." The seeds are used extensively in the cuisines of Asia, China, Latin America, and Spain. The flavor of coriander combines nicely with those of beets, onions, potatoes, and lentils.

Dill

Dill (*Anethum graveolens*) is a member of the same plant family (Umbelliferae) as carrot, celery, and parsley. Dill looks a lot like fennel, only dill is smaller. The parts of the plant used are the seeds and the leaves.

Key Health Benefits

Dill has a long history of folk use. Its name comes from the Norse word *dilla*, which means "to lull"; this commemorates the fact that dill was used as a mild sedative. Like other aromatic herbs, dill provides its prime health benefit as a carminative in the elimination of flatulence and digestive disturbance.

Selection

Fresh dill leaves and seeds are preferable to the dried forms. Dill is also quite easy to grow.

Uses

Dill is a familiar flavor thanks largely to the popularity of dill pickles. Dill is a versatile herb that combines well with fruits, vegetables, fish, and poultry. The seeds are slightly stronger in flavor than the leaves. Here is a recipe for a versatile dill sauce:

Dill Sauce

3 tablespoons olive or canola oil
2 sprigs dill
1 teaspoon dill seeds
1 sprig parsley
1 clove garlic
1 lemon, juice and rind

Simply combine all of the ingredients in a blender and blend. This sauce can be served over potatoes and steamed vegetables.

Ginger

Ginger is an erect perennial herb that has thick tuberous rhizomes (underground stems and root). Ginger originated in southern Asia, although it is now extensively cultivated throughout the tropics (for example, in India, China, Jamaica, Haiti, and Nigeria). Exports from Jamaica to all parts of the world amount to more than 2 million pounds annually. Ginger has been used for thousands of years in China to treat numerous health conditions.

Key Health Benefits

Historically, the majority of complaints for which ginger was used involved the gastrointestinal system. It is generally regarded as an excellent carminative (a substance that promotes the elimination of intestinal gas) and intestinal spasmolytic (a substance that relaxes and soothes the intestinal tract).

A clue to ginger's success in eliminating gastrointestinal distress is offered by recent double-blind studies that demonstrated ginger's effectiveness in preventing the symptoms of motion sickness, especially seasickness. In fact, in one study ginger was shown to be far superior to Dramamine, a commonly used over-the-counter and prescription drug for motion sickness. Ginger reduces all symptoms associated with motion sickness, including dizziness, nausea, vomiting, and cold sweating.

Ginger has also been used to treat the nausea and vomiting associated with pregnancy. Recently, the benefit of ginger was confirmed in treating hyperemesis gravidarum, the most severe form of pregnancy-related nausea and vomiting. This condition usually requires hospitalization. Ginger root powder at a dose of 250 mg four times a day brought about a significant reduction in both the severity of the nausea and the number of attacks of vomiting.

Ginger has also been shown to be very potent in inhibiting the formation of inflammatory compounds (prostaglandin and thromboxanes). This could explain some of ginger's historical use as an anti-inflammatory agent. However, ginger also has strong antioxidant abilities and contains a protease (a protein-digesting enzyme) that may act similarly to bromelain in response to inflammation.

In one clinical study, seven patients with rheumatoid arthritis, for whom conventional drugs had provided only temporary or partial relief, were treated with ginger. One patient took 50 grams per day of lightly cooked ginger, while the remaining six took either 5 grams of fresh or 0.1 to 1 gram of powdered ginger daily. All patients reported substantial improvement, including pain relief, increased joint mobility, and decreased swelling and morning stiffness. Ginger, like garlic, has also been shown to reduce serum cholesterol and to improve liver function significantly.

Although most scientific studies have used powdered ginger root as the test substance, fresh ginger root at an equivalent dosage should yield even better results because it contains active enzymes. Most studies utilized a dosage of 1 gram of powdered ginger root. This would be equivalent to approximately 10 grams or ⅓ ounce of fresh ginger root—roughly a ¼-inch slice. Fresh ginger root is available at most grocery stores.

Selection

Fresh ginger can now be purchased in the produce section of most supermarkets. The bronze root should look fresh, with no signs of decay such as soft spots, mold, or a dry, wrinkled skin. Store fresh ginger in the refrigerator. If fresh ginger is not available, use dried ginger, which is widely available.

Uses

Ginger is an important spice, but it can also be used as a fantastic addition to fresh fruit and vegetable juices—especially pineapple, carrot, and apple. Ginger tea is another option. The recipe for cinnamon–ginger tea is given on page 202; the cinnamon can be omitted for a plainer ginger tea, or nutmeg or cardamom can be substituted for the cinnamon.

Horseradish

Horseradish (*Armoracia rusticana*), like mustard and radish, is a member of the cabbage family. It is valued for its pungent, long, white, tapered root, which has quite a sharp bite. This effect can be put to good use as a flavoring and as a medicinal agent.

Key Health Benefits

Horseradish contains mustard oil (allylisothiocyanate), which can act as a counterirritant. This means that, when it is applied to the skin, it causes local irritation and increased blood flow. The net effect is that the internal or preexisting pain is relieved. A horseradish poultice has long been used as a folk remedy for treating arthritis and sore muscles. Internally, horseradish has been used as a nasal decongestant and as a diuretic. Eating some horseradish promotes nasal discharge, a beneficial effect in cases of sinusitis or upper-respiratory-tract infection. Horseradish is believed to be one of the more potent herbal diuretics.

Selection

Horseradish is available as a whole fresh root or in commercial preparations. The whole fresh root stays fresh in the refrigerator for months;

however, once grated, horseradish spoils quite rapidly. The commercial preparations are most often made by mixing fresh grated horseradish with vinegar. Horseradish is also available as a dried powder.

Uses

Horseradish provides a sharp, mustardlike taste. It is most often used on roast beef, salmon, and beets. Horseradish also combines with lemon and tomato paste to make an excellent tangy dip—the so-called cocktail sauce of shrimp and other seafood—for raw zucchini, carrots, and other crudités. The dried powder can be mixed with water to form a flavorful paste (wasabi) that is a popular condiment in Japanese dishes.

Mint

The mint family is among the most useful medicinal and culinary herb families. The reason for this is the valuable oils produced by the hairlike oil glands on the surfaces of the leaves and stems of these plants. One member of the mint family—basil—has already been described. Other members of this family include lemon balm, marjoram, peppermint, sage, savory, spearmint, oregano, rosemary, and thyme.

Key Health Benefits

Mints have a wide range of applications. Like other aromatic plants they are primarily applied as carminatives and digestants. Peppermint oil has been shown to relieve spasms of the gastrointestinal tract, and it also relieves gas. The U.S. Dispensatory notes that peppermint "is generally regarded as an excellent carminative and gastric stimulant, and is still widely employed in flatulence, nausea and gastralgia." Perhaps this is why after-dinner mints are so popular. An enteric-coated peppermint oil capsule has been used in treating irritable bowel syndrome in Europe. The enteric coating prevents the oil from being released in the stomach.

Mints have demonstrated some antibiotic and immune-enhancing activities. An extract of lemon balm (*Melissa officinalis*) is used in Europe to treat herpes infections. Peppermint, spearmint, and other mint teas are valuable diaphoretics during viral infections. They also can help the person who drinks them become calm and relaxed, making them useful in cases of insomnia, headache, toothache, and mild nervousness.

Selection

Many mints are now widely available in grocery stores fresh. This is the preferred form. If fresh mints are not available in your area, mints can be obtained as dried leaves or extracts. Mints are also relatively easy plants to grow in most climates, thriving on very little care.

Uses

Mints—especially milder varieties such as lemon balm and spearmint—mix quite well with many different foods. Foods that are enhanced by mints include green salads, marinated vegetables, corn, broccoli, asparagus, and legumes.

Mustard Seeds

Mustard greens are discussed in Chapter 5. As a spice, only the seeds are used. Of the several varieties of mustard seeds, white and yellow varieties are most popular in the United States.

Key Health Benefits

Mustard has many of the same applications as horseradish. In addition, the mustard plaster (a type of poultice) has long been used as a treatment to decongest the chest. A mustard plaster is made by mixing one part dry mustard with three parts flour and then adding enough water to make a paste. The paste is then spread on thin cotton (an old pillowcase works well) or cheesecloth, folded, and placed on the chest. It can be left on for up to 20 minutes; however, you must be sure to check its effect periodically, since it will cause blisters if left on too long. Never apply the mustard to the skin directly, because this will definitely cause the skin to blister.

Selection

Mustard seeds can be purchased as whole seeds; as ground, powdered seeds; and as prepared mustard. Alternatively, you can make your own prepared mustard in a blender. Simply boil together 1 cup of apple cider vinegar, 2 tablespoons of honey, ⅛ teaspoon of turmeric, and ½ teaspoon of lite salt. While the mixture is still hot, pour it into a blender, add ½ cup yellow mustard seed, and immediately grind the mixture in a blender.

When the mixture has achieved a smooth consistency, add 1 tablespoon of olive oil.

Uses

Mustard seeds can be used to liven up stir-fries. Prepared mustard can be used as a condiment and as a spread.

Nutmeg

The nutmeg tree (*Myristica fragrans*) is an evergreen tree native to the Spice Islands of Indonesia. Its fruit initially resembles an apricot in structure. Upon drying, the fruit splits in half, revealing a bright red netlike skin wrapped around a dark reddish-brown, brittle shell within which lies the seed. The bright red netlike skin dries to an orange brown color and is the source of mace. The dried brown seed is the nutmeg.

Key Health Benefits

Nutmeg and mace can produce severe toxicity at doses exceeding 1 teaspoon. Nausea, vomiting, and dizziness accompanied by hallucinations, feelings of unreality, and delusions are some of the symptoms that may develop with toxicity. Used in small quantities, nutmeg and mace act as carminatives and digestive aids.

Selection

Nutmeg can be purchased as the whole or ground seed, while mace is available as a ground powder. Whole nutmeg is best, because ground nutmeg rapidly loses its volatile oils, altering its flavor.

Uses

Nutmeg and mace are used primarily in sweet beverages like eggnog and in desserts. But they also can be used with vegetables such as broccoli, spinach, carrots, and Brussels sprouts.

Oregano and Marjoram

Oregano and marjoram are closely related species (*Origanum* spp.) of the mint family. Their appearance and taste are quite similar, although oregano is a bit stronger. Like most other mints, oregano and marjoram are native to the Mediterranean.

Key Health Benefits

Oregano and marjoram provide similar benefits to those offered by other members of the mint family. Because the essential oil content of marjoram and oregano is lower than that of many other mints, these herbs are considered to be slightly weaker in action.

Selection

Oregano and marjoram are often available fresh. This is the preferred form. If the fresh herb is not available, the whole dried leaves are the best remaining alternative.

Uses

Oregano is best known as an ingredient in tomato sauce and pizza. It has a sharp peppery flavor that is used in the cuisines of Italy, Greece, Spain, and Mexico. Marjoram is viewed as a milder oregano. Although either herb adds a delicious flavor to various foods, most often the flavor of oregano or marjoram is combined with garlic, onion, thyme, and basil, which have quite complementary flavors.

Pepper

Black pepper (*Piper nigrum*) and salt are the most widely used seasoning agents in the United States. Pepper accounts for one-quarter of the world's spice production—about 124,000 tons a year. The pepper plant is native to India. It produces a black fruit (peppercorn) that is usually ground. White pepper is produced by removing the black outer skin of the peppercorn.

Key Health Benefits

Many people consider pepper an irritant that is detrimental to health; however, pepper has been used as a medicine for thousands of years. Black pepper has diaphoretic, carminative, and diuretic properties. It also stimulates the taste buds in a way that increases stomach acid secretion, thereby improving digestion. Pepper has demonstrated impressive antioxidant and antibacterial properties. The outer layer of the peppercorn stimulates the breakdown of fat cells.

Selection

Pepper is available as whole peppercorns, or as ground black or white pepper. The whole peppercorn is best, since it retains the volatile oils longer. You can always grind your own.

Uses

For many people, the familiar taste of pepper is a welcome addition to any dish.

Rosemary

Rosemary (*Rosmarinus officinalis*) is another member of the mint family, although it doesn't look like other mints. It grows as an evergreen shrub, with ash-colored scaly bark and short green needlelike leaves. The leaves and flowers of the plant are the portions used.

Key Health Benefits

Due to its high essential oil content, rosemary has many effects similar to those of other mints. Rosemary is considered more of a stimulant than other mints, however, and it can be toxic if taken in large amounts. Rosemary oil contains a potent antioxidant that is being investigated for use as a natural alternative to the synthetic antioxidants that are often added to foods.

Selection

Fresh rosemary is the best. If it is not available, the dried leaves and flowers (either whole or ground) will have to do.

Uses

Rosemary imparts a piney, sweet, somewhat pungent flavor to many foods, particularly roasted meats, soups, and vegetables.

Saffron

Saffron (*Crocus sativus*) is the most expensive common culinary herb. Only the delicate stigma or thread of the saffron flower is used. Dried saffron looks like delicate dark orange thread. It takes some 35,000 flowers to produce just 1 pound of the spice. True saffron costs over $4,500 per pound.

Key Health Benefits

Saffron contains the only water-soluble carotene, crocetin. This dark orange carotene is responsible for much of the color of saffron. Crocetin performs potent antioxidant and anticancer activities, which may explain some of saffron's historical use in treating cancers. Other historical uses of saffron include as a sedative, a diaphoretic, and an aphrodisiac.

Selection

Saffron is available as whole or ground threads. The whole thread is best.

Uses

Saffron is used in numerous cuisines, including Indian, Middle Eastern, North African, Italian, French, and Spanish. It is used with all types of foods, but is especially associated with rice dishes, soups, and vegetable dishes. It is prized both for its delicate flavor and for its ability to color food.

Sage

The silver-green leaves of the sagebrush makes it a popular decorative garden plant. Garden sage (*Salvia officinalis*) is native to the northern Mediterranean coast, where it has been cultivated for centuries. The sagebrush (*Salvia lyrata*) that grows wild in the United States is too bitter to eat. It has been applied to the skin to remove warts, however.

Key Health Benefits

Sage has long been valued as an important medicinal herb. Its Latin name, *Salvia*, comes from *salvus*, which means "healthy." Sage has long been held to promote health and wisdom. It has been said "the young sow wild oats, and the old grow sage." This is a slight pun, since the primary meaning for the word *sage* is "one wise through reflection and experience."

Reported actions of sage include use as an anhydrotic (a substance that prevents perspiration), a blood-sugar-lowering treatment for diabetes; and an antimicrobial agent. It is also known to dry up the flow of milk during lactation, which is why many herbalists recommend that pregnant and nursing women avoid sage.

Selection

Sage is available as fresh or dried (either whole or crumbled) leaves. Dried sage is usually preferred over fresh sage.

Uses

The most popular use of sage is as an ingredient in turkey stuffing at Thanksgiving, but sage has other uses as well. Sage can be added to breads, soups, most vegetables, and legumes.

Tarragon

When fresh tarragon is available, it is a chef's delight. Its licorice-like flavor adds a great deal to many dishes, but it is especially appreciated with fish. The name *tarragon* comes from the French word *esdragon* or "little dragon." This refers to the plant's dragonlike roots, which may strangle the plant if it is not divided often.

Key Health Benefits

Like most aromatic herbs, tarragon exerts a beneficial effect on digestion, acting as a digestant and carminative. Tarragon may also stimulate the appetite during recuperation from illness.

Selection

Fresh tarragon is substantially superior to dried tarragon. Many vinegars are flavored with tarragon, since the two go quite nicely together.

Uses

Tarragon can be overpowering, so use it sparingly on salads, with vegetables, in grain dishes and casseroles, and, of course, with fish.

Thyme

Thyme is a small, evergreen shrub of the mint family that has tiny leaves with a minty, tealike flavor. Native to the western Mediterranean, thyme has been cultivated for centuries.

Key Health Benefits

Thyme has similar benefits to other mints, because of its volatile oil content. Thyme oil has been shown to possess antispasmodic, antibacterial, and carminative actions. Applied topically, it is also reported to have strong fungicidal properties.

Selection

Thyme is available as fresh or dried leaves. Fresh thyme is more aromatic than the dried leaves.

Uses

Thyme works well with many foods and other herbs, especially garlic, basil, and oregano. This can be put to good use in tomato sauces for pasta and pizza. Thyme also adds a great deal to most vegetables, grains, soups, casseroles, and other dishes. It is extremely versatile.

Turmeric

Turmeric (*Curcuma longa*) is a member of the ginger family that is extensively cultivated in India, China, Indonesia, and other tropical countries. The rhizome (root) is the part used; it is usually cured (boiled, cleaned, and sun-dried), polished, and then ground into a powder. Turmeric is the major ingredient of curry powder and is also used in prepared mustard. It is extensively used for both its color and its flavor.

Key Health Benefits

Turmeric is used in the Chinese and Indian systems of medicine as an anti-inflammatory agent and to treat numerous conditions, including flatulence, jaundice, menstrual difficulties, bloody urine, hemorrhage, toothache, bruises, chest pain, and colic. Turmeric poultices are often applied locally to relieve inflammation and pain.

The volatile oil fraction of turmeric has been demonstrated to possess significant anti-inflammatory activity in various experimental models. Even more potent is the yellow pigment of turmeric, curcumin. Curcumin is believed to be the main pharmacological agent in turmeric. Curcumin's effects in these studies were found to be comparable to the potent drugs hydrocortisone and phenylbutazone. While these drugs are associated with significant toxicity (ulcer formation, decreased white blood cell count, and so on), curcumin displays no toxicity.

Clinical studies have substantiated curcumin's anti-inflammatory effect, including a clinical effect in treating rheumatoid arthritis. In this study, curcumin was compared to phenylbutazone. The improvements in shortened duration of morning stiffness, lengthened walking time, and reduced joint swelling were comparable in both groups. In a new human model for evaluating anti-inflammatory drugs, 400 mg of curcumin was comparable to 100 mg of phenylbutazone and 400 mg of ibuprofen (Motrin).

Other beneficial effects noted in scientific studies of either turmeric or curcumin include improved liver function, lowering of cholesterol levels, antioxidant activity, and anticancer effects.

Selection

Turmeric is available as a ground powder. Curcumin-containing products are available at health-food stores.

Uses

Turmeric is used primarily in curries and in chili powders, making it very important in the cuisines of Southeast Asia, India, and Mexico.

PART II

General Principles of Dietary Therapy

11

Designing a Healthful Diet

Most people give very little thought to the design of their diet. They are motivated to eat based on sensual needs rather than on what their body requires. Unfortunately, health is largely a conscious decision. Awareness of what to eat and in what quantities, and of healthful ways to prepare the foods is critical. The American Dietetic Association and the American Diabetes Association, in conjunction with other groups, have developed a convenient tool—the exchange system—for rapidly estimating the calorie, protein, fat, and carbohydrate content of a diet.

Originally designed for use in formulating dietary recommendations for diabetics, the exchange method is now used in calculating and designing virtually all therapeutic diets. Unfortunately, the ADA exchange plan does not place a strong enough focus on the quality of food choices. The Healthy Exchange System presented in this chapter is a more health-conscious version of the ADA's plan, because it emphasizes more healthful food choices and focuses on unprocessed, whole foods. The diet is prescribed by allotting the number of exchanges allowed per list for one day. There are seven exchange lists; however, the milk and meat lists should be considered optional. The list headings are as follows:

THE HEALTHY EXCHANGE SYSTEM

List 1–Vegetables
List 2–Fruits
List 3–Breads, Cereals, and Starchy Vegetables
List 4–Legumes
List 5–Fats
List 6–Milk
List 7–Meats, Fish, Cheese, and Eggs

All food portions within each exchange list provide approximately the same calories, proteins, fats, and carbohydrates per serving. *The Healing*

Table 11.1 Macro-Nutrient Composition per Serving

List	*Protein (g)*	*Fat (g)*	*Carbo-hydrates (g)*	*Fiber (g)*	*Calories (kcal)*
Vegetables	3	0	11	1–3	50
Fruits	0	0	20	1–3	80
Breads, etc.	2	0	15	1–4	70
Legumes	7	0.5	15	6–7	90
Fats	0	5	0	0	45
Milk	8	0	12	0	80
Meats, etc.	7	3	0	0	55

Power of Foods Cookbook is based on the Healthy Exchange System, allowing easy calculation of the number of servings for each list. The exchange lists and the cookbook are very useful for constructing a healthful diet. A healthy person's diet should have the following components:

Carbohydrates: 65 to 75 percent of total calories
Fats: 15 to 25 percent of total calories
Protein: 10 to 15 percent of total calories
Dietary fiber: at least 50 grams

Of the carbohydrates ingested, 90 percent should be complex carbohydrates or naturally occurring sugars. Intake of refined carbohydrate and concentrated sugars (including honey, pasteurized fruit juices, and dried fruit, as well as sugar and white flour) should be limited to less than 10 percent of the total calorie intake from carbohydrates. The intake of polyunsaturated fats should be equal to or greater than the intake of saturated fats. Avoiding food components detrimental to health—sugar, saturated fats, cholesterol, salt, food additives, alcohol, and agricultural residues such as pesticides and herbicides—is strongly recommended.

Constructing a diet that meets these recommendations is simple if you use the exchange lists. In addition, the recommendations ensure a high intake of vital whole foods (particularly vegetables) that are rich in nutritional value. Table 11.1 shows the macro-nutrient composition per serving for each exchange list.

How Many Calories Do You Need?

In determining your calorie needs, it is first necessary to determine your ideal body weight. The most popular height and weight charts are the

Table 11.2 1983 Metropolitan Life Insurance Height and Weight Table

Height	*Small Frame*	*Medium Frame*	*Large Frame*
Men			
5′2″	128–134	131–141	138–150
5′3″	130–136	133–143	140–153
5′4″	132–138	135–145	142–156
5′5″	134–140	137–148	144–160
5′6″	136–142	139–151	146–164
5′7″	138–145	142–154	149–168
5′8″	140–148	145–157	152–172
5′9″	142–151	148–160	155–176
5′10″	144–154	151–163	158–180
5′11″	146–157	154–166	161–184
6′0″	149–160	157–170	164–188
6′1″	152–164	160–174	168–192
6′2″	155–168	164–178	172–197
6′3″	158–172	167–182	176–202
6′4″	162–176	171–187	181–207
Women			
4′10″	102–111	109–121	118–131
4′11″	103–113	111–123	120–134
5′0″	104–115	113–126	122–137
5′1″	106–118	115–129	125–140
5′2″	108–121	118–132	128–143
5′3″	111–124	121–135	131–147
5′4″	114–127	124–138	134–151
5′5″	117–130	127–141	137–155
5′6″	120–133	130–144	140–159
5′7″	123–136	133–147	143–163
5′8″	126–139	136–150	146–167
5′9″	129–142	139–153	149–170
5′10″	132–145	142–156	152–173
5′11″	135–148	145–159	155–176
6′0″	138–151	148–162	158–179

NOTE: Weights are for adults age 25 to 59 years, based on lowest mortality. Weight is expressed in pounds according to frame size in indoor clothing (5 pounds for men and 3 pounds for women), and wearing shoes with 1-inch heels.

tables of "desirable weight" provided by the Metropolitan Life Insurance Company. The most recent edition of these tables, published in 1983, gives weight ranges for men and women at 1-inch increments of height for three body frame sizes (see Table 11.2). Many nutrition experts have been reluctant to use the 1983 table due to its higher weight ranges as compared to earlier tables.

Table 11.3 Elbow Breadth Measurements for Medium-framed Individuals of Different Heights

Height in 1″ Heels	*Elbow Breadth*
Men	
5′2″ to 5′3″	2½″ to 2⅞″
5′4″ to 5′7″	2⅝″ to 2⅞″
5′8″ to 5′11″	2¾″ to 3″
6′0″ to 6′3″	2¾″ to 3⅛″
6′4″	2⅞″ to 3¼″
Women	
4′10″ to 5′3″	2¼″ to 2½″
5′4″ to 5′11″	2⅜″ to 2⅝″
6′0″	2½″ to 2¾″

Determining Frame Size

To make a simple determination of your frame size, first extend your arm and bend your forearm upward at a 90-degree angle. Keep your fingers straight and turn the inside of your wrist away from your body. Place the thumb and index finger of your other hand on the two prominent bones on either side of your elbow. Measure the space between your fingers with a tape measure. Compare the measurement with the measurements in Table 11.3 for medium-framed individuals. A lower reading indicates a small frame; a higher reading indicates a large frame.

After determining your desirable weight in pounds, convert it into kilograms by dividing it by 2.2. Next, take this number and multiply it by the following number of calories, depending on your activity level:

Little physical activity: 30 calories
Light physical activity: 35 calories
Moderate physical activity: 40 calories
Heavy physical activity: 45 calories

Weight (in kg) × Activity level = Appropriate calorie requirements
_____ × _____ = _________

Using this calculation, a 70-kg (154-pound) man whose physical activity level is moderate would need 2,800 calories to maintain that weight. A sedentary 50-kg (110-pound) woman would require only 1,500 calories to maintain her weight. This formula can be used to determine the rate of weight loss to be expected from calorie restriction. For example, to lose 1 pound of fat by diet alone in one week, an individual needs to have a negative calorie intake of 500 calories per day or 3,500 calories per week. To lose 1 pound of fat, a person must take in 3,500 fewer calories than he or she expends. To lose 2 pounds of fat each week, the person must maintain a negative caloric balance of 1,000 calories a day. This can be achieved by decreasing the amount of calories ingested and/or by exercising to burn up additional calories. To reduce one's caloric intake by 1,000 calories is often difficult, as is burning an additional 1,000 calories per day by exercise (a person would have to jog for 90 minutes, play tennis for 2 hours, or take a brisk (2½-hour walk). The most sensible approach to weight loss is to decrease caloric intake and to exercise simultaneously. This is discussed in greater detail in Chapter 12.

Examples of Exchange Recommendations

1,500-CALORIE VEGAN DIET

List 1–Vegetables: 5 servings
List 2–Fruits: 2 servings
List 3–Breads, Cereals, and Starchy Vegetables: 9 servings
List 4–Beans: 2.5 servings
List 5–Fats: 4 servings

The preceding recommendation would result in a daily intake of approximately 1,500 calories, of which 67 percent are derived from complex carbohydrates and naturally occurring sugars, 18 percent from fat, and 15 percent from protein. The protein intake is entirely from plant sources, but it still provides approximately 55 grams—a number well above the recommended daily allowance of protein intake for a person requiring a diet of 1,500 calories. At least half of the fat servings should be from nuts, seeds, and other whole foods from the Fat Exchange List. The dietary fiber intake would be approximately 31 to 74.5 grams. Thus, to summarize, the numbers are as follows:

Percentage of calories as carbohydrates: 67%
Percentage of calories as fats: 18%
Percentage of calories as protein: 15%
Protein content: 55 g
Dietary fiber content: 31 to 74.5 g

1,500-CALORIE OMNIVORE DIET

List 1–Vegetables: 5 servings
List 2–Fruits: 2.5 servings
List 3–Breads, Cereals, and Starchy Vegetables: 6 servings
List 4–Beans: 1 serving
List 5–Fats: 5 servings
List 6–Milk: 1 serving
List 7–Meats, Fish, Cheese, and Eggs: 2 servings

Percentage of calories as carbohydrates: 67%
Percentage of calories as fats: 18%
Percentage of calories as protein: 15%
Protein content: 61 g (75% from plant sources)
Dietary fiber content: 19.5 to 53.5 g

2,000-CALORIE VEGAN DIET

List 1–Vegetables: 5.5 servings
List 2–Fruits: 2 servings
List 3–Breads, Cereals, and Starchy Vegetables: 11 servings
List 4–Beans: 5 servings
List 5–Fats: 8 servings

Percentage of calories as carbohydrates: 67%
Percentage of calories as fats: 18%
Percentage of calories as protein: 15%
Protein content: 79 g
Dietary fiber content: 48.5 to 101.5 g

2,000-CALORIE OMNIVORE DIET

List 1–Vegetables: 5 servings
List 2–Fruits: 2.5 servings
List 3–Breads, Cereals, and Starchy Vegetables: 13 servings
List 4–Beans: 2 servings
List 5–Fats: 7 servings
List 6–Milk: 1 serving
List 7–Meats, Fish, Cheese, and Eggs: 2 servings

Percentage of calories as carbohydrates: 66%
Percentage of calories as fats: 19%

Percentage of calories as protein: 15%
Protein content: 78 g (72% from plant sources)
Dietary fiber content: 32.5 to 88.5 g

2,500-CALORIE VEGAN DIET

List 1–Vegetables: 8 servings
List 2–Fruits: 3 servings
List 3–Breads, Cereals, and Starchy Vegetables: 17 servings
List 4–Beans: 5 servings
List 5–Fats: 8 servings

Percentage of calories as carbohydrates: 69%
Percentage of calories as fats: 15%
Percentage of calories as protein: 16%
Protein content: 101 g
Dietary fiber content: 33 to 121 g

2,500-CALORIE OMNIVORE DIET

List 1–Vegetables: 8 servings
List 2–Fruits: 3.5 servings
List 3–Breads, Cereals, and Starchy Vegetables: 17 servings
List 4–Beans: 2 servings
List 5–Fats: 8 servings
List 6–Milk: 1 serving
List 7–Meats, Fish, Cheese, and Eggs: 3 servings

Percentage of calories as carbohydrates: 66%
Percentage of calories as fats: 18%
Percentage of calories as protein: 16%
Protein content: 102 g (80% from plant sources)
Dietary fiber content: 40.5 to 116.5 g

3,000-CALORIE VEGAN DIET

List 1–Vegetables: 10 servings
List 2–Fruits: 4 servings
List 3–Breads, Cereals, and Starchy Vegetables: 17 servings
List 4–Beans: 6 servings
List 5–Fats: 10 servings

Percentage of calories as carbohydrates: 70%
Percentage of calories as fats: 16%
Percentage of calories as protein: 14%
Protein content: 116 g
Dietary fiber content: 50 to 84 g

3,000-CALORIE OMNIVORE DIET

List 1–Vegetables: 10 servings
List 2–Fruits: 3 servings
List 3–Breads, Cereals, and Starchy Vegetables: 20 servings
List 4–Beans: 2 servings
List 5–Fats: 10 servings
List 6–Milk: 1 serving
List 7–Meats, Fish, Cheese, and Eggs: 3 servings

Percentage of calories as carbohydrates: 67%
Percentage of calories as fats: 18%
Percentage of calories as protein: 15%
Protein content: 116 g (81% from plant sources)
Dietary fiber content: 45 to 133 g

Use these recommendations as the basis for calculating other calorie diets. For example, for a 4,000-calorie diet, add the 2,500-calorie diet to the 1,500-calorie diet. For a 1,000-calorie diet, divide the 2,000-calorie diet in half.

The Healthy Exchange Lists

Exchange List 1–Vegetables

Vegetables are excellent sources of vitamins, minerals, and health-promoting fiber compounds. Vegetables are fantastic "diet" foods, because they are very high in nutritional value but low in calories. Notice that starchy vegetables such as potatoes and yams are included in List 3 (Breads, Cereals, and Starchy Vegetables). In addition to eating vegetables whole, you can consume vegetables as fresh juice. There is also a list of "free" vegetables. These vegetables are termed "free foods" and can be eaten in any desired amount because the calories they contain are offset by the number of calories your body burns in the process of digesting them. These foods are especially valuable diet foods as they help keep you feeling satisfied between meals.

As the recommended consumption levels for vegetables in the Healthy

Exchange System are quite high, many individuals may find it necessary (or convenient) to juice their fresh, raw vegetables. Juicing allows for easy absorption of the health-giving components of fresh fruits and vegetables in larger amounts.

The list that follows shows the vegetables to use for 1 vegetable exchange. In each case, 1 cup of cooked vegetables or of fresh vegetable juice, or 2 cups of raw vegetables equals 1 exchange:

- Artichoke (1 medium)
- Asparagus
- Bean sprouts
- Beets
- Broccoli
- Brussels sprouts
- Carrots
- Cauliflower
- Eggplant
- Greens:
  - Beet
  - Chard
  - Collard
  - Dandelion
  - Kale
  - Mustard
  - Spinach
  - Turnip
- Mushrooms
- Okra
- Onions
- Rhubarb
- Rutabaga
- Sauerkraut
- String beans, green or yellow
- Summer squash
- Tomatoes, tomato juice, vegetable juice cocktail
- Zucchini

The following vegetables may be eaten as often as desired, especially in their raw form:

- Alfalfa sprouts
- Bell peppers
- Bok choy (Chinese cabbage)
- Cabbage
- Chicory
- Celery
- Cucumber
- Endive
- Escarole
- Lettuce
- Parsley
- Radishes
- Spinach
- Turnips
- Watercress

List 2–Fruits

Fruits make excellent snacks because they contain fructose (fruit sugar). This sugar is absorbed slowly into the bloodstream, thereby allowing the body time to utilize it. Fruits are also excellent sources of vitamins, minerals, and health-promoting fiber compounds. However, fruits are not as nutrient-dense as vegetables are, because they are typically higher in calories. That is why vegetables are favored over fruits in weight-loss plans and in overall healthful diets.

Each of the following equals 1 fruit exchange:

Juice, fresh	1 cup (8 oz)
Juice, pasteurized	⅔ cup
Apple	1 large
Applesauce (unsweetened)	1 cup
Apricots, fresh	4 medium
Apricots, dried	8 halves
Banana	1 medium
Berries	
Blackberries	1 cup
Blueberries	1 cup
Cranberries	1 cup
Raspberries	1 cup
Strawberries	1½ cup
Cherries	20 large
Dates	4
Figs, fresh	2
Figs, dried	2
Grapefruit	1
Grapefruit juice	1 cup
Grapes	20
Mango	1 small
Melons	
Cantaloupe	½ small
Honeydew	¼ medium
Watermelon	2 cups
Nectarine	2 small
Orange	1 large
Papaya	1½ cup
Peach	2 medium
Persimmon, native	2 medium
Pineapple	1 cup
Plums	4 medium
Prunes	4 medium
Prune juice	½ cup
Raisins	4 tbsp
Tangerine	2 medium

Additional fruit exchanges are as follows (no more than one of these should be consumed per day):

Honey	1 tbsp
Jams, jellies, preserves	1 tbsp
Sugar	1 tbsp

List 3–Breads, Cereals, and Starchy Vegetables

Breads, cereals, and starchy vegetables are classified as complex carbohydrates. Chemically, complex carbohydrates are made up of long chains of simple carbohydrates or sugars. To utilize these, the body has to digest or break down the large sugar chains into simple sugars. Therefore, the sugar from complex carbohydrates enters the bloodstream relatively slowly. This in turn means that blood-sugar levels and appetite are better controlled.

Complex carbohydrate foods such as breads, cereals, and starchy vegetables are higher in fiber and nutrients but lower in calories than are foods that contain large quantities of simple sugars, like cakes and candies. Each of the following equals 1 complex carbohydrate exchange:

Breads	
Bagel, small	½
Dinner roll	1
Dried bread crumbs	3 tbsp
English muffin, small	½
Tortilla (6-inch)	1
Whole-wheat, rye, or pumpernickel	1 slice
Cereals	
Bran flakes	½ cup
Cornmeal (dry)	2 tbsp
Cereal (cooked)	½ cup
Flour	2½ tbsp
Grits (cooked)	½ cup
Pasta (cooked)	½ cup
Puffed cereal (unsweetened)	1 cup
Rice or barley (cooked)	½ cup
Wheat germ	¼ cup
Other unsweetened cereal	¾ cup
Crackers	
Arrowroot	3
Graham (2½″ square)	2
Matzo (4″ × 6″)	½

Rye wafers (2″ × 3½″)	3
Saltines	6
Starchy vegetables	
Corn	⅓ cup
Corn on cob	1 small
Parsnips	⅔ cup
Potato, mashed	½ cup
Potato, white	1 small
Yam or sweet potato	¼ cup
Prepared foods	
Biscuit, 2″ diameter (omit 1 fat exchange)	1
Corn bread, 2″ × 2″ × 1″ (omit 1 fat exchange)	1
French fries, 2 to 3″ long (omit 1 fat exchange)	8
Muffin, small (omit 1 fat exchange)	1
Popcorn (airpopped, uncooked)	½ cup
Potato or corn chips (omit 2 fat exchange)	15
Pancake, 5″ × ½″ (omit 1 fat exchange)	1
Waffle, 5″ × ½″ (omit 1 fat exchange)	1

List 4–Legumes

Legumes (beans) are fantastic foods, rich in important nutrients and health-promoting compounds. Legumes help improve liver function, lower cholesterol levels, and improve blood-sugar control. Since obesity and diabetes have been linked to loss of blood-sugar control (insulin insensitivity), legumes apear to be extremely important in weight-loss plans and in the dietary management of diabetes.

In each case, ½ cup of the following cooked or sprouted beans equals 1 legume exchange:

Black-eyed peas
Chick-peas (garbanzos)
Kidney beans
Lentils
Lima beans
Pinto beans
Soybeans, including tofu (omit 1 fat exchange)
Split peas
Other dried beans and peas

List 5–Fats and Oils

Animal fats are typically solid at room temperature and are referred to as "saturated fats," while vegetable fats are liquid at room temperature and are referred to as "unsaturated fats" or "oils." Vegetable oils provide the greatest dietary source of the essential fatty acids linoleic acid and linolenic acid. These fatty acids function in our bodies as components of nerve cells, cellular membranes, and hormonelike substances. Fats also provide energy to the body.

While fats are important to human health, too much fat in the diet—especially saturated fat—is linked to numerous cancers, heart disease, and strokes. Most nutritional experts strongly recommend that total fat intake in the diet be kept below 30 percent of total calories. They also recommend that at least two times more unsaturated fats be consumed than saturated fats.

Each of the following equals 1 fat exchange:

POLYUNSATURATED

Vegetable oils	1 tsp
Canola	
Corn	
Flax	
Safflower	
Soy	
Sunflower	
Avocado (4″ diameter)	⅛
Almonds	10 whole
Pecans	2 large
Peanuts	
Peanut butter	2 tbsp
Spanish	20 whole
Virginia	10 whole
Seeds	1 tbsp
Flax	
Pumpkin	
Sesame	
Sunflower	
Walnuts	6 small

MONOUNSATURATED

Olive oil	1 tsp
Olives	5 small

SATURATED (USE SPARINGLY)

Butter	1 tsp
Bacon	1 slice

Cream, light or sour	2 tbsp
Cream, heavy	1 tbsp
Cream cheese	1 tbsp
Salad dressings	2 tsp
Mayonnaise	1 tsp

List 6–Milk

Is milk for "everybody"? Definitely not. Many people are allergic to milk or lack the necessary enzymes to digest milk. Drinking cow's milk is a relatively new dietary practice for humans. This may be the reason why so many people have difficulty with milk. Certainly milk consumption should be limited to no more than two servings per day.

In each case, 1 cup equals 1 milk exchange:

Nonfat milk or yogurt
2% milk (omit 1 fat exchange)
Low-fat yogurt (omit 1 fat exchange)
Whole milk (omit 2 fat exchanges)
Yogurt (omit 2 fat exchanges)

List 7–Meats, Fish, Cheese, and Eggs

When selecting from this list, choose primarily from the low-fat group and remove the skin of poultry. This will limit the amount of saturated fat consumed. Although many people advocate vegetarianism, the following exchange list provides high concentrations of certain nutrients that are difficult to obtain in an entirely vegetarian diet, including the full range of amino acids, vitamin B_{12}, and heme iron. The most important recommendation may be to use these foods in small amounts as "condiments" in the diet, rather than as mainstays.

Each of the following equals 1 meat exchange:

LOW-FAT (LESS THAN 15% FAT CONTENT)

Beef: baby beef, chipped beef, chuck, steak (flank, plate), tenderloin plate ribs, round (bottom, top), all cuts rump, spare ribs, tripe	1 oz
Cottage cheese, low-fat	¼ cup
Fish	1 oz
Lamb: leg, rib, sirloin, loin (roast and chops), shank, shoulder	1 oz

Poultry: chicken or turkey without skin	1 oz
Veal: leg, loin, rib, shank, shoulder, cutlet	1 oz

MEDIUM-FAT (FOR EACH, OMIT ½ FAT EXCHANGE)

Beef: ground (15% fat), canned corned beef, rib eye, round (ground commercial)	1 oz
Cheese: mozzarella, ricotta, farmer's, parmesan	1 oz
Eggs	1
Organ meats	1 oz
Pork: loin (all tenderloin), picnic & boiled ham, shoulder, Boston butt, Canadian bacon	1 oz

HIGH-FAT (FOR EACH, OMIT 1 FAT EXCHANGE)

Beef: brisket, corned beef, ground beef (more than 20% fat), hamburger, roasts (rib), steaks (club and rib)	1 oz
Cheese: cheddar	1 oz
Duck or goose	1 oz
Lamb: breast	1 oz
Pork: spareribs, loin, ground pork, country-style ham, deviled ham	1 oz

12

Achieving Ideal Body Weight

It is estimated that from 30 to 50 percent of the adult population are obese.[1] The simplest definition of *obesity* is the condition of having an excessive amount of body fat. It must be distinguished from the term *overweight,* which refers to an excess of body weight relative to height. For example, a muscular athlete may be overweight, yet have a very low body-fat percentage. What causes him or her to be overweight is muscle or lean body mass. Despite the fact that body weight alone does not always reflect body-fat percentage, *obesity* is often defined as a weight greater than 20 percent more than the average desirable weight for men and women of a given height. The most popular height and weight charts are the tables of "desirable weight" issued by the Metropolitan Life Insurance Company. These are provided in Table 11.2 in Chapter 11.

Many physicians and nutritionists utilize more precise estimations of body fat percentage, such as skinfold thickness, bioelectric impedance, and ultrasound. These techniques provide much greater accuracy in determining whether a person has too much fat on his or her body. With these techniques, obesity is better defined as a body-fat percentage greater than 30 percent for women and greater than 25 percent for men.[2]

What Causes Obesity?

While psychological factors are important, more and more research is supporting the notion of there being a biological basis for obesity. Biological models of obesity are closely tied to the metabolism of the fat cells.[3] These models support the idea that obesity is not just a matter of overeating, and they explain why some people can eat very large quantities of calories and not increase their weight substantially, while for the obese just the reverse is the case.

Research has found that each person has a physiologically programmed "set point" weight. Individual fat cells may control this set point: When the fat cell becomes smaller, it sends a message to the brain to eat.[4] Since obese individuals often have both more and larger fat cells, the result is an overpowering urge to eat.

This explains why most diets don't work. While obese individuals can fight off the impulse for a time, eventually the signal becomes too strong to ignore. The result is rebound overeating, with individuals often exceeding their previous weight. In addition, their set point becomes reset at a higher level, making it even more difficult for them to lose weight.[5] This is known as the "yo-yo" or "ratchet" effect.

The set point seems to be tied to the sensitivity of fat cells to insulin, a hormone secreted by the pancreas. Its primary function is to help regulate blood-sugar levels by promoting the uptake of blood glucose by cells of the body. Obesity leads to insulin insensitivity and vice versa. When cells become insensitive to insulin, blood-sugar levels reach higher-than-normal levels. This is known as diabetes. Both obesity and diabetes are strongly linked to the so-called "Western diet," presumably because of the harmful effects refined sugar has on insulin and blood-sugar-control mechanisms.[6]

The key to overcoming the fat cell's set point appears to be to increase the sensitivity of the fat cells to insulin. The set-point theory suggests that a weight-loss plan that does not improve insulin sensitivity will likely fail to provide long-term results. Insulin sensitivity can be improved, and the set point lowered, by exercise and a specially designed program like the one outlined here.

How to Lose Weight

Weight loss is among the most challenging health goals. Few people want to be overweight, yet only 5 percent of markedly obese individuals and only 66 percent of people who are just a few pounds overweight are able to attain and maintain "normal" body weight.

A program for successful permanent weight loss must incorporate high nutrition, adequate exercise, and a positive mental attitude. All of these components are critical and interrelated; no single element is more important than the others. Improvement in one facet may be enough to result in some positive changes, but addressing all three yields the greatest results.

Hundreds of diets and diet programs claim to be the answer to the problem of obesity. Dieters are constantly bombarded with reports of new "wonder" diets to follow. However, the basic equation for losing weight never changes. For an individual to lose weight, calorie intake must be less than calories burned. This can be done by decreasing food intake and/or by exercising.

To lose 1 pound of fat, a person must take in 3,500 fewer calories than he or she expends. To lose 2 pounds of fat each week, a person must maintain a negative caloric balance of 1,000 calories per day. This can be achieved by decreasing the amount of calories ingested and/or by exercising. To reduce one's caloric intake by 1,000 calories is often difficult, as is burning an additional 1,000 calories per day by exercise (a person would need to jog for 90 minutes, play tennis for 2 hours, or take a brisk 2½-hour walk). The most sensible approach to weight loss is to decrease caloric intake and simultaneously to exercise.

A successful weight-loss program should provide a diet with approximately 1,200 to 1,500 calories per day. This, along with aerobic exercise for 15 to 20 minutes three or four times per week will produce optimum weight loss at a rate of approximately 1 to 3 pounds per week. Starvation and crash diets usually result in rapid weight loss (largely in the form of muscle and water loss), but cause rebound weight gain and a higher set point. The most successful approach to weight loss is gradual weight reduction through long-standing dietary and lifestyle modifications.

Building a Positive Mental Attitude

Obese individuals have experienced much psychological trauma to their self-esteem. Fashion trends, insurance programs, college placements, and employment opportunities all discriminate against obese people. Consequently, obese people learn many self-defeating and self-degrading attitudes. They are led to believe that fat is "bad," which often results in a vicious cycle of low self-esteem, depression, overeating for consolation, increased fatness, social rejection, and further lowering of self-esteem. Counseling is often necessary to change attitudes about being obese and to aid in the improvement of self-esteem. If this underlying need is not dealt with, even an otherwise perfect diet and exercise plan will fail. Improving the way overweight people feel about themselves assists them in changing their eating behaviors.

Increasing self-esteem and promoting a healthy positive mental attitude are critical factors in a successful weight-loss program. To achieve these goals, you need to exercise or condition your attitude similarly to how you condition your body. To help you, I have developed some exercises designed to help you achieve the kind of permanent results you really want by conditioning you for success. You will need to get a notebook that you can write in. This will become your personal journal. A journal is a powerful tool to help you stay in touch with your feelings, thoughts, and emotions. The exercises are designed to help you learn how to adopt healthier attitudes. The exercises provide the foundation, and you will build on this with your daily personal journal.

EXERCISE 1

CREATING A POSITIVE GOAL STATEMENT

Learning to set goals in a way that yields a positive experience is critical to your success. The following guidelines can be used to set any goal, including your desired weight. You can use goal setting to create a "success cycle." Achieving goals helps you feel better about yourself, and the better you feel about yourself, the more likely you are to achieve further goals. Here are the guidelines:

1. State the goal in positive terms; do not use any negative words in your goal statement. For example, it is better to say "I enjoy eating healthy, low-calorie, nutritious foods" than to say "I will not eat sugar, candy, ice cream, and other fattening foods." Remember, always state the goal in positive terms, and do not use any negative words in the goal statement.
2. Make your goal attainable and realistic. Again, goals can be used to create a success cycle and a positive self-image. Little things add up to make a major difference in the way you feel about yourself.
3. Be specific. The clearer your goal is defined, the more likely you are to reach it. What is the weight you desire? What is the body-fat percentage or measurements you desire? Clearly define what it is you want to achieve.
4. State the goal in present tense, not future tense. To reach your goal, you have to believe you have already attained it. As noted psychologist Dr. Wayne Dyer says "You'll see it, when you believe it." You must program yourself to achieve the goal. See and feel yourself as having already achieved the goal, and success will be yours. Remember, always state your goal in the present tense.

Goal Statement

Use the preceding guidelines above to construct a positive goal statement.

EXAMPLE: "My body is strong and beautiful. I have a 23 percent body-fat percentage and I weigh 125 pounds. I feel good about myself and my body. I am losing 2 pounds a week, and I feel fantastic!"

Short-term Goals

Any journey begins with one step, followed by many other steps. Short-term goals can be used to help you achieve the long-term results described in your positive goal statement. Get in the habit of asking yourself the following question each morning and evening: "What must I do today to achieve my long-term goal?"

Exercise 2

Why Are You Ready to Lose Weight Now?

Now that you have created your positive goal statement, how committed are you to achieving your goal? Without commitment, there can be no success. If you can absolutely commit to achieving your goal, nothing can stand in your way.

Here is one of my favorite quotes from Goethe:

> Until one is committed there is hesitancy, the chance to draw back, always ineffectiveness. Concerning all acts of initiative (and creation), there is one elementary truth, the ignorance of which kills countless ideas and splendid plans: that the moment one definitely commits oneself, then Providence moves too. All sorts of things occur to help one that would never have otherwise occurred. A whole stream of events issues from the decision, raising in one's favor all manner of unforeseen incidents and meeting and material assistance which no man could have dreamed would have come his way. Whatever you can do, or dream you can, begin it. Boldness has genius, power, and magic in it. Begin it now!

Right now you must be absolutely committed to reaching your desired weight right now. To reinforce this commitment you will need to write the answers to the following questions:

- What is the pleasure you have gotten by not losing weight?
- What is the pain that has kept you from losing weight?
- What pain would you experience in the future if you didn't lose the weight you desire to lose?
- What do you have to gain by losing weight?
- Give 10 reasons why you absolutely must lose weight right now.
- Give 10 reasons why you absolutely can lose weight right now.

Exercise 3

The Power of Questions

According to Anthony Robbins, author of the bestsellers *Unlimited Power* and *Awakening the Giant Within*, the quality of your life is equal to the quality of the questions you habitually ask yourself. This is based on the belief that—whatever question you ask your brain—you will get an answer.

Consider the following example: An individual faces a particular challenge or problem. In this situation, he or she can ask a number of questions. Questions many people ask under such circumstances include: "Why does this always happen to me?" and "Why am I always so stupid?" Do they get answers to these questions? Do the answers build self-esteem? Does the problem keep reappearing? What would constitute a higher-quality question? How about, "This is a very interesting situation; what do I need to learn from this situation so that it never happens again?" Or, how about "What can I do to make this situation better?"

If you want to have a better life, ask better questions. It sounds simple, because it is. To help you achieve not only your desired weight, but also a happier life, ask yourself the following questions on a regular basis.

The Morning Questions

1. What am I most happy about in my life right now?
   Why does that make me happy?
   How does that make me feel?
2. What am I most excited about in my life right now?
   Why does that make me excited?
   How does that make me feel?
3. What am I most grateful about in my life right now?
   Why does that make me grateful?
   How does that make me feel?
4. What am I enjoying most in my life right now?
   What about that do I enjoy?
   How does that make me feel?
5. What am I committed to in my life right now?
   Why am I committed to that?
   How does that make me feel?
6. Whom do I love [Starting close and moving out]
   Who loves me?
7. What must I do today to achieve my long-term goal?

The Evening Questions

1. What have I given today?
   In what ways have I been a giver today?
2. What did I learn today?
3. In what ways was today a perfect day?
4. Repeat the morning questions.

The Problem or Challenge Questions

1. What is right/great about this problem?
2. What is not perfect yet?
3. What am I willing to not do to make it the way I want?
4. How can I enjoy doing the things necessary to make it the way I want it?

Exercise 4

Affirmations

An affirmation is a positive statement. Affirmations can make imprints on the subconscious mind to create a healthy, positive self-image. In addition, affirmations can actually fuel the changes you desire. In creating your own affirmations, observe some simple guidelines. Always phrase an affirmation in the present tense. Always phrase the affirmation in a positive way, and totally associate yourself with the positive feelings that it generates. Keep the affirmation short and simple, but full of feeling. Be creative. Imagine yourself really experiencing what you are affirming. Make the affirmation personal and meaningful.

Here are some examples of positive affirmations:

1. I am a whole and complete person.
2. I am in control of my life.
3. I am an open channel of love and joy.
4. I am filled with peace and wisdom.
5. I am good to my body.
6. I am growing stronger every day.
7. I am healthier and thinner.

Using the preceding guidelines and examples, write down five affirmations about eating healthfully and five affirmations about physical activity. State these affirmations aloud for a total of 5 minutes each day. Choose a location that is comfortable and quiet, and a time when you will not be interrupted or disturbed. Sit or lie in a comfortable position. Begin by taking 10 deep breaths—inhaling to a count of one, holding for a count of two, and exhaling to a count of four.

Your Personal Journal

Your personal journal will serve as a testimonial record to your success. In your journal, you will need to enter a daily diary and make sure you performed all of the daily exercises. Construct a Daily Diary and Check List.

Make sure that you ask the morning and evening questions, write down your current weight, rewrite your goal statement, and perform your affirmations. Also write down everything that you ate for breakfast, lunch, snacks, dinner, as well as your physical activities, little things that made this day special, and your greatest triumph of the day.

The Importance of Exercise

The health benefits of regular exercise cannot be overstated. The immediate effect of exercise is stress on the body; with a regular exercise program, however, the body adapts. The body's response to regular stress is to become stronger, to function more efficiently, and to develop greater endurance. Exercise is a vital component in a successful permanent weight-loss plan.[7]

Physical inactivity may be a major cause of obesity in the United States. Indeed, childhood obesity seems to be associated more closely with inactivity than with overeating, and strong evidence suggests that 80 to 86 percent of adult obesity begins in childhood. In the adult population, obese adults are less active than are their leaner counterparts.[8] Regular exercise is a necessary component of a weight-loss program for the following reasons:

1. When weight loss is achieved by dieting without exercise, a substantial portion of the total weight loss comes from the lean tissue (primarily as water loss).[9]
2. When exercise is included in a weight-loss program, there is usually an improvement in body composition due to a gain in lean body weight (because of an increase in muscle mass) and a concomitant decrease in body fat.[10]
3. Exercise helps counter the reduction in basal metabolic rate (BMR) that usually accompanies calorie restriction alone.[11]
4. Exercise increases the BMR for an extended period of time following the exercise session.[12]
5. Moderate to intense exercise may have an appetite-suppressing effect.[13]
6. Subjects who exercise during and after weight reduction are better able to maintain the weight loss than those who do not exercise.[14]

Physical Benefits of Exercise

The entire body benefits from regular exercise, largely as a result of improved cardiovascular and respiratory function. Simply stated, exercise enhances the transport of oxygen and nutrients into cells. At the same time, exercise enhances the transport of carbon dioxide and waste products from the tissues of the body to the bloodstream and ultimately to the eliminative organs.

Regular exercise is particularly important in reducing the risk of heart disease. It does this by lowering cholesterol levels, improving the supplies of blood and oxygen to the heart, increasing the functional capacity of the heart, reducing blood pressure, reducing obesity, and exerting a favorable effect on blood clotting.

Psychological and Social Benefits of Exercise

Regular exercise makes people not only look better, but also feel better. Tensions, depressions, feelings of inadequacy, and worries diminish greatly with regular exercise. The value of an exercise program in the treatment of depression cannot be overstated. Exercise alone has been demonstrated to have a tremendous impact on improving mood and the ability to handle stressful life situations.

In a recent study published in the *American Journal of Epidemiology*, increased participation in exercise, sports, and physical activities was found to be strongly associated with decreased symptoms of depression (feelings that life is not worth while, low spirits, and so on), anxiety (restlessness, tension, and so on), and malaise (rundown feeling, insomnia, and so on).[15]

How to Start an Exercise Program

First make sure that you are fit enough to start an exercise program. If you have been mostly inactive for a number of years or have a previously diagnosed illness, see your physician before attempting anything strenuous.

If you are fit enough to begin, select an activity that you feel you would enjoy. The best exercises are the kind that get your heart moving. Aerobic activities such as walking briskly, jogging, bicycling, cross-country skiing, swimming, aerobic dance, and racquet sports are good examples. Brisk walking (5 miles per hour) for approximately 30 minutes may be the very best form of exercise for weight loss. Walking can be done anywhere; it doesn't require expensive equipment—just comfortable clothing and well-fitting shoes—and the risk for injury is extremely low.

The concept of "spot reduction" is a myth. Exercise draws from all of the fat stores in the body, not just from local deposits. While aerobic exercise generally enhances weight-loss programs, weight-training programs can also substantially alter body composition, by increasing lean body weight and decreasing body fat.[16] Thus, weight training may be just as effective as, or more so than, aerobic exercise in maintaining or increasing lean body weight and, therefore, improving the metabolic rate of individuals undergoing weight reduction.[17]

Intensity of Exercise

Exercise intensity is determined by measuring your heart rate (the number of times your heart beats per minute). This can be quickly done by placing the index and middle finger of one hand on the side of the neck just below the angle of the jaw or on the opposite wrist. Beginning with zero, count the number of heartbeats for 6 seconds. Then simply add a zero to this number, and you have your pulse. For example, if you counted 14 beats, your heart rate was 140. Is this a good number? It depends on your training zone.

A quick and easy way to determine your maximum training heart rate is simply to subtract your age from 185. For example, if you are 40 years old, your maximum heart rate is 145. To determine the bottom of your training zone, simply subtract 20 from this number. In the case of a 40-year-old, this number is 125. So the training range would be at a heart rate of between 125 and 145 beats per minute. For maximum health benefits, you must stay within this range and never exceed it.

Duration and Frequency

A minimum of 15 to 20 minutes of exercising at your training heart rate at least three times a week is necessary to gain any significant benefits from exercise. It is better to exercise at the lower end of your training zone for longer periods of time than to exercise at a higher intensity for shorter periods of time. It is also desirable to make exercise a part of your daily routine.

Eat to Lose Weight

We have discussed the importance of attitude and exercise in a successful weight-loss plan. Now let's review some key dietary recommendations. First of all, it is extremely important to provide the body the high-quality nutrition it needs, especially during weight loss. If the body is not fed, it feels that it is starving. As a result, metabolism will slow down; and this means that less fat will be burned. Eating or drinking the juice of raw fruits and vegetables is extremely important in achieving permanent weight loss.

Diets containing a high percentage of uncooked foods are significantly associated with weight loss, improved blood-sugar control, and lower blood pressure.[18] Researchers seeking to determine why raw food diets produce these effects have reached the following three conclusions:

1. A raw food diet is much more satisfying to the appetite. Cooking can cause the loss of up to 97 percent of water-soluble vitamins (B-vitamins and vitamin C) and up to 40 percent of fat-soluble vitamins (A, D, E, and K). Since uncooked foods such as juices contain more vitamins and other nutrients, they are more satisfying to the body. The result is reduced calorie intake and improved weight loss in obese individuals.
2. The blood-pressure-lowering effect of raw foods is most likely due to more healthful food choices, fiber, and potassium. However, the effect of cooking the food cannot be ruled out. When patients are switched from a raw food diet to a cooked diet (without altering the content of calories or sodium), there is a rapid increase in blood pressure relative to prestudy values.
3. A diet composed of an average of 60 percent of the calories ingested from raw foods reduces stress on the body. Specifically, the presence of enzymes in raw foods, the reduced allergenicity of raw foods, and the effects of raw foods on our gut-bacteria ecosystem are thought to be much more healthful than the effects of cooked foods.

Raw foods appear to help reset the body's appetite control center by providing the body the high-quality nutrition it needs. This is vitally important at all times, but especially so during weight loss. If the body is not fed, it feels that it is starving. In response, metabolism slows down, which means that less fat is burned. Juicing fresh fruits and vegetables is an excellent way to supply key nutrients to the body in a fresh, raw, and natural way, boosting energy levels and promoting weight loss.

Preparing Your Body for Weight Loss

During the first week of a weight-loss program, it is often recommended that an individual prepare the body by going on a "juice fast" consisting of three or four 8- to 12-ounce juice meals spread throughout the day. During this week your body will begin ridding itself of stored toxins. Drinking fresh juice for cleansing reduces some of the side effects associated with a water fast, such as light-headedness, tiredness, and headaches. While on a "fresh juice fast," individuals typically experience an increased sense of well-being, renewed energy, clearer thought, and a sense of purity.

Although a short juice fast can be started at any time, it is best to begin on a weekend or during a time period when adequate rest can be assured. The greater the rest, the better the results, as energy can be directed toward healing instead of toward other body functions.

Prepare for a fast on the day before solid food is to be stopped by having the last meal consist exclusively of fresh fruits and vegetables. (Some authorities recommend a full day of raw food to start a fast—even a juice fast.)

Only fresh fruit and vegetable juices (ideally prepared from organic produce) should be consumed for the next 3 to 5 days. Four 8- to 12-ounce glasses of fresh juice should be consumed throughout the day. In addition to the fresh juice, pure water should be consumed. The quantity of water should be dictated by thirst, but at least four 8-ounce glasses should be consumed every day during the fast.

No coffee, commercially prepared juice, soft drinks, cigarettes, or anything else by mouth should be taken except water. Herbal teas can be quite supportive of a fast, but they should not be sweetened.

Exercise is not usually recommended during a fast. It is a good idea to conserve energy and allow maximal healing. Short walks or light stretching are useful, but heavy workouts tax the system and inhibit repair and elimination.

Rest is one of the most important aspects of a fast. A nap or two during the day is recommended. Less sleep will usually be required at night, since daily activity is lower. Body temperature usually drops during a fast, as does blood pressure, and pulse and respiratory rate—all measures of the slowing of the metabolic rate of the body. It is important, therefore, to stay warm.

In breaking a fast, as outlined in Table 12.1, an individual is encouraged to eat slowly, chew thoroughly, limit quantities, and eat foods at room temperature. While breaking a fast and in the days that follow, it can be very helpful to carefully record what is eaten and note any adverse effects. Many of today's health problems are due to food allergies and overeating.

Table 12.1 Breaking Your Fast

	Breakfast	*Lunch*	*Dinner*
Day 1	One of the following: melon, nectarine, pineapple	A different fruit from the breakfast list	8 oz of any fruit
Day 2	12 oz of one type of fresh fruit	14 oz of whole pears or citrus fruit	Raw vegetable salad with leafy greens, tomato, celery, and cucumber, or 2 pears, 2 apples, and avocado
Day 3	Resume healthful diet (raw fresh fruits, raw/steamed vegetables, whole grains, nuts, seeds, and legumes)		

The Importance of Fiber

A fiber-deficient diet is an important factor in the development of obesity.[19] Dietary fiber plays a role in preventing obesity by various means: (1) slowing the eating process; (2) increasing excretion of calories in the feces; (3) altering digestive hormone secretion; (4) improving glucose tolerance; and (5) inducing satiety by increased gastric filling, stimulating the release of appetite-suppressing hormones such as cholecystokinin, and intestinal bulking action.[20]

Perhaps the primary effects of fiber on obesity are related to improving glucose metabolism. Blood-sugar problems (hypoglycemia and diabetes) appear to be among the problems most clearly related to inadequate dietary fiber intake.[21] Numerous clinical trials have demonstrated the beneficial effects of several water-soluble fibers (including guar gum, gum karaya, and pectin) on blood-sugar control. In the treatment of obesity, dietary fiber supplementation has been shown to promote weight loss.[22] Fiber's main action appears to be in reducing calorie consumption by increasing the feeling of fullness and decreasing the feeling of hunger. These data suggest that, in addition to eating a high-fiber diet, supplementing the diet with additional fiber (especially water-soluble fibers) may provide additional benefits.

Using Meal Replacement Formulas

Meal replacement formulas that mix with water, juice, or milk are popular weight-loss aids. The drink mixture is used to replace a meal. While these formulas can provide short-term benefit, in the long run a successful program must incorporate more healthful food choices. Numerous meal replacement formulas are available on the market. Here are five guidelines for choosing a healthful version:

1. Look for a product that contains high-quality protein from grains and legumes, or hydrolyzed lactalbumin. Avoid casein-based formulas. Casein, a milk protein, is often difficult for people to digest; many people are allergic to it; and it has been shown to raise blood cholesterol levels. Casein is used in many meal replacement formulas, as well as in glues, molded plastics, and paints.
2. The formula should contain at least 5 grams of a combination of soluble and insoluble dietary fibers.
3. Look for balanced, high-quality nutrition with enhanced levels of nutrients critical to weight loss such as chromium.

4. The formula should have a low total fat content, but should supply some essential fatty acids.
5. The formula should not contain sweeteners, artificial flavors, or other artificial food additives. Refined sugar leads to loss of blood-sugar control, diabetes, and obesity. Sucrose (white table sugar) is the first ingredient in many meal replacement formulas.

For Permanent Results

Permanent results require permanent changes in choosing what foods to eat and when to eat them. The healthful diet component of an effective weight-loss program must stress fresh fruits and vegetables, along with grains and beans. These foods contain not only valuable nutrients, but also dietary fiber compounds that have important weight-loss-promoting properties. Avoiding food components that are detrimental to health—sugar, saturated fats, cholesterol, salt, food additives, alcohol, and agricultural residues such as pesticides and herbicides—is strongly recommended.

In closing, here are 10 weight-loss tips that really seem to work:

1. Avoid snacking. Eat regular, planned meals. If you feel a need to have a snack, drink a glass of fresh vegetable juice, eat a piece of fruit, or have a salad.
2. Reduce intake of fatty foods, spreads, salad dressings, butter, and other sources of fat. Keep fat intake to a minimum.
3. At all your meals, eat large quantities of fresh vegetables and salads to fill you up.
4. Eat high-fiber whole-grain cereals instead of white bread and refined cereals.
5. Eliminate desserts and sweets by substituting fresh fruits.
6. Avoid alcohol and soft drinks.
7. Drink a glass of fresh fruit juice 30 to 45 minutes before your main meal. The fructose (fruit sugar) in the fresh juice will dampen your appetite, resulting in fewer calories being consumed.
8. When eating out, choose restaurants that offer low-fat choices. Avoid fast-food restaurants.
9. Learn to eat slowly. Enjoy your meals, and allow your body time to realize that it has been fed.
10. Avoid eating late at night, since the calories consumed then tend to be stored rather than burned for energy.

13

Finding and Controlling Food Allergies

The recognition of food allergy was first recorded by the famous Greek physician Hippocrates, who observed that milk could cause gastric upset and hives (urticaria). He wrote, "to many this has been the commencement of a serious disease when they have merely taken twice in a day the same food which they have been in the custom of taking once. . . ."[1]

A food allergy occurs when the body has an adverse reaction to the ingestion of a food. The reaction may or may not be mediated by the immune system. The reaction may be caused by a food protein, by a starch, by some other food component, or by a contaminant or additive found in the food (a coloring, a preservative, or the like). A classic food allergy occurs when an ingested food molecule acts as an antigen—a substance that can be bound by an antibody—and is bound by allergic antibodies known as IgE. IgE then binds to specialized white blood cells known as "mast cells" and "basophils." This binding causes the release of substances such as histamine that cause swelling and inflammation.

Other terms often used to refer to a food allergy include *food hypersensitivity, food anaphylaxis, food idiosyncrasy, food intolerance, pharmacologic* [drug like] *reaction to food, metabolic reaction to food,* and *food sensitivity.* From a clinical perspective, naturopaths, clinical ecologists, and preventive- and nutrition-oriented physicians recognize two basic types of food allergies—cyclic and fixed. Cyclic allergies account for 80 to 90 percent of all food allergies. The sensitivity is slowly developed over the course of repeated consumption of a food. If the allergenic food is avoided for a period of time (typically over 4 months), it may be reintroduced and once again tolerated unless it is eaten too frequently. Fixed allergies occur whenever a food is eaten, no matter what the time span between instances of ingestion. Long-term avoidance may reestablish tolerance, but it is no guarantee.

Signs and Symptoms of Food Allergies

Food allergies have been implicated as a contributing factor in a wide range of conditions; no part of the human body is immune from being a target cell or organ. The actual symptoms of an allergic response depend on the location of the immune system activation, the mediators of inflammation involved, and the sensitivity of the tissues to specific mediators. As Table 13.1 shows, food allergies have been linked to many common symptoms and health conditions.[2]

The number of people suffering from food allergies has increased dramatically during the last 15 years. Some physicians claim that food allergies are the leading cause of most undiagnosed symptoms and that at least 60 percent of the American population suffers from symptoms associated with food reactions. Various theories seek to explain why the incidence has increased: increased stresses on the immune system (such as greater chemical pollution in the air, water, and food); earlier weaning and earlier introduction of solid foods to infants; genetic manipulation of plants, resulting in food components with greater allergenic tendencies; and increased ingestion of fewer foods. Probably all of these and more have contributed to the increased frequency and severity of symptoms.

Food allergies and respiratory tract allergies are characterized by the following signs:

Dark circles under the eyes (allergic shiners)
Puffiness under the eyes

Table 13.1 Symptoms and Diseases Commonly Associated with Food Allergies

System	*Symptoms and Diseases*
Gastrointestinal	canker sores, celiac disease, chronic diarrhea, stomach ulcer, gas, gastritis, irritable colon, malabsorption, ulcerative colitis
Genitourinary	bed-wetting, chronic bladder infections, kidney disease
Immune	chronic infections, frequent ear infections
Mental/Emotional	anxiety, depression, hyperactivity, inability to concentrate, insomnia, irritability, mental confusion, personality change, seizures
Musculoskeletal	bursitis, joint pain, low back pain
Respiratory	asthma, chronic bronchitis, wheezing
Skin	acne, eczema, hives, itching, skin rash
Miscellaneous	arrythmia, edema, fainting, fatigue, headache, hypoglycemia, itchy nose or throat, migraines, sinusitis

Horizontal creases in the lower lid
Chronic noncyclic fluid retention
Chronic swollen glands

It is often unclear whether a symptom is due to a food allergy or to something else. This appears to be due to the body's adaptation to chronic exposure to allergenic foods. The symptom process may involve three stages:

Stage 1 – Hypersensitivity (preadapted): Obvious allergic response following exposure to allergenic food.

Stage 2 – Adaptive: Less recognizable response after eating the allergenic food, and an increase in chronic symptoms. This can be considered an addictive phase, since ingestion of the allergenic food(s) may actually temporarily relieve symptoms. This stage typically involves food cravings and withdrawal responses. It is also known as "masked allergies."

Stage 3 – Maladaptive: The body is in a constant state of biochemical dysfunction. The allergic person is totally unaware of sensitivities as a cause of his or her ill health.[3]

What Causes Food Allergies?

Food allergy is often inherited. When both parents have allergies, each child has a 67 percent chance of also having allergies. Where only one parent is allergic, a child's chance of being prone to allergies drops to 33 percent.[4] The actual expression of an allergy can be triggered by various stressors that may disrupt the immune system, such as physical and emotional trauma, excessive use of drugs, immunization reactions, excessively frequent consumption of specific foods, and/or environmental toxins.

Most food allergies are mediated by the immune system as a result of interactions between ingested food, the digestive tract, white blood cells, and food-specific antibodies (immunoglobulins), such as IgE and IgG. Food molecules (and other foreign bodies) capable of being bound by antibodies are known as antigens. Food represents the largest antigenic challenge confronting the human immune system.[5] When the immune system is activated by food antigens, white blood cells and antibodies cooperate in an immune response that, under certain circumstances, can have negative effects.

There are five major families of antibodies: IgE, IgD, IgG, IgM, and IgA. IgE is involved primarily in the classic immediate reaction, while the others seem to be involved in delayed reactions, such as those seen in the cyclic type of food allergy. Although the function of the immune system is to protect the host from infections and cancer, abnormal immune responses can lead to tissue injury and disease (food allergy reactions being only one expression of these). There are four distinct types of immune-mediated reactions: immediate hypersensitivity, cytotoxic reactions, immune complex–mediated reactions, and T-cell-dependent reactions.

Type I – Immediate Hypersensitivity

Reactions of this type occur in less than 2 hours. Antigens bind to preformed IgE antibodies that are attached to the surface of the mast cell or the basophil and cause release of mediators—histamine, leukotrienes, and the like. A variety of allergic symptoms may result, depending on the location of the mast cell: in the nasal passages, it causes sinus congestion; in the bronchioles, constriction (asthma); in the skin, hives and eczema; in the synovial cells that line the joints, arthritis; in the intestinal mucosa, inflammation with resulting malabsorption; and in the brain, headaches, loss of memory, and "spaciness." It has been estimated that Type I reactions account for only 10 to 15 percent of all food allergy reactions.[6]

Type II – Cytotoxic Reactions

Cytotoxic reactions involve the binding of either IgG or IgM antibodies to cell-bound antigens. Antigen–antibody binding activates factors that result in the destruction of the cell to which the antigen is bound. Examples of tissue injury include immune hemolytic anemia. It has been estimated that at least 75 percent of all food allergy reactions are accompanied by cell destruction.[7]

Type III – Immune Complex–Mediated Reactions

Immune complexes are formed when antigens bind to antibodies. They are usually cleared from the circulation by the phagocytotic system. If these complexes are deposited in tissues, however, they can produce tissue injury. Two important factors promote tissue injury: increased quantities of circulating complexes; and the presence of histamine and other amines, which increase vascular permeability and favor the deposition of immune complexes in tissues.

These responses are of the delayed type, often occurring 2 hours after exposure. This type of allergy has been shown to involve IgE and IgG immune complexes.[8] It is estimated that 80 percent of food allergy reactions involve IgG.[9]

Type IV – T-cell-dependent Reactions

This delayed type of reaction is mediated primarily by T-lymphocytes. It results when an allergen contacts the skin, respiratory tract, gastrointestinal tract, or other body surface. Within 36 to 72 hours of contact, the contact can cause inflammation by stimulating sensitized T-cells. Type IV does not involve any antibodies. Examples include poison ivy (contact dermatitis), allergic colitis, and regional ileitis.

Immune System Disorders and Food Allergies

Several immune system disorders can play a major role in food allergies.[10] Some studies have shown that individuals who have a tendency to develop asthma and eczema also have abnormalities in the number and ratios of special white blood cells known as T-cells. Specifically, these individuals have nearly 50 percent more helper T-cells than do nonallergic persons.[11] These cells help other white blood cells make antibodies.

An emerging theory suggests that individuals prone to asthma and eczema have a lower allergic set point. With more helper T-cells in circulation, the level of attack required to trigger an allergic response is lower. Other T-cell abnormalities have been noted in patients with migraines and in asthmatic children; both groups commonly suffer from food allergies.[12]

Food-sensitive people have been observed to have unusually low levels of serum IgA.[13] On the lining of the mucosal membrane surfaces of the intestinal tract, IgA plays an important role in helping protect against the entrance of foreign substances into the body. In other words, IgA acts as a barricade against the entry of food antigens. When insufficient IgA is present in the lining of the intestines, the absorption of food allergens (and microbial antigens) increases dramatically. It has been suggested that even a relatively short-term IgA deficiency predisposes a person to develop allergies, especially during the first months of life.[14]

There is also evidence that stress can impair immune function and lead to decreased secretory IgA.[15] These findings might explain the relationship that many observers report between food allergies and stress. During stress, food allergies tend to be more severe.

Other Factors

Repetitious exposure to a food, improper digestion, and poor integrity of the intestinal barrier are additional factors that can lead to food allergies. When properly chewed and digested, 98 percent of ingested proteins are absorbed as amino acids and small peptides. However, partly digested dietary protein has been documented to cross the intestinal barrier and be absorbed into the bloodstream. It then causes a food-allergic response, directly at the intestinal barrier, at distant sites, or throughout the body.[16]

Gastric acidity and pancreatic enzymes limit the passage of organisms into the intestinal tract and are important in the digestion of protein. Low hydrochloric acid and pancreatic enzyme levels in the stomach are associated with an increased incidence of intestinal infections and increased circulation of antibodies to foods. An individual with food allergies must often be supported with supplemental levels of hydrochloric acid and/or pancreatic enzymes; research has shown that incompletely digested proteins can impair the immune system, leading to long-term allergies.[17]

Besides lack of digestive factors, other causes of increased intestinal absorption of large protein molecules include immaturity of the gastrointestinal system, abnormal bacteria in the gut, vitamin A deficiency, inflammation of the intestinal tract, intestinal ulceration, and diarrhea. Proper functioning of the liver is also very important, because of its role in removing foreign proteins.

Premature newborn infants absorb much larger quantities of ingested food proteins than do older children.[18] This suggests that the weaning of infants to solid foods should be done slowly and carefully, to lessen their exposure to potentially allergenic foods. Breastfeeding has been shown to protect against the development of allergies.

Nonimmunological Mechanisms

Many adverse reactions to foods are not triggered by the immune system. Instead, the reaction is caused by inflammatory mediators (prostaglandins, leukotrienes, SRS-A, serotonin, platelet-activating factor, histamine, kinins, and so on). Foods may also produce a pseudo-allergic reaction due to their histamine content or histamine-releasing effects and to compounds in foods known as biogenic amines (see Table 13.2).

Diagnosis

Two basic categories of tests are commonly used: food challenge and laboratory methods. Each has its advantages. Food challenge methods require no additional expense, but they require a great deal of motivation. Laboratory procedures (such as blood tests) can provide immediate identification of suspected allergens, but they are more expensive.

Table 13.2 Mechanisms Responsible for Pseudo-allergic Reactions

- Increased production of inflammatory mediators
- Activation of platelets, resulting in serotonin release
- Enhanced reactivity of mast cells and/or basophils to various triggering stimuli
- Excessive intake of histamine-containing foods: sausage, sauerkraut, tuna, wine, preserves, spinach, tomato
- Excessive intake of histamine-releasing foods: mollusks, crustaceans, strawberry, tomato, chocolate, protease-containing fruits (bananas, papaya), lectin-containing nuts, peptones, alcohol
- Intolerance to foods containing vasoactive amines: tyramine (cabbage, cheese, citrus, seafood, potato), serotonin (banana), phenylethylamine (chocolate)

Food Challenge

Many physicians believe that oral food challenge is the best way of diagnosing food sensitivities. There are two broad categories of food challenge testing: elimination (also known as oligoantigenic) diet, followed by food reintroduction; and pure water fast, followed by food challenge. Food challenge testing should NOT be used in people with potentially life-threatening symptoms (such as airway constriction of severe allergic reactions).

In the elimination diet method, the person is placed on a limited diet; commonly eaten foods are eliminated and replaced with either hypoallergenic foods rarely eaten, or special hypoallergenic formulas.[19] The fewer the allergenic foods involved, the greater the ease of establishing a diagnosis with an elimination diet. The standard elimination diet consists of lamb, chicken, potatoes, rice, banana, apple, and a cabbage family vegetable (cabbage, Brussels sprouts, broccoli, or the like). Some variations of the elimination diet are suitable; however, it is extremely important that no allergenic foods be consumed.

The individual stays on this limited diet for at least 1 week and for up to 1 month. If the symptoms are related to food sensitivity, they will typically disappear by the fifth or sixth day of the diet. If the symptoms do not disappear, a reaction to one of the foods in the elimination diet may be responsible, in which case an even more restricted diet must be utilized.

After 1 week, individual foods are reintroduced according to some plan by which a particular food is reintroduced every 2 days. Methods range from reintroducing only one food every 2 days to reintroducing one every one or two meals. Usually after the 1-week "cleansing" period, the patient will develop an increased sensitivity to offending foods.

Reintroduction of an allergenic food typically produces a more severe or recognizable symptom than before. A careful, detailed record must be maintained, describing when foods were reintroduced and what symptoms appeared upon reintroduction.[20] It can be very useful to track the wrist pulse during reintroduction, since pulse changes may occur when an allergenic food is consumed.[21]

For many people, elimination diets offer the most viable means of detection. Because one can sometimes dramatically experience the effects of food reactions, motivation to eliminate the food can be high. The down side of this procedure is that it is time-consuming and requires personal discipline and motivation.

A refinement that often yields even better results than the simple elimination diet is the 5-day water fast with subsequent food challenge. Proponents of this approach believe that a patient must fast for at least 5 days in order to "clear" the body of allergic responses.[22] During the fast, "withdrawal" symptoms are likely to be experienced. These symptoms usually subside by the fourth day. As in the elimination diet, symptoms caused by the food allergy diminish or disappear after the fourth day.

After the 5-day fast, individual foods are singly reintroduced, with continuous monitoring of symptoms and pulse. Due to the hyperreactive state, symptoms tend to be more acute and pronounced than they were before the fast. This method can produce dramatic results, greatly motivating future avoidance of the offending foods.

This method is only advisable for people who are physically and mentally capable of a 5-day water fast. Close monitoring by a physician with experience in fasting is highly recommended. At times, careful interpretation of results is needed, due to the possible occurrence of delayed reactions.

Laboratory Methods

Skin Tests The skin prick test or skin scratch test commonly employed by many allergists only tests for IgE-mediated allergies. But since only about 10 to 15 percent of all food allergies are mediated by IgE, this test is of little value in diagnosing most food allergies. Nonetheless, skin tests are often performed.

Food extracts are placed on the patient's skin with a scratch or prick method. If the patient is allergic to the food through IgE mediation, a welt will form immediately as the allergen reacts with IgE-sensitized cells in the patient's skin.

Blood Tests Despite a tremendous amount of scientific support, the diagnosis of food allergies by blood testing is still somewhat controversial. These tests are convenient, but they tend to be relatively expensive. Various blood tests are available to physicians, with the RAST (radio-allergo-sorbent test) and the ELISA (enzyme-linked immunosorbent assay) test currently the best laboratory methods available.

Dealing with Food Allergies

Avoidance and Elimination

The simplest and most effective method of treating food allergies consists of avoiding allergenic foods. Eliminating the offending antigens from the diet will begin to alleviate associated symptoms as the body clears itself of the antigen/antibody complexes and after the intestinal tract rids itself of any remaining food (usually 3 to 5 days). The allergic person must not only avoid the food in its most identifiable state (for examples, eggs in an omelet), but also in its hidden state (for example, eggs in bread). In the case of severe reactions, closely related foods with similar antigenic components may also have to be eliminated (for example, rice and millet in patients with a severe wheat allergy).

Avoiding allergenic foods may not be simple or practical, however, for several reasons:

1. Common allergenic foods such as wheat, corn, and soy are found as components of many processed foods.
2. When eating away from home, a person may find it difficult to determine what ingredients were used in purchased foods and prepared meals.
3. The number of foods that single individuals are allergic to has dramatically increased. This condition represents a syndrome that may indicate broad immune system dysfunction. It may be difficult (psychologically, socially, and nutritionally) to eliminate a large number of common foods from a person's diet.

Rotary Diversified Diet

Many experts believe that the key to dietary control of food allergies is the "Rotary Diversified Diet." The diet was first developed by Dr. Herbert J. Rinkel in 1934.[23] The diet is made up of a highly varied selection of foods that are eaten in a definite rotation or order to prevent the formation of new allergies and to control existing ones.

Tolerated foods are eaten at regularly spaced intervals of 4 to 7 days. For example, a person who has wheat on Monday must wait until Friday to have anything with wheat in it again. This approach is based on the principle that infrequent consumption of tolerated foods is not likely to induce new allergies or to intensify existing mild allergies, even in highly sensitized and immune-compromised individuals. As tolerance for eliminated foods returns, they may be added back into the rotation schedule without reactivating the allergy. (This of course applies only to cyclic food allergies; fixed allergenic foods may never be eaten again.)

It is not simply a matter of rotating tolerated foods. Food families must be rotated as well. Foods, whether animal or vegetable, come in families. The reason it is important to rotate food families is that foods in one family can "cross-react" with allergenic foods. Steady consumption of foods that are members of the same family can lead to allergies. Food families need not be as strictly rotated as individual foods. Authorities usually recommend avoiding eating members of the same food family 2 days in a row. Table 13.3 lists family classifications for edible plants and animals, while a simplified 4-day rotation diet plan is provided in Table 13.4.

Final Comments

While there is no known simple "cure" for food allergies, a number of measures will help avoid and lessen symptoms and correct the underlying causes. First, all allergenic foods should be identified through one of the previously discussed methods. After identifying allergenic foods, the best approach is clearly to avoid all major allergens and to rotate all other foods for at least the first few months. As the patient improves, the dietary restrictions can be relaxed, although some individuals may require a rotation diet indefinitely. In the case of strongly allergenic foods, all members of the food family should be avoided.

Table 13.3 Edible Plant and Animal Kingdom Taxonomic List

Vegetables

Legumes	**Mustard**	**Parsley**	**Potato**	**Grass**	**Lily**
Beans	Broccoli	Anise	Chili	Barley	Asparagus
Cocoa bean	Brussels sprout	Caraway	Eggplant	Corn	Chives
Lentil	Cabbage	Carrot	Peppers	Oat	Garlic
Licorice	Cauliflower	Celery	Potatoes	Rice	Leek
Peanut	Mustard	Coriander	Tomato	Rye	Onions
Peas	Radish	Cumin	Tobacco	Wheat	
Soybean	Turnip	Parsley			
Tamarind	Watercress				

Laurel	**Sunflower**	**Beet**	**Buckwheat**
Avocado	Artichoke	Beet	Buckwheat
Camphor	Lettuce	Chard	Rhubarb
Cinnamon	Sunflower	Spinach	

Fruits

Gourds	**Plums**	**Citrus**	**Cashew**	**Nuts**	**Beech**
Cantaloupe	Almond	Grapefruit	Cashews	Brazil nut	Beechnut
Cucumber	Apricot	Lemon	Mango	Pecan	Chestnut
Honeydew	Cherry	Lime	Pistachio	Walnut	Chinquapin nut
Melons	Peach	Mandarin			
Pumpkin	Plum	Orange			
Squash	Persimmon	Tangerine			
Zucchini					

Banana	**Palm**	**Grape**	**Pineapple**	**Rose**	**Birch**
Arrowroot	Coconut	Grape	Pineapple	Blackberry	Filberts
Banana	Date	Raisin		Loganberry	Hazelnuts
Plantain	Date sugar			Raspberry	
				Rosehips	
				Strawberry	

Apple	**Blueberry**	**Pawpaws**
Apple	Blueberry	Papaya
Pear	Cranberry	Pawpaw
Quince	Huckleberry	

Animals

Mammals (Meat/Milk)	**Birds (Meat/Egg)**	**Fish**		**Crustaceans**	**Mollusks**
Cow	Chicken	Catfish	Salmon	Crab	Abalone
Goat	Duck	Cod	Sardine	Crayfish	Clams
Pig	Goose	Flounder	Snapper	Lobster	Mussels
Rabbit	Hen	Halibut	Trout	Prawn	Oysters
Sheep	Turkey	Mackerel	Tuna	Shrimp	Scallops

Table 13.4 Four-day Rotation Diet

Food Family	*Food*
Day 1	
Citrus	Lemon, orange, grapefruit, lime, tangerine, kumquat, citron
Banana	Banana, plantain, arrowroot (musa)
Palm	Coconut, date, date sugar
Parsley	Carrots, parsnips, celery, celery seed, celeriac, anise, dill, fennel, cumin, parsley, coriander, caraway
Spices	Black and white pepper, peppercorn, nutmeg, mace
Subucaya	Brazil nut
Bird	All fowl and game birds, including chicken, turkey, duck, goose, guinea, pigeon, quail, pheasant, eggs
Juices	Juices (preferably fresh) may be made and used from any fruits and vegetables listed above, in any combination desired, without adding sweeteners.
Day 2	
Grape	All varieties of grapes, raisins
Pineapple	Juice-pack, water-pack, or fresh
Rose	Strawberry, raspberry, blackberry, loganberry, rose hips
Gourd	Watermelon, cucumber, cantaloupe, pumpkin, squash, other melons, zucchini, pumpkin or squash seeds
Beet	Beet, spinach, chard
Legume	Pea, black-eyed pea, dry beans, green beans, carob, soybeans, lentils, licorice, peanut, alfalfa
Cashew	Cashew, pistachio, mango
Birch	Filberts, hazelnuts
Flaxseed	Flaxseed
Swine	All pork products
Mollusks	Abalone, snail, squid, clam, mussel, oyster, scallop
Crustaceans	Crab, crayfish, lobster, prawn, shrimp
Juices	Juices (preferably fresh) may be made and used without added sweeteners from any fruits, berries, or vegetables listed above, in any combination desired, including fresh alfalfa and some legumes.
Day 3	
Apple	Apple, pear, quince
Gooseberry	Currant, gooseberry
Buckwheat	Buckwheat, rhubarb
Aster	Lettuce, chicory, endive, escarole, globe artichoke, dandelion, sunflower seeds, tarragon
Potato	Potato, tomato, eggplant, peppers (red and green), chili pepper, paprika, cayenne, ground cherries
Lily (onion)	Onion, garlic, asparagus, chives, leeks
Spurge	Tapioca
Herb	Basil, savory, sage, oregano, horehound, catnip, spearmint, peppermint, thyme, marjoram, lemon balm

Table 13.4 *(continued)*

Food Family	*Food*
Day 3 (continued)	
Walnut	English walnut, black walnut, pecan, hickory nut, butternut
Pedalium	Sesame
Beech	Chestnut
Saltwater fish	Herring, anchovy, cod, sea bass, sea trout, mackerel, tuna, swordfish, flounder, sole
Freshwater fish	Sturgeon, salmon, whitefish, bass, perch
Juices	Juices (preferably fresh) may be made and used without added sweeteners from any fruits and vegetables listed above, in any combination.
Day 4	
Plum	Plum, cherry, peach, apricot, nectarine, almond, wild cherry
Blueberry	Blueberry, huckleberry, cranberry, wintergreen
Pawpaws	Pawpaw, papaya, papain
Mustard	Mustard, turnip, radish, horseradish, watercress, cabbage, Chinese cabbage, broccoli, cauliflower, Brussels sprouts, kale, kohlrabi, rutabaga
Laurel	Avocado, cinnamon, bay leaf, sassafras, cassia buds or bark
Sweet potato or yam	
Grass	Wheat, corn, rice, oats, barley, rye, wild rice, cane, millet, sorghum, bamboo sprouts
Orchid	Vanilla
Protea	Macadamia nut
Conifer	Pine nut
Fungus	Mushrooms and yeast (brewer's yeast, etc.)
Bovid	Milk products—butter, cheese, yogurt, beef and milk products, oleomargarine, lamb
Juices	Juices (preferably fresh) may be made and used without added sweeteners from any fruits and vegetables listed above, in any combination desired.

PART III

Food as Medicine

14

Food for Specific Diseases

"The doctor of the future will give no medicine, but will interest his patient in the care of the human frame, in diet and in the cause and prevention of disease."

—*Thomas Edison*

Are Edison's words prophetic? I believe so. In fact, the doctor of the future may very well be the naturopathic physician of today. Naturopathic doctors are trained in the use of many natural therapies, but nutrition serves as the foundation.

There is an ever-growing body of knowledge on the use of foods and nutrients to prevent and treat disease. Many common medical conditions respond quite well to diet therapy. They respond because nutrition often addresses the underlying cause of the illness.

You have undoubtedly heard the expression, "You are what you eat." Is there any truth to this statement? What determines the composition of your body? Genetics certainly plays a role, but the foods you eat are utilized by the body every day. You certainly are what you eat. Whether you are in a state of poor health or simply desire better health, improving the quality of the foods you regularly consume is essential.

Simply following the recommendations given for designing a healthful diet using the Healthy Exchange System, along with those offered in Chapter 13, has the potential to be quite therapeutic for most common illnesses. However, many common medical conditions can be further ameliorated by more specific recommendations for dietary treatment. The purpose of this chapter is to provide such recommendations.

Diet is just one natural method of treating illness, but it may be the most important. If you desire more information about any health condition described in this chapter, I urge you to consult *The Encyclopedia of Natural Medicine*, which I co-authored with Joseph Pizzorno, N.D., the President of the Bastyr College of Natural Health Sciences.

These recommendations are not designed to substitute for proper individual medical treatment. In all cases involving a physical or medical complaint, ailment, or therapy, please consult a physician. Proper medical care and advice can significantly improve the quality and duration of your life. Readers are strongly urged to develop a good relationship with a physician knowledgeable in the art and science of natural and preventive medicine, such as naturopathic physicians (see Epilogue). References from the medical literature are cited so that physicians unfamiliar with dietary treatment will recognize that these recommendations are based on scientific understanding and will work with their patient to arrive at a cure.

Acne

Acne is the most common of all skin problems. It occurs mostly on the face and, to a lesser extent, on the back, chest, and shoulders. It is more common in males and typically begins at puberty. It occurs in two forms: acne vulgaris, which affects the hair follicles and oil-secreting glands of the skin and manifests itself as blackheads (comedones), whiteheads (pustules), and inflammation (papules); and acne conglobata, which is a more severe form, with deep cyst formation and subsequent scarring.[1]

Dietary Considerations

In addition to the general healthful diet that is recommended, a few specifics are in order. All refined carbohydrates and fried foods must be eliminated, and foods containing trans-fatty acids (milk, milk products, margarine, shortening, and other synthetically hydrogenated vegetable oils) or oxidized fatty acids (fried oils) should be avoided, since these foods may aggravate acne. Milk consumption should also be limited because of its high hormone content. Specific nutrients that have been shown to exert a positive effect include: vitamin A, zinc, chromium, selenium, and vitamin E.[2]

Zinc is vitally important in the treatment of acne. Zinc supplementation in the treatment of acne has been the subject of much controversy and many double-blind studies. The inconsistency of the results may be due to differences in the body's absorption of the various zinc salts used. For example, studies using effervescent zinc sulfate show a level of effectiveness similar to that of the antibiotic tetracycline (with fewer side effects from chronic use), while those using plain zinc sulfate have shown less beneficial results.[3] Most patients required 12 weeks of supplementation before good results were achieved, although some showed dramatic improvement immediately. Zinc levels are lower in 13- and 14-year-old males than in any other age group.[4] Foods rich in zinc include nuts, whole grains, and legumes.

Also important are dietary antioxidants, as male acne patients have significantly decreased levels of antioxidant enzymes.[5] This normalizes when vitamin E and selenium are supplemented in the diet. The acne of both men and women improves with this treatment, probably due to inhibition of lipid peroxide formation, which suggests the use of other antioxidants. A diet rich in plant foods should provide adequate levels of a wide range of antioxidants, including vitamin E and selenium.

Other Recommendations

Here are six additional recommendations that should provide additional benefit:

1. Avoid medications that contain bromides or iodides.
2. Avoid exposure to oils and greases.
3. Avoid the use of greasy creams and cosmetics.
4. Thoroughly cleanse the face daily with a sulfur-containing soap or suitable alternative such as calendula soap.
5. Extract blackheads every 2 to 3 days and have cystic lesions incised and drained by a physician every 2 weeks.
6. Supplementation with high doses of vitamin A, zinc, and other nutrients (under the supervision of a physician) may prove beneficial.

Anemia

Anemia refers to a condition in which the blood is deficient in red blood cells or in the hemoglobin (iron-containing) portion of red blood cells. The primary function of the red blood cell (RBC) is to transport oxygen from the lungs to the tissues of the body and to exchange it there for carbon dioxide. The symptoms of anemia, such as extreme fatigue, reflect a lack of oxygen being delivered to tissues and a consequent buildup of carbon dioxide.

The most common cause of anemia is deficient red blood cell production due to nutritional deficiencies. Although deficiencies in various vitamins and minerals can produce anemia, the most common ones are of iron and vitamin B_{12}.

Iron deficiency is the most common cause of anemia; however, anemia is the last stage of an iron-deficient state. Studies in several developed countries, including the United States, have found evidence of iron deficiency in 30 to 50 percent of the population. The groups at highest risk for iron deficiency are infants under 2 years of age, teenage girls, pregnant women, and the elderly. Iron deficiency may be due to an increased iron requirement, decreased dietary intake, diminished iron absorption or utilization, blood loss, or a combination of factors.[6]

The diagnosis of iron deficiency can best be made by measuring serum ferritin, the iron storage protein. This is by far the most sensitive test for iron deficiency. Other measures of iron stores such as serum iron, total iron binding capacity, and RBC hemoglobin are less sensitive but are often performed on a routine basis. Long-term iron deficiency is characterized by low RBC levels, low hematocrit (volume of red blood cells), small RBCs, and low serum ferritin levels.[7]

Vitamin B_{12} Deficiency Anemia

Vitamin B_{12} deficiency is most often due to a defect in absorption and not to a dietary lack of the vitamin. To be absorbed, vitamin B_{12} must be liberated from food by hydrochloric acid and must bond to a substance known as intrinsic factor within the small intestine. Lack of intrinsic factor results in a condition known as pernicious anemia. The defect is rare in individuals before the age of 35, and it is more common in people of Scandinavian, English, and Irish descent. It is much less common in southern Europeans, Asians, and Blacks. Pernicious anemia is frequently associated with iron deficiency as well.[8]

A dietary lack of vitamin B_{12} is most often associated with a strict vegetarian diet. Since normal body stores of vitamin B_{12} may last an individual 3 to 6 years, deficiency of vitamin B_{12} is usually not apparent in a vegetarian until after many years. Fermented foods such as soy sauce, miso, and tempeh may contain some vitamin B_{12}, but strict vegetarians should supplement their diet with additional B_{12}.

Dietary Considerations

Perhaps the best food for an individual with any kind of anemia is calf liver. It is rich in iron and in all B-vitamins. However, no more than 4 ounces of liver should be eaten regularly because of its high content of vitamin A. Hydrolyzed (liquid) liver extracts are perhaps an even better source of highly bio-available nutrients than regular liver; and since they are free of the fat portion, these extracts offer the benefits of liver without the fats, cholesterol, and fat-soluble vitamins.

The use of liver or liver extracts has fallen out of favor in mainstream medicine. Instead, isolated vitamin B_{12}, folic acid, or iron is used. The use of liver therapy in the treatment of anemia has come to be viewed as a "shotgun" approach, since liver contains such a large number of factors that can stimulate normal RBC production in addition to vitamins and minerals. In my opinion, liver or hydrolyzed liver extracts still represent an effective natural treatment for all types of anemia.

Green leafy vegetables are also of great benefit to individuals with any kind of anemia. These vegetables contain natural fat-soluble chlorophyll, as well as other important nutrients including iron and folic acid. The chlorophyll molecule is very similar to the hemoglobin molecule.

Other foods rich in iron include dried beans, blackstrap molasses, lean meat, organ meats, dried apricots and other dried fruits, almonds, and shellfish. Vitamin C supplementation has been shown to greatly enhance the absorption of dietary iron. In fact, vitamin C is regarded as the most potent enhancer of iron absorption.[9] A vitamin C supplement alone will often increase the body's iron stores; 500 mg with each meal is a suitable dose for this effect.

Several foods and beverages contain substances that inhibit iron absorption, including tea, coffee, wheat bran, and egg yolk. Antacids and overuse of calcium supplements also decrease iron absorption. These items should be avoided in the diets of individuals with iron deficiency.[10]

For an individual with pernicious anemia or a vegetarian with vitamin B_{12} deficiency, the standard approach involves injecting vitamin B_{12} at a dose of 1 μg (microgram) daily for 1 week followed by a daily oral dose of 1,000 μg or 1 mg, preferably as a sublingual tablet or liquid.

Asthma and Hayfever

Asthma is an allergic disorder characterized by spasm of the bronchial tubes and excessive excretion of a viscous mucus in the lungs that can lead to difficult breathing. It occurs in recurrent attacks that may range from mild wheezing to life-threatening inability to breathe.

Hayfever (seasonal allergic rhinitis) is an allergic reaction to windborne pollens. Ragweed pollen accounts for about 75 percent of the hayfever in the United States. Other significant pollens capable of inducing hayfever include various grass and tree pollens. If the hayfever develops in the spring, it is usually due to tree pollens; if it develops in the summer, grass and weed pollens are usually the culprits.

Dietary Considerations

Food Allergies Many studies have indicated that food allergies play an important role in asthma and hayfever.[11] Adverse reactions to food may be immediate or delayed. Double-blind food challenges in children have shown that immediate onset sensitivities are usually due (in decreasing order of frequency) to eggs, fish, shellfish, nuts, and peanuts; while foods most commonly associated with delayed onset reactions include (in decreasing order of frequency) milk, chocolate, wheat, citrus, and food colorings.[12] Elimination diets have been successful in treating asthma, particularly in infants and children (see Chapter 13).

Vitally important in the control of asthma is the elimination of food additives.[13] Tartrazine (FD&C yellow dye #5), benzoates, sulphur dioxide, and (in particular) sulfites have been reported to cause asthma attacks in susceptible individuals.[14] Tartrazine is found in most processed foods and can even be found in vitamin preparations and antiasthma prescription drugs (such as theophylline). An estimated 2 to 3 mg of sulfites are consumed each day by the average U.S. citizen, while an additional 5 to 10 mg are ingested by wine and beer drinkers.[15]

Vegetarian Diet A long-term trial of a vegan diet (elimination of all animal products) provided significant improvement in 23 of the 25 treated patients (92 percent) who completed the study (9 dropped out—all within the first 2 months).[16] The researchers also found a reduction in the tendency to contract infectious disease. However, while 91 percent of the patients responded within 4 months, 1 year of therapy was required before the 92 percent level was reached.

The diet excluded all meat, fish, eggs, and dairy products. Drinking water was limited to spring water (chlorinated tap water was specifically prohibited); and coffee, ordinary tea, chocolate, sugar, and salt were excluded. Herbal spices were allowed, as were up to 1½ liters per day of water and herbal teas. Vegetables used freely were lettuce, carrots, beets, onions, celery, cabbage, cauliflower, broccoli, nettles, cucumber, radishes, Jerusalem artichokes, and all beans except soybeans and green peas. Potatoes were allowed in restricted amounts. A number of fruits were also used freely: blueberries, cloudberries, raspberries, strawberries, black currants, gooseberries, plums, and pears. Apples and citrus fruits were not allowed, and grains were either very restricted or eliminated.

The beneficial effects of this dietary regime are probably related to two areas: elimination of common food allergens, and altered fatty acid metabolism. Leukotrienes, which contribute to the allergic and inflammatory reactions found in asthma, are derivatives of arachidonic acid, a fatty acid found exclusively in animal products. In addition, several of the foods consumed (such as onions and berries) have exerted antiasthmatic effects in experimental studies. Onions are particularly beneficial (see page 122).

Antioxidants Vitamin C and other antioxidants are thought to provide an important defense, since oxidizing agents can both stimulate bronchoconstriction and increase allergic reactions to other agents.[17] Both treated and untreated asthmatic patients have been shown to have significantly lower levels of ascorbic acid in their serum and white blood cells.[18] Vitamin C inhibits induced bronchial constriction in both normal and asthmatic subjects.[19] Vitamin C appears to normalize fatty acid metabolism and reduce histamine production. Carotenes, vitamin E, and selenium are also important, due to their powerful antioxidant activity.

Other Recommendations

Jonathan Wright, M.D., believes "B_{12} therapy is the mainstay in childhood asthma."[20] In one clinical trial, weekly intramuscular injections of 1,000 μg of vitamin B_{12} produced definite improvement in asthmatic patients. Of 20 patients, 18 showed less shortness of breath on exertion, as well as improved appetite, sleep, and general condition.[21] Vitamin B_{12} appears to be especially effective in sulfite-sensitive individuals. It offers the best protection when taken orally prior to challenge, compared to drugs like cromolyn sodium, atropine, and doxepin.[22] The mode of action is formation of a sulfite-cobalamin complex, which blocks sulfite's effect.

The old-time herbal treatment of asthma and hayfever involves the use of ephedra plants in combination with herbal expectorants. Expectorants are herbs that modify the quality and quantity of secretions of the respiratory tract, resulting in the expulsion of the secretions and improvement in respiratory tract function. Examples of commonly used expectorants include: lobelia (*Lobelia inflata*), licorice (*Glycyrrhiza glabra*), and grindelia (*Grindelia camporum*). In ephedra preparations, the dosage should be equivalent to 12.5 to 25 mg of ephedrine three times daily.

Bladder Infection (Cystitis)

Bladder infections are very common in women, as 21 percent of all women have urinary tract discomfort at least once a year. Bladder infections in males are much less common and in general indicate an anatomical abnormality or a prostate infection. The body has many defenses against bacterial growth in the urinary tract: urine flow tends to wash away bacteria; the surface of the bladder has antimicrobial properties; the pH of the urine inhibits the growth of many bacteria; the body quickly secretes white cells to control the bacteria; and in men, prostatic fluid has many antimicrobial substances.

Dietary Considerations

If inadequately treated, bladder infections can become chronic or can lead to kidney infections; the care of a physician is strongly encouraged. Avoid all simple sugars, refined carbohydrates, and food allergens. Drink large amounts of fluids (at least 3 quarts per day), including at least 16 ounces of unsweetened cranberry juice per day. (The role of cranberry juice as a urinary tract antiseptic was discussed on pages 139, 140.) Blueberry juice may be a suitable alternative. In addition, the liberal consumption of garlic and onions is recommended for their antimicrobial and immune-enhancing effects.

Other Recommendations

The herb uva ursi or bearberry (*Arctostaphylos uva-ursi*) has a long folk use as a urinary tract antiseptic and may prove useful in assisting the body during a bladder infection.[23]

Candidiasis (Chronic)

The common yeast *Candida albicans* is present in every individual. Normally, the yeast lives harmlessly in the gastrointestinal tract. However, occasionally the yeast overgrows, leading to significant disease. Candida overgrowth is believed to cause a wide range of symptoms, as part of a complex medical syndrome known as the yeast syndrome or chronic candidiasis. The major body systems most sensitive to yeast are the gastrointestinal, genitourinary, endocrine, nervous, and immune systems.[24] Allergies have also been attributed to candida overgrowth. Here are some of the more common signs and symptoms of chronic candidiasis:

- Overgrowth of *Candida albicans* in stool culture
- Presence of high levels of antibodies against *Candida albicans*
- General symptoms: chronic fatigue, loss of energy, general malaise, decreased libido
- Gastrointestinal symptoms: thrush (candida overgrowth of the mouth), bloating, gas, intestinal cramps, rectal itching, and altered bowel function
- Genitourinary system complaints: vaginal yeast infection and frequent bladder infections
- Endocrine system complaints: primarily menstrual complaints such as premenstrual syndrome
- Nervous system complaints: depression, irritability, and inability to concentrate
- Immune system complaints: allergies, chemical sensitivities, and low immune function

Candida overgrowth is most often associated with chronic antibiotic use. Antibiotics kill off the friendly bacteria that help keep candida in check. When antibiotic use first became widespread, physicians noticed immediately that yeast infections increased. Initially, antifungal drugs were commonly given along with the antibiotic to prevent this problem, but for some reason the practice fell out of favor.

The yeast syndrome or chronic candidiasis has been around for a long time. However, it was not until Orion Truss published *The Missing Diagnosis* and William Crook published *The Yeast Connection* that the public and many physicians became aware of the magnitude of the problem. Individuals with chronic candidiasis have different symptoms due to such factors as age, sex, host resistance, and environmental exposure to various factors promoting candida overgrowth.

Dietary Considerations

A number of dietary factors appear to promote the overgrowth of candida; therefore, a special diet must be employed in treating candidiasis.[25] The diet should be free of refined sugar—including sucrose, fructose, commercial fruit juices, honey, and maple syrup—since candida thrives in a high-sugar state. Foods with a high content of yeast or mold—including alcoholic beverages, cheeses, dried fruits, and peanuts—are also thought to promote candida overgrowth and should also be eliminated.

Milk and milk products should be avoided because of their high content of lactose (milk sugar) and their trace levels of antibiotics. All known allergens should also be eliminated, since allergies can weaken the immune system and provide a more hospitable environment for the yeast.

Foods that can be eaten freely include all vegetables, protein sources (legumes, fish, poultry, and meat), and whole grains. Two to three 1-cup servings of the following fruits can be eaten per day as well: apples, blueberries, cherries, other berries, and pears.

A special food for the candidiasis sufferer is garlic. Garlic has demonstrated significant antifungal activity against a wide range of fungi.[26] Garlic is especially active against *C. albicans,* having been found to be more potent than nystatin, gentian violet, and six other reputed antifungal agents.[27]

Other Recommendations

As thoroughly discussed in *The Encyclopedia of Natural Medicine,* there are seven important steps in the successful control of *Candida albicans:*[28]

1. Eliminate the use of antibiotics, steroids, immune-suppressing drugs, and birth control pills (unless required to do otherwise by absolute medical necessity).

2. Follow the candida control diet previously discussed.
3. Enhance digestion with the use of digestive aids, if necessary.
4. Enhance immune function through high-quality nutrition and, if necessary, herbal substances.
5. Enhance liver function by eating a high-fiber, low-fat diet.
6. Use nutritional and herbal supplements that help prevent yeast overgrowth and promote a healthy bacterial flora.
7. Eliminate candida toxins by using a water-soluble fiber source such as guar gum, psyllium husks, or pectin, which can bind to toxins in the gut and promote their excretion.

Canker Sores

Recurrent canker sores (aphthous stomatitis) is an extremely common condition that is estimated to affect 20 percent of the population. Recurrent canker sores, based on studies of initiating factors, appear to be related to food allergies, stress, and/or nutrient deficiency.[29]

Dietary Considerations

Food Allergies The association of recurrent canker sores with food allergies is widely accepted. A diet that eliminates allergenic foods usually prevents further recurrences. The most common offending foods are milk products and wheat.[30] Gluten appears to be a major causative factor for many individuals, and the rate of recurrent canker sores is increased in patients with celiac disease—a condition caused by sensitivity to wheat gluten.[31] Biopsies of the small intestine in 33 patients with recurrent canker sores showed 8 to have the intestinal damage typical of celiac disease, along with signs of allergic reactions to food antigens.[32] The remaining patients also exhibited these types of signs, but to a lesser degree.

An underlying gluten sensitivity can also contribute to nutritional deficiencies. Withdrawing gluten from the diet results in complete remission of recurrent canker sores in patients with celiac disease and usually some improvement in the remaining patients.[33]

Nutrient Deficiencies A study of 330 patients with recurrent canker sores found that 47 (14.2 percent) were deficient in iron, folate, or vitamin B_{12}, or in a combination of these nutrients.[34] When these patients' deficiencies were corrected by supplementation, the majority experienced complete remission. Other studies have shown similar deficiency rates for the same nutrients and equally good response to supplementation.[35] For foods rich in these nutrients, see the discussion of anemia on pages 266, 267.

Other Recommendations

Stress is often a precipitating factor in recurrent canker sores, because stress greatly increases the likelihood of developing allergies. During times of stress, it may be particularly important to avoid suspected allergens. DGL (see page 341) may also be of benefit.

Carpal Tunnel Syndrome

Carpal tunnel syndrome is a common and painful disorder caused by compression of the median nerve as it passes between the bones and ligaments of the wrist. Compression of the nerve causes weakness, pain when gripping, and burning, tingling, or aching, which may radiate to the forearm and shoulder. Symptoms may be occasional or constant, and they usually occur most noticeably at night. Carpal tunnel syndrome is found most often in people who perform repetitive, strenuous work with their hands (such as carpenters). It may also follow injuries of the wrist; more frequently, however, there is no history of significant trauma.[36]

Dietary Considerations

Vitamin B_6 deficiency is a common finding in patients with carpal tunnel syndrome. In fact, except when the syndrome was traceable to direct trauma or systemic disease, Ellis and coworkers never found an exception to this correlation.[37] Several clinical studies have conclusively demonstrated that vitamin B_6 supplementation (usually 50 to 100 mg/day) relieves all symptoms of the carpal tunnel syndrome in patients with low levels of vitamin B_6.[38] Even Phalen (who pioneered the surgical treatment for carpal tunnel syndrome) agrees that, in the future, pyridoxine (in doses of 100 to 200 mg/day) may be the treatment of choice.[39] A therapeutic response may require up to 3 months of supplementation. Foods rich in B_6 include sunflower seeds, soybeans, walnuts, lentils and other legumes, brown rice, and bananas. Table 3.9 on page 55 provides a complete listing of foods rich in vitamin B_6.

The increased rate of carpal tunnel syndrome since its initial description by Phalen in 1952 parallels the increased levels of vitamin B_6 antagonists found in the food supply and in drugs during the same period.[40] These antagonists include tartrazine (FD&C yellow #5), many drugs, oral contraceptives, and excessive protein intake. Although no particular diet has been tested for the treatment of carpal tunnel syndrome, it seems appropriate to increase foods rich in vitamin B_6, to avoid foods containing yellow dyes, and to limit protein consumption to 50 grams per day.

Other Recommendations

During flare-ups, fresh pineapple juice and fresh ginger may help, thanks to their anti-inflammatory activity. Curcumin (from turmeric) is perhaps nature's most potent anti-inflammatory agent. Curcumin preparations available at health-food stores may be useful during episodes of inflammation associated with this syndrome.

Cataracts

Cataracts are the leading cause of impaired vision and blindness in the United States. Approximately 4 million people have some degree of vision-impairing cataract, and at least 40,000 people in the United States are blind because of cataracts. Cataracts are a source of a tremendous financial burden on our society; cataract surgery is the most common major surgical procedure done in the United States for persons on Medicare (600,000 per annum, at a cost of over $4 billion).[41]

Cataract formation is ultimately related to free-radical damage to some of the sulfur-containing proteins in the lens. As with most diseases, prevention or treatment at an early stage is most effective. Since free-radical damage appears to be the primary factor in senile cataracts, individuals with cataracts should avoid direct sunlight and other bright light, and should wear protective lenses (sunglasses) when outdoors. They should also greatly increase their intake of antioxidant nutrients by eating legumes (high in sulfur-containing amino acids), whole grains (vitamin E), and fresh fruits and vegetables (rich in carotenes, flavonoids, and numerous other antioxidants).

Progression of the disease process can be stopped and early-stage cataracts can be reversed. However, significant reversal of well-developed cataracts does not appear to be possible at this time.

Dietary Considerations

In cataract formation, the normal protective mechanisms are unable to prevent free-radical damage. This appears to be closely tied to nutritional status.[42] Specifically, individuals with higher dietary intakes of vitamins E and C and carotenes are at lower risk for developing cataracts, while individuals with low levels of these nutrients in their diets are at increased risk. Thus, individuals who consume more fruits and vegetables are much less likely to develop cataracts than are individuals who consume fewer fruits and vegetables.[43]

Particularly important in the prevention of cataracts may be the consumption of fresh fruits and vegetables, due to the higher content of glutathione in them than in their cooked counterparts.[44] Glutathione is found in very high concentrations in the lens, where it plays a vital role in maintaining the lens's health. Specifically, glutathione functions as an antioxidant, maintains the structure of the lens proteins, acts in various enzyme systems, and participates in amino acid and mineral transport.[45] Glutathione levels are diminished in virtually all forms of cataracts.[46]

In the initial stages, cataracts can often be corrected or at least halted with proper nutrition. For example, clinical studies have demonstrated that vitamin C supplementation can halt cataract progression.[47] In one study, 450 patients with cataracts were placed on a nutritional program that included 1 gram of vitamin C per day; the result was a significant reduction in cataract development.[48] More recent information indicates that a dose of at least 1,000 mg (that is, 1 gram) of vitamin C is needed to increase levels of vitamin C in the aqueous humor and lens.[49]

Other Recommendations

In addition to eating a diet rich in antioxidants by focusing on fresh fruits and vegetables, you should consider antioxidant supplements when cataracts are already apparent. Specifically, it may be worth while to supplement the diet with vitamin C (1 gram three times daily), vitamin E (600 I.U. per day), and selenium (400 μg per day).

Celiac Disease

Celiac disease—also known as nontropical sprue, gluten-sensitive enteropathy, or celiac sprue—is characterized by malabsorption and an abnormal small intestine structure that reverts to normal on removal of dietary gluten. The protein gluten and its derivative, gliadin, are found primarily in wheat, barley, and rye grains.

Symptoms of celiac disease most commonly appear during the first 3 years of life, after cereals are introduced into the diet. A second peak incidence occurs during the third decade of life. Breastfeeding appears to have a preventive effect, since breast-fed babies have a decreased risk of developing celiac disease.[50]

The early introduction of cow's milk is also believed to be a major causative factor.[51] Research in the past few years has clearly indicated that breastfeeding, along with delayed administration of cow's milk and cereal grains, can greatly reduce an infant's risk of developing celiac disease.

Celiac disease also appears to have a genetic cause.[52] The frequency of individuals having the genetic trait for celiac disease is much higher in northern and central Europe and in the northwest Indian subcontinent than elsewhere (for example, 1:300 in southwest Ireland compared with 1:2,500 in the United States [estimated]).[53] Wheat cultivation in these areas is a relatively recent development (1000 B.C.).

Dietary Considerations

Gluten, a major component of the wheat endosperm, is composed of gliadins and glutenins. Only the gliadin portion has been demonstrated to activate celiac disease. In rye, barley, and oats, the proteins that appear to activate the disease are termed *secalins, hordeins,* and *avenins,* respectively, and *prolamines* collectively. Cereal grains belong to the family Gramineae. The closer a grain's taxonomic (classification) relationship to wheat, the greater its likelihood of activating celiac disease. Rice and corn, two grains that do not appear to activate celiac disease, contain very little gliadin.[54]

Once the diagnosis of celiac disease has been established, a gluten-free diet is indicated. This diet disallows any wheat, rye, barley, triticale, or oats. Buckwheat and millet are often excluded as well. Although buckwheat is not in the grass family, and millet appears to be more closely related to rice and corn, they do contain prolamines that are similar to alpha-gliadin of wheat. Following modification of the diet, a person usually shows improvement within a few days or weeks (30 percent respond within 3 days; another 50 percent within 1 month, and 10 percent within another month). However, 10 percent of individuals only respond after 24 to 36 months of avoiding gluten.[55]

Maintaining a strictly gluten-free diet is quite difficult in the United States, due to the wide distribution of gliadin and other activators of celiac disease in processed foods. Individuals with celiac disease must read labels carefully to avoid hidden sources of gliadin in such unexpected places as some brands of soy sauce, modified food starch, ice cream, soup, beer, wine, vodka, whisky, and malt. Consult the following resources for patient education and information on gluten-free recipes:

American Celiac Society
45 Gifford Avenue
Jersey City, NJ 07304

American Digestive Disease Society
7720 Wisconsin Avenue
Bethesda, MD 20014

Gluten Tolerance Group of North America
P.O. Box 23053
Seattle, WA 98102

National Digestive Disease Education and Information Clearing House
1555 Wilson Boulevard, Suite 600
Rosslyn, VA 22209

Other Recommendations

Papain, the protein-digesting enzyme from papaya, has been shown to be able to digest wheat gluten and render it harmless in celiac disease subjects.[56] Taking a papain supplement (500 to 1,000 mg) with meals may allow some individuals to tolerate small amounts of gluten.[57]

Constipation

The frequency of defecation and the consistency and volume of stools vary so greatly from individual to individual that it is difficult to determine what is normal. In general, most nutritionally oriented physicians recommend two to three bowel movements per day, as this is the number typically found in healthy people eating a high-fiber diet and getting adequate exercise.

Dietary Considerations

It is well established that a low-fiber diet causes constipation. Equally clear is the efficacy of dietary changes that increase fiber in the treatment of chronic constipation. Increased dietary fiber increases the frequency and quantity of bowel movements, decreases the transit time of stools, decreases the body's absorption of toxins from the stool, and appears to be a preventive factor in several diseases. Particularly effective are foods containing water-insoluble fibers such as cellulose (for example, wheat bran), which increase stool weight as a result of their water-holding properties. When high-fiber foods are to be used to increase bulk, the typical recommendation is ½ cup of bran cereal, increasing to 1½ cups over several weeks. Corn bran is more effective than wheat bran for this purpose, while oat bran is less irritating and a better absorber of fats. For best results, adequate amounts of fluids must be consumed. If bran alone is being used, ¼ to ½ cup per day is the recommended dosage.

Table 14.1 Rules for Bowel Retraining

- Never repress an urge to defecate.
- Eat a high-fiber diet, particularly fruits and vegetables.
- Drink six to eight glasses of fluid per day.
- Sit on the toilet at the same time every morning (even when the urge to defecate is not present), preferably immediately after breakfast or exercise.
- Exercise at least twenty minutes, three times per week.
- Stop using laxatives (except as directed below) and enemas.

  WEEK ONE: Every night before bed, take 3 (determine actual number needed by amount needed to ensure a bowel movement every morning) herbal laxative tablets.

  WEEKLY: Each week, decrease dosage by ½ tablet. If constipation recurs, go back to the previous week's dosage. Decrease by 1 tablet if diarrhea occurs.

Other Recommendations

If constipation has been a chronic problem and laxatives have been used frequently, the bowels must be retrained. Table 14.1 lists recommended rules for reestablishing bowel regularity. The recommended procedure takes 4 to 6 weeks.

Crohn's Disease and Ulcerative Colitis

Crohn's disease and ulcerative colitis are the two major categories of inflammatory bowel disease (IBD)—a general term for a group of chronic inflammatory disorders. IBD is characterized by recurrent inflammation of specific intestinal segments, resulting in diverse clinical manifestations. Crohn's disease is characterized by an inflammatory reaction throughout the entire thickness of the bowel wall. Although Crohn's disease most often affects the ileum or terminal portion of the small intestine, the same inflammatory process may involve the mouth, esophagus, stomach, duodenum, jejunum, and colon. Ulcerative colitis involves a nonspecific inflammatory response that is mostly limited to the lining of the colon. Crohn's disease and ulcerative colitis share many common features.

The rates of the two diseases differ slightly, with most studies showing ulcerative colitis to be more common than Crohn's disease. The current estimate of the yearly rate of newly diagnosed cases of ulcerative colitis in Western Europe and the United States is approximately 6 to 8 cases per 100,000, and the estimated rate of the total number of cases is approximately 70 to 150 cases per 100,000. In contrast, the estimate of the yearly rate of newly diagnosed cases of Crohn's disease is approximately 2 cases per 100,000, while the total number of cases is estimated at 20 to 40 cases per 100,000. The rate of Crohn's disease is increasing in Western cultures.[58]

Theories about the cause of IBD can be divided into several groups: genetic predisposition; infectious agent or agents; immunologic abnormality; dietary factors; and various miscellaneous concepts implicating psychosomatic, vascular, traumatic, and other mechanisms.[59]

Although possible dietary causes of Crohn's disease are hardly considered (if mentioned at all) in most standard medical and gastroenterology texts, several lines of evidence strongly support dietary factors as being the most important causative factor.[60]

The incidence of Crohn's disease is increasing in cultures consuming the "Western" diet, while it is virtually nonexistent in cultures consuming a more primitive diet.[61] Since food is the preeminent factor in determining the intestinal environment, the considerable change in "Western" dietary habits over the last century could explain the rising rates of Crohn's disease.

Dietary Considerations

Pre-illness Several studies analyzing the pre-illness diet of patients with Crohn's disease have found that people who develop Crohn's disease habitually eat more refined sugar, and less raw fruit and vegetables and dietary fiber, than do healthy people.[62] In one study, the pre-illness intake of refined sugar in Crohn's disease patients was nearly twice that of controls (122 g/day versus 65 g/day).[63] One researcher found that, before the onset of disease, Crohn's disease patients had eaten cornflakes more frequently than had controls.[64] Although other researchers could not verify this specific finding, cornflakes are high in refined carbohydrates and are derived from a very common allergen (corn).

Another important dietary factor that standard texts entirely overlook is the role of food allergy. Support for this hypothesis is offered in clinical studies that have utilized an allergy elimination diet with great success in treating Crohn's disease and ulcerative colitis.[65]

General Nutrition Many nutritional complications occur during the course of IBD. The major mechanisms contributing to nutritional depletion in these patients are listed in Table 14.2.

A decreased level of food intake is the most important mechanism of nutritional deficiency in IBD patients, and deficient calorie intake is the most common nutritional deficit in patients requiring hospitalization (see Table 14.3). Often the patient feels significant pain, diarrhea, nausea, and/or other symptom after a meal, resulting in a subtle diminution in dietary intake. Weight loss is prevalent in 65 to 75 percent of IBD patients.[66]

As shown in Table 14.3, the number of nutritional deficiencies is quite

Table 14.2 Causes of Malnutrition in Inflammatory Bowel Disease

- Decreased oral intake
- Disease-induced (pain, diarrhea, nausea, anorexia)
- Doctor-induced (restrictive diets without supplementation)
- Malabsorption
- Decreased absorptive surface due to disease or resection
- Bile salt deficiency after surgical resection
- Bacterial overgrowth
- Drugs (corticosteroids, sulfasalazine, cholestyramine)
- Increased secretion and nutrient loss
- Protein-losing enteropathy
- Electrolyte, mineral, and trace mineral loss in diarrhea
- Increased utilization and increased requirements
- Inflammation, fever, or infection
- Increased intestinal cell turnover

high in patients hospitalized with IBD.[67] In addition to these deficiencies, low levels of vitamin K, copper, niacin, and vitamin E have been reported.[68] The importance of correcting nutritional deficiencies in patients with IBD cannot be overstated. Nutrient deficiencies lead to altered gastrointestinal function and structure, which may draw the patient into a vicious cycle.

The foremost task in nutritional therapy is to provide adequate calorie intake. It should be assumed that the majority of patients suffer from nutrient deficiency, although often the deficiency is subclinical and can only be detected by appropriate laboratory investigation.

Table 14.3 Prevalence of Nutritional Deficiency in Patients Hospitalized with Inflammatory Bowel Disease

Deficiency	*Prevalence (%)*
Hypoalbuminemia	25–80
Anemia	60–80
Iron deficiency	40
Low serum vitamin B_{12}	48
Low serum folate	54–64
Low serum magnesium	14–33
Low serum potassium	6–20
Low serum retinol	21
Low serum ascorbate	12
Low serum vitamin D	25–65
Low serum zinc	40–50

In general, patients with inflammatory bowel disease should be placed on therapeutic vitamin supplements of at least five times the RDA. Since the drug sulfasalazine interferes with folic acid metabolism, the diet must be supplemented with at least 400 μg of folic acid per day if an individual is on this drug. Several minerals may also need to be supplemented at equally high levels.

Allergy Elimination Diets Both elemental and elimination diets have proved themselves effective in the treatment of IBD.[69] An elemental diet involves being fed a formula that contains all essential nutrients, with protein being provided only as predigested or free-form amino acids. Hospitalization is often required for satisfactory administration of elemental diets. Relapse is quite common when patients resume normal eating. A standard allergy elimination diet may be a more acceptable alternative in the treatment of IBD, particularly when chronic IBD is involved.

Although food allergy has long been considered an important causative factor in the development of IBD, studies have only recently begun examining the use of elimination diets in the treatment of IBD.[70] These studies demonstrate that elimination of food allergies is the therapy of choice in the treatment of chronic IBD. An alternative approach is to determine the actual allergens by laboratory methods—preferably a method that measures both IgG- and IgE-mediated reactions (see Chapter 13). Then either the allergens are avoided or a rotary diversified diet is used, as appropriate.

Studies found that the most common offending foods were wheat and dairy products. Dairy products containing carrageenan may be especially troublesome for patients with IBD. Carrageenan, a thickening agent isolated from red seaweeds, is widely used in dairy products like ice cream, cottage cheese, and yogurt. Indeed, researchers investigating ulcerative colitis often use carrageenan experimentally to induce the disease in animals. Carrageenan compounds are used by the food industry as stabilizing and suspending agents, and are especially popular in milk products because of carrageenan's ability to stabilize milk proteins. While carrageenan may be very safe for most people, in an individual with IBD it may be a problem. Strict avoidance of carrageenan seems warranted by individuals with IBD until further research clarifies its safety.

Dietary Recommendations After elimination of food allergens, the patient's diet should be rich in plant foods. Treatment with a high-fiber diet has been shown to have a favorable effect on the course of Crohn's disease.[71] This is in direct contrast to one of the oldest medical treatments of IBD—namely, a low-fiber diet. Dietary fiber has a profound effect on the intestinal environment and is thought to promote a more beneficial intestinal flora composition.[72] Although some foods may be too "rough" to handle, the dietary treatment of IBD should utilize an unrefined-carbohydrate, fiber-rich diet combined with an avoidance or rotary diversified diet (see Chapter 13). The latter combination is much more effective than a high-fiber diet alone.[73]

As in other inflammatory conditions, manipulation of dietary oils is indicated. Dietary intake of arachidonic acid should be reduced considerably, while consumption of omega-3 oils (linolenic acid and eicosapentaenoic acid, as found in flaxseed oil and fish oils, respectively) should be encouraged. The omega-3 oils lead to significantly fewer inflammatory leukotrienes and have been shown to reduce inflammatory processes.

The effect of fish oil on the course of ulcerative colitis was recently investigated in a well-designed clinical trial.[74] In the study, 87 patients received supplements of 20 ml of fish oil (4.5 grams of eicosapentaenoic acid) or of olive oil (placebo) daily for 1 year. Treatment with the fish oil resulted in measurable improvements, with a trend toward achieving remission (off corticosteroids).

Other Recommendations

Cabbage juice, due to its ability to soothe irritated membranes and promote healing, should be used to treat IBD as well as to treat peptic ulcers. A gel-forming fiber supplement containing such fibers as psyllium seed husks, pectin, guar gum, or oat bran should be used at night to help regulate bowel function and to bind toxins that might irritate the bowels.

Detoxification and Liver Support

The liver is an intricate, complex, and truly remarkable organ. It is, without question, the most important organ of metabolism. To a large extent, an individual's health and vitality are determined by the health and vitality of his or her liver. Since the liver is responsible for detoxifying harmful chemicals in the body, every effort should be made to promote optimal liver function.

Fasting

Fasting, which was briefly discussed in Chapter 12, is often used as a detoxification method. It is one of the quickest ways to increase elimination of wastes and to enhance the healing processes of the body. Fasting is defined as abstinence from all food and drink except water for a specific period of time, usually for a therapeutic or religious purpose.

Although therapeutic fasting is probably one of the oldest known therapies, it has been largely ignored by the modern scientific community. The most recent development in the study and promotion of fasting involves the formation of the International Association of Professional Natural Hygienists (IAPNH, 204 Staumbaugh Building, Youngstown, OH 44503). This organization comprises doctors specializing in therapeutic fasting as an integral part of total health care.

Research into fasting has been reported since 1880. Since then, medical journals have carried articles on the use of fasting to treat obesity, chemical poisoning, arthritis, allergies, psoriasis, eczema, thrombophlebitis, leg ulcers, irritable bowel syndrome, impaired or deranged appetite, bronchial asthma, depression, neurosis, and schizophrenia.[75]

A most encouraging use of fasting was published in the *American Journal of Industrial Medicine* in 1984.[76] This study involved patients who had ingested rice oil contaminated with polychlorinated-biphenyls or PCBs. All patients reported improvement in symptoms—and some observed "dramatic" relief—after undergoing 7- to 10-day fasts. This research supports earlier studies conducted by Imamura of PCB-poisoned patients and indicates the therapeutic effects of fasting. Caution must be used, however, when planning to fast after significant contamination with fat-soluble toxins such as pesticides. The pesticide DDT has been shown to be mobilized during a fast and may then reach blood levels that are toxic to the nervous system.[77]

If a person is particularly toxic, it is a good idea to support detoxification reactions while fasting. This is partly done by undertaking a fresh juice fast instead of a water fast, but many people may still need additional support as toxins previously stored in fat cells are released into the system. Here are some suggestions:

- Take a high-potency multiple vitamin and mineral formula to provide general support.
- Take a lipotropic formula—a special formula for supporting the liver. These formulas, which are available at health-food stores, are typically rich in choline and methionine, two important nutrients for the liver. Your dosage of the lipotropic formula should provide 1 gram of each of these nutrients.
- Take 1 gram of vitamin C three times daily.
- Take 1 to 2 tablespoons of a fiber supplement at night before retiring. The best fiber sources are water-soluble fibers such as powdered psyllium seed husks, guar gum, and oat bran.

- If you need additional liver support, take a special extract of milk thistle known as *silymarin.* The proper dosage is 70 to 210 mg of silymarin three times daily.

After the fast, be sure to follow the guidelines given on pages 244, 245.

Dietary Considerations

Detoxification of harmful substances is a continual process in the body. It does not have to be an unpleasant experience, and it does not have to be performed only while on a fast. Actually, the best approach may be to detoxify gradually.

A rational approach to aiding the body's detoxification mechanisms might include the use of periodic short juice fasts (of 3 to 5 days' duration) or longer, medically supervised fasts. However, to support the body's detoxification processes effectively, a long-term detoxification program is recommended. This involves adopting three things: a healthful diet that focuses on fresh fruits and vegetables, whole grains, legumes, nuts, and seeds; a healthful lifestyle that includes regular exercise; and a healthy attitude or positive mental outlook.

A healthful diet and lifestyle will promote detoxification largely as a result of improved food intake and use. A diet rich in dietary fiber and plant foods, low in refined sugar and fat, and as free as possible from pesticides and pollutants is preferred. Consumption of saturated fats, sugar, alcohol, drugs, and other substances toxic to the liver is undesirable.

A diet high in antioxidants is essential to protect the liver from damage as it performs its vital functions. Optimum tissue concentrations of these compounds should be maintained in the treatment of hepatic disease as well as in the promotion of liver health. Once again, a diet that concentrates on fresh fruits, vegetables, grains, legumes, nuts, and seeds provides the answers to health.

Several nutrients are especially critical to liver function. Choline, methionine, betaine, and folic acid are often referred to as *lipotropic agents*—compounds that promote the flow of fat and bile to and from the liver. In essence, lipotropic agents produce a "decongesting" effect on the liver and promote improved fat metabolism. Formulas containing lipotropic agents have been used for a wide range of conditions by naturopathic physicians. These agents have been used in treating numerous liver disorders, including hepatitis, cirrhosis, and alcohol-induced fatty infiltration of the liver.[78]

Foods especially rich in lipotropic compounds or other compounds that promote healthy liver function include artichokes, beets, carrots, dandelion, cabbage-family vegetables, whole grains, legumes, and many herbs and spices like turmeric, cinnamon, and licorice.

Other Recommendations

Perhaps the most effective natural remedy for liver disorders is silymarin, a group of compounds found in the common milk thistle. In fact, silymarin is one of the most potent liver medicines known. In human studies, silymarin has been shown to have positive effects in treating several types of liver disease, including cirrhosis, hepatitis, fatty infiltration of the liver caused by chemicals or alcohol, and gallbladder inflammation.[79] The standard dosage is 70 to 210 mg of silymarin three times daily.

Diabetes

Diabetes or high blood sugar occurs when the pancreas does not secrete enough insulin or when the cells of the body become resistant to insulin. Diabetes is an extremely common problem in the United States. It is a chronic disorder of carbohydrate, fat, and protein metabolism, characterized by fasting elevations of blood glucose levels and a greatly increased risk of atherosclerosis, kidney disease, and loss of nerve function.[80]

There are two primary subclasses of diabetes:

- Insulin-dependent Diabetes Mellitus (IDDM or Type 1) – This type of diabetes is associated with juvenile onset and with complete destruction of the beta-cells of the pancreas, which manufacture insulin.
- Non-insulin-dependent Diabetes Mellitus (NIDDM or Type 2) – NIDDM usually has an adult onset. It is subdivided into two subgroups: obese NIDDM and nonobese NIDDM.

The percentage of individuals with diabetes in the United States is estimated at 4 percent, of which 90 percent are NIDDM and the rest IDDM. The prevalence of diabetes is rising and is now the seventh leading cause of death in the United States. At the current rate of increase (6 percent per year), the total number of diabetics would double every 15 years.[81]

Diabetic individuals must be monitored carefully, particularly if they are on insulin or have relatively uncontrolled diabetes. Careful attention to symptoms, home glucose monitoring, and other blood tests are essential in monitoring the progress of the diabetic individual. It is important to recognize that, as the diabetic individual employs some of the suggestions made here, drug dosages will have to be altered; a good working relationship with the prescribing doctor will greatly aid the healing process.

Dietary Considerations

Diabetes, perhaps more than any other disease, is strongly associated with Western culture and diet. It is quite uncommon in cultures where a more "primitive" diet is consumed.[82] However, as cultures switch from their native diets to the "foods of commerce," their rate of diabetes increases, eventually reaching the same proportions seen in Western societies. The evidence indicting the "Western" diet and lifestyle as the ultimate causative factor in diabetes is overwhelming.[83]

Dietary modification and treatment are fundamental to the successful treatment of diabetes. Clinical trials of dietary treatment with a more primitive diet—high in fiber and complex carbohydrates, and low in fat and animal products—have consistently demonstrated superior therapeutic effects over drugs, insulin (when less than 30 units per day), and other previously recommended dietary plans (carbohydrate restriction, high protein, and the American Diabetes Association or ADA diet).[84]

Use of the high-carbohydrate, high-plant-fiber (HCF) diet to treat diabetes was popularized by Dr. James Anderson.[85] It has substantial support and validation in the scientific literature as the diet of choice in the treatment of diabetes. It is high in cereal grains, legumes, and root vegetables; and it restricts simple sugar and fat intake. The caloric intake consists of 70 to 75 percent complex carbohydrates, 15 to 20 percent protein, and only 5 to 10 percent fat. The total fiber content is almost 100 grams per day. The positive metabolic effects of the HCF diet are many: reduced elevations in blood-sugar levels after meals; increased tissue sensitivity to insulin; reduced cholesterol and triglyceride levels, with increased HDL cholesterol levels; and progressive weight reduction. If patients resume a conventional ADA diet, their insulin requirements return to prior levels.

Some patients try to increase the fiber content of their diet through supplementation rather than through diet. Although fiber-supplemented diets are beneficial, they are less effective than the HCF diet. Insulin dosages on fiber-supplemented diets can usually be reduced to one-third those used on control (ADA) diets. Indeed, the HCF diet has led to discontinuation of insulin therapy in approximately 60 percent of NIDDM patients, and to significantly reduced doses in the other 40 percent.[86]

The dietary guidelines provided in Chapter 11 allow the diabetic to incorporate complex carbohydrates and fiber along with higher levels of legumes. In essence, an even more healthful version of Anderson's HCF diet is produced. Consumption of legumes should be encouraged because a high-carbohydrate, legume-rich, high-fiber diet has been shown to improve all aspects of diabetic control.[87] The beneficial effects of legumes are primarily due to their water-soluble, gel-forming fiber components, which have effects similar to those of guar gum and pectin in producing a positive effect on blood-sugar control.[88]

The Importance of Ideal Body Weight Body weight is a significant factor in blood-sugar control. Even in normal individuals, significant weight gain results in carbohydrate intolerance, higher insulin levels, and insulin insensitivity in fat and muscle tissue.[89] Progressive development of insulin insensitivity is believed to be the underlying factor in the genesis of NIDDM. Weight loss corrects all of these abnormalities and significantly improves the metabolic disturbances of diabetes.[90] In other words, since 90 percent of people with NIDDM are obese, the majority of Americans with diabetes could cure themselves simply by achieving their ideal body weight.

Special Foods for the Diabetic Some specific foods have been shown to produce positive effects on blood-sugar control. In addition to whole grains, legumes, and other high-fiber foods, certain foods contain compounds that exert beneficial effects in cases of diabetes. For example, in addition to the high-chromium foods listed in Table 3.17 on page 69, refer to the discussions in this book of the following foods: artichoke, bitter melon, garlic, Jerusalem artichoke, and onion.

Other Recommendations

Exercise is critical to achieving good blood-sugar control. A graded exercise program should be developed, based on the individual's fitness level and interest, that elevates the person's heart rate to at least 60 percent of maximum for ½ hour three times a week.

For individuals who have had diabetes for many years, consult *The Encyclopedia of Natural Medicine* for additional recommendations on how to reduce the risk of major complications of diabetes.

Diarrhea

Diarrhea is a common symptom whose presence usually indicates a mild functional disorder. However, it may also be the first suggestion of a serious underlying disease. Diarrhea that lasts longer than a few days should not be taken lightly; its cause must be determined and treated appropriately.

Dietary Considerations

Chronic diarrhea is one of the most common symptoms of food allergy. After the food allergens have been diagnosed, significant allergens should be avoided, and milder allergens should be rotated on a 4-day cycle. This topic is fully discussed in Chapter 13.

Another common dietary cause of diarrhea is a deficiency in the enzyme lactase, which is responsible for digesting the lactose from dairy products. This deficiency is common worldwide. It has been estimated that 70 to 90 percent of Oriental, Black, Native American, and Mediterranean adults lack this enzyme. The incidence of deficiency is 10 to 15 percent among northern and western Europeans.[91] Acute illness, such as viral and bacterial intestinal infections, frequently injure the mucosal cells of the small intestine, resulting in a temporary deficiency of lactase and other disaccharide enzymes. This is one reason why many physicians of natural medicine recommend fasting during acute infections. Symptoms may range from minor abdominal discomfort and bloating to severe diarrhea in response to even small amounts of lactose. The deficiency is confirmed by the lactose challenge test.

To help solidify stools, pectin-rich fruits and vegetables (such as pears, apples, grapefruit, carrots, potatoes, and beets) may offer some benefit. Also, fresh blueberries have a long historical use in counteracting diarrhea. Vegetable broths and dilute fruit and vegetable juices should be consumed to maintain proper electrolyte levels.

Other Recommendations

Since most acute diarrheal states are self-limited and are due to dietary indiscretions or mild gastrointestinal infections, simple dietary approaches should be used first. If no response follows, more detailed diagnostic procedures should be used. If significant illness (for example, fever or debility) accompanies the diarrhea or if it lasts for more than a few days, a physician should be consulted.

Ear Infection (Otitis Media)

A middle-ear infection (otitis media) is characterized by a sharp, stabbing, dull, and/or throbbing pain in the ear. The pain is due to inflammation, swelling, or infection of the middle ear, and is a common affliction of childhood. Chronic ear infections affect 20 to 40 percent of children under the age of 6, and ear infections are the most frequent diagnosis of children in a clinical practice. It has been estimated that approximately $2 billion is spent annually on medical and surgical treatment of earache in the United States.[92]

Since an ear infection can be quite serious, any individual with symptoms of an acute ear infection should be seen by a physician. The recommendations that follow are intended to be used along with proper medical care.

Dietary Considerations

Recurrent ear infection is strongly associated with early bottle feeding, while prolonged breastfeeding (minimum of 6 months) has a protective effect.[93] Whether this is due to an allergy to formula or to the protective effect of human milk against infection has not yet been determined. It is probably a combination of both. In addition, prolonged breastfeeding prevents food allergies, particularly if the mother avoids consuming sensitizing foods (that is, those to which she is allergic) during pregnancy and lactation.[94] Another worthwhile step is to exclude the foods to which children are most commonly allergic—wheat, egg, fowl, and dairy—particularly during the first 9 months after birth.

Since a child's digestive tract is quite permeable to food antigens, especially during the first 3 months, careful control of the child's eating patterns (no frequent repetitions of any food, avoiding the common allergenic foods, and introducing foods in a controlled manner—that is, introducing one food at a time and carefully watching for a reaction) will reduce or prevent the development of food allergies.

The role of allergy as the major cause of chronic otitis media has been firmly established in the medical literature.[95] Most studies show that 85 to 93 percent of these children have allergies: 16 percent to inhalants, 14 percent to food, and 70 percent to both.

One illustrative study of 153 children with earaches demonstrated that 93.3 percent of the children (using the RAST test for diagnosis) were allergic to foods, inhalants, or both.[96] The 12-month success rate for 119 of the children, when treated for inhalant sensitivities and an elimination diet for food allergens, showed that 92 percent improved. This compares favorably with the surgically treated control group (ear tubes and, as indicated, tonsillectomy and adenoidectomy), which showed only a 52 percent response.

Other Recommendations

Locally applied heat is often very helpful in reducing discomfort. It can be applied as a hot pack, with warm oil (especially mullein oil), by blowing hot air into the ear, and so on. Also of value is putting hygroscopic anhydrous glycerine (available at pharmacies) into the ear. This helps pull fluids out and reduces the pressure in the middle ear.

Eczema

Eczema (atopic dermatitis) is an intensely itchy, allergic disease of the skin. It is commonly found on the face, the wrists, and the insides of the elbows and knees. Although it may occur at any age, it is most common in infants and it completely clears in half of these cases by the time the child is 18 months of age. Eczema is a very common condition affecting 2.4 to 7 percent of the population. It is often associated with asthma.

Dietary Considerations

The role of food allergy as a major cause in childhood eczema is well established.[97] In infants, milk appears to be the most common allergenic food.[98] Controlling eczema critically depends on finding and eliminating all (or at least most) of the food allergens. A recent study conducted at the Middlesex Hospital in London provides additional support for the role of food allergies as a cause of childhood eczema.[99] In this study, based on their results, the researchers estimated that simply eliminating cow's milk, eggs, tomatoes, artificial colors, and food preservatives would help up to 75 percent of children afflicted with moderate to severe eczema. For additional recommendations about how to deal with food allergies, see Chapter 13.

Patients with eczema also appear to have an essential fatty acid deficiency. This results in decreased synthesis of anti-inflammatory prostaglandins. Treatment with evening primrose oil has been shown to normalize the essential fatty acid abnormalities and to relieve the symptoms of eczema in many patients.[100] Supplementation with other medicinal oils may provide similar benefits. It may be particularly important to increase the dietary intake of omega-3 oils, either by eating more fatty fish (such as mackerel, herring, and salmon) or by consuming nuts, seeds, flaxseed oil, or fish oil supplements. Foods rich in vitamin A and zinc are also important, since these nutrients are critical to healthy skin and have been shown to be of value in treating eczema.[101]

Other Recommendations

A number of herbal substances have demonstrated effects equal to or superior to cortisone when applied topically. *Glycyrrhiza glabra* (licorice) and *Matricaria chamomilla* (German chamomile) are the most active.[102] Proprietary formulas containing essences of these botanical species may be quite beneficial in temporarily relieving eczema.

Fibrocystic Breast Disease

Fibrocystic breast disease (FBD), also known as cystic mastitis, is a mildly uncomfortable to severely painful benign cystic swelling of the breasts. It is typically cyclic, and it usually precedes a woman's menses. It is the most common disease of the breast, afflicting 20 to 40 percent of all premenopausal women. It is usually a component of the premenstrual syndrome (PMS) and is considered a risk factor for breast cancer.

Both FBD and breast cancer rates are on the rise. An estimated one in seven American women will develop breast cancer in their lives. Breast cancer is the most common cancer among women. Suggested causes for this astounding statistic are a high-fat, low-fiber diet; smoking; and environmental factors.

One suggested environmental factor is pesticide residues. Widespread environmental contamination has occurred with a group of compounds known as "halogenated hydrocarbons." Included in this group are the toxic pesticides DDT, DDE, PCB, PCP, dieldrin, and chlordane. Their molecules are difficult to break down and are stored in fat cells. These chemicals are known to cause cancer in animals, but direct evidence of their causing cancer in humans is scant. Nonetheless, these compounds have been shown to suppress immune function, to possess estrogenic activity, and to alter hormone levels; and all of these effects could lead to breast cancer.

To evaluate the possible role of pesticides and pollutants in breast cancer, researchers have measured the levels of these compounds in the fat cells of the breast in women with malignant cancers and compared these findings to those for women with nonmalignant growths. The results? Elevated levels of pesticide residues were found in the women with breast cancer compared to the women with benign breast disease. Although these results must still be confirmed, there now appears to be a strong association between pesticide levels in breast tissue and breast cancer.[103] This constitutes another strong case for choosing organically grown foods.

Dietary Considerations

Breast diseases, including FBD and breast cancer, have been linked to the "Western" diet and to bowel dysfunction. There is an interesting association between cellular abnormalities in breast fluid and the frequency of bowel movements.[104] Women who have fewer than three bowel movements per week have a risk of fibrocystic breast disease 4.5 times greater than do women who have at least one bowel movement per day.

This association is probably due to the actions of bacterial flora in the large intestine, which are capable of transforming colon contents into various toxic metabolites, including cancer-causing compounds.[105] Fecal microorganisms are capable of liberating estrogen from previously excreted and detoxified estrogen. Dietary fiber plays a major role in determining the colon microflora, the transit time, and the concentration of absorbable bowel toxins and metabolites.

Women on a vegetarian diet excrete two to three times more detoxified estrogens than do women on an omnivorous diet; the latter also reabsorb more estrogens.[106] Furthermore, meat-eating women have 50 percent higher mean levels of undetoxified estrogens. Plant lignans (see page 88) exert a healthful influence on the levels of sex hormones in the body.

Very strong evidence supports an association between consumption of caffeine, theophylline, and theobromine—as found in coffee, tea, cola, chocolate, and caffeinated medications—and fibrocystic breast disease.[107] In one study, limiting these compounds in the diet resulted in improvement in 44 of the 45 women (97.5 percent) who completely abstained and in 21 of the 28 (75 percent) who limited their consumption of coffee, tea, cola, chocolate, and caffeinated medications. Those who continued with little change in their methylxanthine consumption showed little improvement.[108] According to this study, women may have varying thresholds of response to methylxanthines.

Other Recommendations

Several double-blind clinical studies have shown vitamin E to relieve many premenstrual symptoms, including FBD.[109] The mode of action remains obscure, although vitamin E has been shown to normalize circulating hormones in PMS and FBD patients. Try taking 600 I.U. of vitamin E per day.

Gallstones

Gallstones are an extremely common occurrence in the United States. This year alone at least 1 million more Americans will develop gallstones, and some 300,000 gallbladders will be removed. As is typical of most diseases and conditions, gallstones are much easier to prevent than to reverse. Once gallstones have formed, therapeutic intervention involves avoiding aggravating foods and employing measures that increase the solubility of cholesterol in bile. If symptoms persist or worsen, removal of the gallbladder is indicated. If no symptoms are apparent, however, surgery should be avoided.

The critical factor in gallstone formation is the solubility of the bile within the gallbladder. Bile solubility is based on the relative concentrations of cholesterol, bile acids, phosphatidylcholine (lecithin), and water.

Dietary Considerations

The belief that the main cause of gallstones is the consumption of fiber-depleted refined foods has considerable research support. Gallstones, like most chronic diseases, are associated with the "Western" diet in population studies.[110] Such a diet—high in refined carbohydrates and fat, and low in fiber—leads to a reduction in the synthesis of bile acids by the liver and consequently to a lower bile acid concentration in the gallbladder. A diet high in fiber (especially fibers capable of binding to deoxycholic acid—that is, predominantly the water-soluble fibers found in vegetables, fruits, pectin, oat bran, and guar gum) is extremely important in the prevention and reversal of most gallstones.

A vegetarian diet has been shown to protect against gallstone formation. A study performed in England compared a large group of healthy nonvegetarian women to a group of vegetarian women. Ultrasound diagnosis showed that gallstones occurred significantly less frequently in the vegetarian group.[111]

While this may simply be a result of the increased fiber content of the vegetarian diet, other factors may be equally important. Animal proteins, such as casein from dairy products, have been shown to encourage the formation of gallstones in animals; while vegetable proteins, such as soy, were shown to oppose gallstone formation. (This is discussed in more detail in Chapter 3.)

Obesity Obesity causes increased secretion of cholesterol in the bile, as a result of increased cholesterol synthesis. Therefore, obesity is associated with gallstones. It is important to recognize that, during active weight reduction, bile cholesterol saturation initially increases. This is because, although secretion of all bile components is reduced during weight loss, secretion of bile acids decreases more than does that of cholesterol. It is a good idea for people on weight-loss programs to support liver function with high-fiber foods and plenty of liquids. Consumption of six to eight glasses of liquids is necessary each day to maintain the water content of bile. Pure water or fresh fruit and vegetable juices are the preferred ways to meet your body's water requirements.

Once the person's weight stabilizes, bile acid output returns to normal levels, while cholesterol output remains low. The net effect of weight loss is a significant reduction in cholesterol saturation.

Food Allergies Since 1948, Dr. J. C. Breneman, author of *Basics of Food Allergy,* has used a very successful therapeutic regimen to prevent gallbladder attacks: allergy elimination diets. The scientific literature offers some support for the idea that food allergies cause gallbladder pain. A 1968 study revealed that 100 percent of a group of patients were free of symptoms while they were on a basic elimination diet (beef, rye, soybean, rice, cherry, peach, apricot, beet, and spinach).[112]

Foods inducing symptoms, in decreasing order of their occurrence, were egg, pork, onion, fowl, milk, coffee, citrus, corn, beans, and nuts. Adding eggs to the diet caused gallbladder attacks in 93 percent of the patients.[113]

Several mechanisms have been proposed to explain the association of food allergy and gallbladder attacks. Dr. Breneman believes that ingestion of allergy-causing substances causes swelling of the bile ducts, resulting in impairment of bile flow from the gallbladder.

Other Recommendations

The naturopathic approach to the treatment of gallstones has typically involved the use of nutritional formulas rich in lipotropic factors (choline, methionine, inositol, and so on). These can be used to improve liver function and to increase the solubility of the bile.

Gout

Gout is a common type of arthritis caused by an increased concentration of uric acid in biological fluids. Uric acid is the final breakdown product of purine metabolism. Purines are made in the body and are also ingested in foods. In gout, uric acid crystals are deposited in joints, tendons, kidneys, and other tissues, where they cause considerable inflammation and damage.[114]

Gout is associated with affluence and is often called the "rich man's disease." Throughout history, the sufferer of gout has been depicted as a portly, middle-aged man sitting in a comfortable chair with one foot resting painfully on a soft cushion as he consumes great quantities of meat and wine. In fact, the traditional picture does have some basis in reality, since meats (particularly organ meats) are high-purine foods, while alcohol inhibits uric acid secretion by the kidneys. Furthermore, even today, gout is primarily a disease of adult men; over 95 percent of gout sufferers are men over the age of 30. The incidence of gout is approximately 3 adults in 1,000, although as much as 10 to 20 percent of the adult population may have elevated uric acid levels in the blood.[115]

Dietary Considerations

Several dietary factors are known to cause gout: consumption of alcohol, high-purine containing foods (organ meats, meat, yeast, poultry, and so on), fats, and refined carbohydrates, and overconsumption of calories.[116] The dietary treatment of gout involves the following guidelines, each of which will be briefly summarized:

1. Elimination of alcohol intake
2. Introduction of a low-purine diet
3. Achievement of ideal body weight
4. Liberal consumption of complex carbohydrates
5. Low fat intake
6. Low protein intake
7. Liberal fluid intake

Alcohol Alcohol increases uric acid production and reduces uric acid excretion by increasing lactate production (as a result of the breakdown of alcohol), which impairs kidney function. The net effect is a significant increase in serum uric acid levels. This explains why alcohol consumption is often a precipitating factor in acute attacks of gout. In many individuals, elimination of alcohol is all that is needed to reduce uric acid levels and prevent gout.[117]

Low-purine Diet For many years, a low-purine diet has been the mainstay of the dietary therapy for gout. However, with the advent of potent drugs that lower uric acid levels, many physicians lower the serum urate levels without subjecting the patient to the inconvenience and deprivation people may associate with a purine-free diet. Dietary restriction of purines is, however, recommended to reduce metabolic stress. Foods with high purine levels should be entirely omitted. These include organ meats, meats, shellfish, yeast (brewer's and baker's), herring, sardines, mackerel, and anchovies.

Weight Reduction Individuals with gout are typically obese, prone to high blood pressure and diabetes, and at relatively high risk for cardiovascular disease. Weight reduction in obese individuals significantly reduces serum uric acid levels. For these people, achieving ideal body weight may be the most important dietary goal.[118]

Carbohydrates, Fats, and Protein Refined carbohydrates and saturated fats should be kept to a minimum; the former increase uric acid production, while the latter decrease uric acid excretion. Protein intake should not exceed 0.8 g/kg of body weight per day. It has been shown that uric acid synthesis may be accelerated in both normal and gouty patients by a high protein intake. Adequate protein (0.8 g/kg of body weight) is necessary, however, since amino acids decrease the reabsorption of uric acid in the kidney, thus increasing uric acid excretion and reducing serum uric acid concentrations.[119]

Fluid Intake Liberal fluid intake keeps the urine dilute and promotes the excretion of uric acid. Furthermore, dilution of the urine reduces the individual's risk of developing kidney stones.[120]

Flavonoids Consuming the equivalent of ½ pound of fresh cherries per day has been shown to be very effective in lowering uric acid levels and preventing attacks of gout.[121] As discussed previously, cherries, hawthorn berries, blueberries, and other dark red-blue berries are rich sources of anthocyanidins and proanthocyanidins. These flavonoid molecules give the fruits their deep red-blue color and are remarkable in their ability to prevent collagen destruction.

Other flavonoids are of benefit to individuals with gout as well. For example, the flavonoid quercetin has demonstrated several effects in experimental studies that indicate its possible benefit to individuals with gout. Quercetin may offer significant protection by inhibiting uric acid production in a similar fashion to the drug allopurinol, as well as by inhibiting the manufacture and release of inflammatory compounds.[122] Quercetin is widely found in fruits and vegetables.

Other Recommendations

A secondary type of gout, sometimes called saturnine gout, can result from lead toxicity.[123] Historically, saturnine gout was due to consuming alcoholic beverages stored in containers containing lead (for example, leaded crystal). Use of such containers for storage of foods should be avoided.

Headache (Migraine Type)

Migraine headache is a surprisingly common disorder, affecting 15 to 20 percent of men and 25 to 30 percent of women.[124] The symptoms of a classic migraine include severe throbbing pain on one or both sides of the head; head pain accompanied by nausea, with or without vomiting; and (in half of all sufferers) warning symptoms (auras) before the onset of pain, such as blurring or bright spots in the vision, anxiety, fatigue, disturbed thinking, and numbness or tingling on one side of the body. The migraine attack typically starts in the morning, peaks within an hour, lasts 4 to 24 hours, and happens several times a month. The peak incidence occurs when the sufferer is between 20 and 35 years of age; then the frequency of attacks gradually declines. More than half of the patients have a family history of the illness.

Dietary Considerations

There is little doubt that food allergy/intolerance is the major cause of migraine headache. Many careful, double-blind, placebo-controlled studies have demonstrated that detecting and removing allergenic/untolerated foods will eliminate or greatly reduce migraine symptoms in the majority of sufferers.[125] The most common allergens are milk, wheat, chocolate, food additives, tomatoes, and fish.

Foods such as chocolate, cheese, beer, and wine precipitate migraine attacks in many people not only because of allergies, but also because these foods contain compounds known as *vasoactive amines* that can trigger migraines in sensitive individuals. Many migraine sufferers have been found to have significantly lower levels of a particular platelet enzyme (phenolsulphotransferase) that normally breaks down these dietary amines.[126] Since red wine contains substances that are potent inhibitors of this enzyme, it often triggers migraines in these individuals—especially if it is consumed along with foods high in vasoactive amines, like cheese.[127]

Other Recommendations

A double-blind study done at the London Migraine Clinic demonstrated that the herb feverfew (*Tanacetum parthenium*) offered significant protection against migraine attacks.[128] Feverfew has subsequently been shown to exert many beneficial effects in the treatment of migraine headaches. While the dose used in the study was 50 mg per day of the dried leaf, the optimum dose for feverfew has not yet been determined.

Heart Disease

The term *heart disease* usually refers to a disease of the coronary arteries, which supply the heart with oxygen and nutrients. If the blood flow through these arteries is restricted or blocked, severe damage or death to the heart muscle may occur; this results in what is known as a heart attack. In most cases, the condition that blocks the blood and oxygen supply is

Figure 14.1 Structure of an artery.

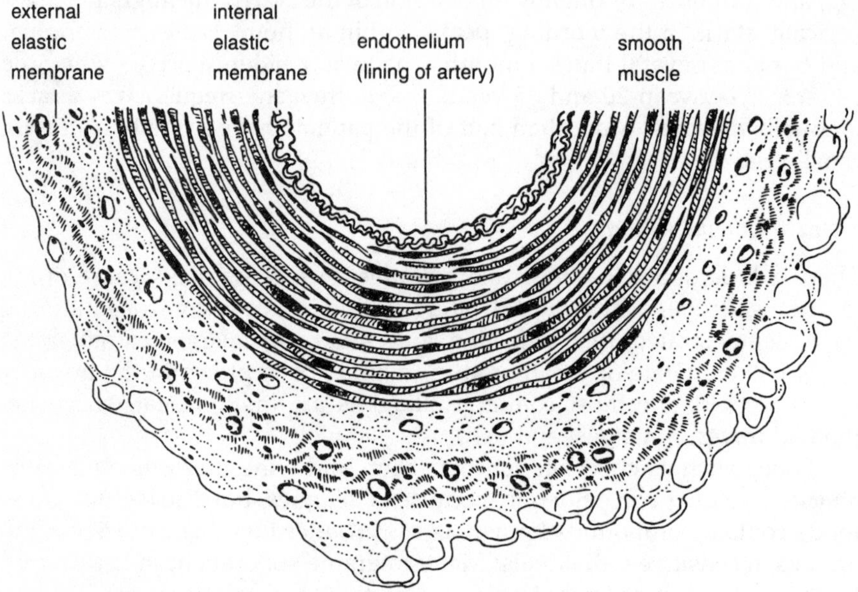

atherosclerosis or hardening of the artery walls due to a buildup of plaque containing cholesterol, fatty material, and cellular debris.

Atherosclerosis and its complications are the major causes of death in the United States, and they have reached epidemic proportions throughout the Western world. Heart attacks alone account for 20 percent of all deaths in the United States, while cerebral vascular disease, another complication of atherosclerosis, is the third most common cause of death. Altogether, cardiovascular disease is responsible for 43 percent of all deaths in the United States. It has been estimated that the healthcare costs attributable to atherosclerosis now exceed $60 billion dollars per year in the United States.

Atherosclerosis is a degenerative condition of the arteries characterized by accumulation of lipids (mainly cholesterol—usually complexed to proteins—and cholesterol esters) within the artery. The atherosclerotic plaque, or atheroma, represents the endpoint of a complex, insidious process. Although any artery may be affected, the aorta and the coronary and cerebral vascular systems are the pathways most frequently involved.[129]

To understand the development of atherosclerosis, we must closely examine the structure of an artery (see Figure 14.1). An artery is divided into three major layers:

1. The intima of the artery consists of a layer of endothelial cells lining the vessel's interior surface. Beneath the surface cells is a layer of ground substance compounds that provides support to the endothelial cells and separates the intima from the media. The ground substance is composed of collagen, mucopolysaccharides, and glycosaminoglycans.

2. The media consists primarily of smooth muscle cells. Interposed among the cells are ground substance structures that provide support and elasticity to the artery.

3. The adventitia consists primarily of connective tissue that provides structural support and elasticity to the artery.

No single theory explaining the development of atherosclerosis has yet been formulated that satisfies all investigators. However, the most widely accepted theory is the "reaction to injury hypothesis," which theorizes that the lesions of atherosclerosis are initiated as a response to injury to the cells lining the inside of the artery—the arterial endothelium.[130] Details of the progression of atherosclerosis, according to the reaction to injury hypothesis, are illustrated in Figure 14.2. The steps are as follows:

Step 1. The initial step in the development of atherosclerosis is damage to the endothelium by free radicals. Immune, physical, mechanical, viral, chemical, and drug factors have all been shown to induce damage to the endothelium that can lead to plaque development.

Step 2. Once the endothelium has been damaged, sites of injury become more permeable to plasma constituents, especially lipoproteins (fat-carrying proteins). The binding of lipoproteins to glycosaminoglycans leads to a breakdown in the integrity of the ground substance matrix and causes an increased affinity for cholesterol.

When significant damage has occurred, monocytes (large white blood cells) and platelets begin adhering to the damaged area, where they release growth factors that stimulate smooth muscle cells to migrate from the media into the intima and to replicate there.

Step 3. The local concentration of lipoproteins, monocytes, and platelets leads to the migration of smooth muscle cells from the media into the intima, where they undergo proliferation. The smooth muscle cells dump cellular debris into the intima, contributing to further development of plaque.

Step 4. A fibrous cap consisting of collagen, elastin, and glycosaminoglycans forms over the intimal surface. Fat and cholesterol deposits accumulate.

Figure 14.2 Stages in the development of atherosclerosis.

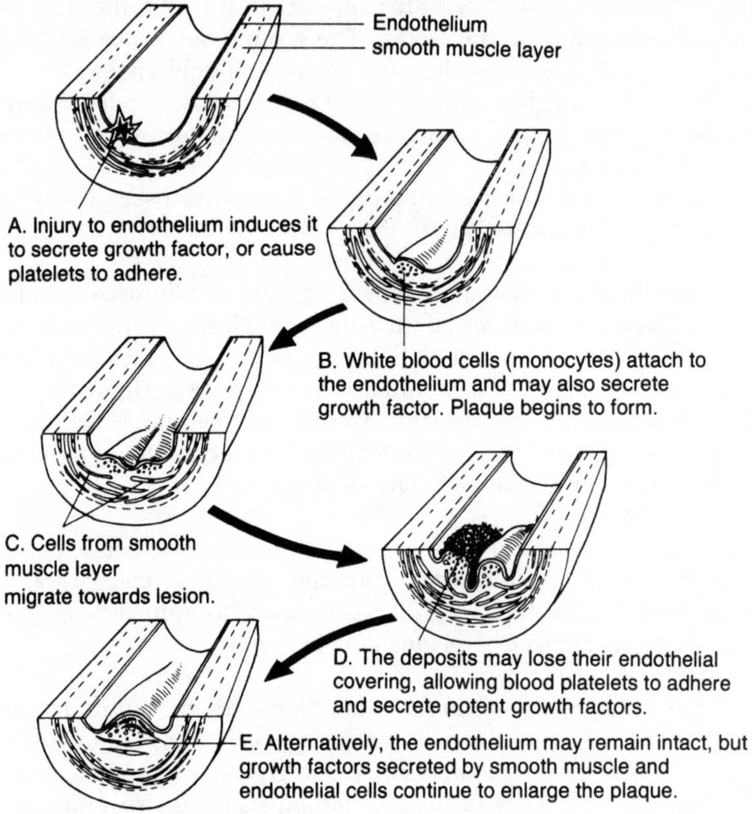
Endothelium
smooth muscle layer
A. Injury to endothelium induces it to secrete growth factor, or cause platelets to adhere.
B. White blood cells (monocytes) attach to the endothelium and may also secrete growth factor. Plaque begins to form.
C. Cells from smooth muscle layer migrate towards lesion.
D. The deposits may lose their endothelial covering, allowing blood platelets to adhere and secrete potent growth factors.
E. Alternatively, the endothelium may remain intact, but growth factors secreted by smooth muscle and endothelial cells continue to enlarge the plaque.

Step 5. The plaque continues to grow until eventually it blocks the artery. Blockage is usually around 90 percent before symptoms of atherosclerosis are apparent.

Dietary Considerations

Preventing or reversing atherosclerosis through diet requires a comprehensive approach that addresses all factors involved in the initiation and progression of atherosclerosis. Specifically this involves eating foods that reduce LDL cholesterol while raising HDL cholesterol, prevent initial damage to the endothelium, inhibit platelet aggregation, and support the integrity of connective tissue components of the artery. All of these goals can be achieved by increasing the dietary intake of fruits, vegetables, whole grains, legumes, nuts, and seeds.

Table 14.4 Recommended Blood Cholesterol Levels

Type	*Level*
Total cholesterol	less than 200 mg/dl
LDL cholesterol	less than 130 mg/dl
HDL cholesterol	greater than 35 mg/dl

Cholesterol and Atherosclerosis The foremost concern in preventing and treating heart disease is to reduce blood cholesterol levels. The evidence overwhelmingly demonstrates that elevated cholesterol levels greatly increase a person's risk of dying from heart disease. Cholesterol is transported in the blood by molecules known as lipoproteins. Cholesterol bound to low-density lipoprotein or LDL is often referred to as the "bad" cholesterol, while cholesterol bound to high-density lipoprotein or HDL is referred to as the "good" cholesterol. This is because LDL cholesterol increases a person's level of risk for heart disease, strokes, and high blood pressure, while HDL cholesterol actually protects against heart disease. Research has shown that, for every 1 percent drop in cholesterol level, the risk of having a heart attack drops by 2 percent.[131] Table 14.4 lists recommended blood cholesterol levels.

LDL transports cholesterol to the tissues. But HDL transports cholesterol to the liver for metabolism and excretion. Therefore, the body's HDL-to-LDL ratio largely determines whether cholesterol is being broken down or deposited into tissues. A person's risk for heart disease can be reduced dramatically by lowering the LDL cholesterol level while simultaneously raising the HDL cholesterol level. This can be done quite easily in just a few weeks by making changes in diet and lifestyle. The dietary changes are simple: eat less saturated fat and cholesterol, by reducing or eliminating the amounts of animal products in the diet; increase the consumption of fiber-rich plant foods (fruits, vegetables, grains, and legumes); and lose weight if necessary. The lifestyle changes include getting regular aerobic exercise; stopping smoking; and reducing or eliminating the consumption of coffee (both caffeinated and decaffeinated), to remove the roasted hydrocarbons in it from the diet.

More and more evidence indicates that increasing the HDL-to-LDL ratio through diet and lifestyle not only protects against heart disease, but also can dramatically reverse the blockage of coronary arteries.[132] This is perhaps best illustrated in the now famous Lifestyle Heart Trial conducted by Dr. Dean Ornish.[133] In this study, subjects with heart disease were divided into a control group and an experimental group. The control group received regular medical care, while the experimental group was asked to eat a low-fat vegetarian diet for at least 1 year. The diet included fruits, vegetables, grains, legumes, and soybean products. Subjects were allowed to consume as many calories as they wished. The only animal products allowed were egg white and 1 cup per day of nonfat milk or yogurt. The diet contained approximately 10 percent fat, 15 to 20 percent protein, and 70 to 75 percent carbohydrate (predominantly in the form of complex carbohydrate). The experimental group was also asked to perform stress reduction techniques such as breathing exercises, stretching exercises, meditation, imagery, and other relaxation techniques for 1 hour each day and to exercise for at least 3 hours each week. At the end of the year, the subjects in the experimental group showed significant overall regression of atherosclerosis of the coronary blood vessels. In contrast, subjects in the control group, who were being treated with regular medical care and were following the standard American Heart Association diet actually showed progression of their disease; that is, the control group actually got worse. Ornish and his collaborators state: "This finding suggests that conventional recommendations for patients with coronary heart disease (such as a 30% fat diet) are not sufficient to bring about regression in many patients."

Although most authorities now agree that the level of plasma cholesterol is largely determined by the dietary intake of total calories of cholesterol, saturated fat, and polyunsaturated fat, the results of Ornish's study and others suggest that other factors are also important. Strict vegetarianism may not be as important as consuming a diet that is high in fiber and complex carbohydrates, low in fat, and low in cholesterol; but vegetarians are recognized to have a much lower risk of developing heart disease, and a vegetarian diet has been shown to be quite effective in lowering cholesterol levels and reducing the risk for atherosclerosis.[134] Such a diet is rich in such protective factors as fiber, antioxidants, essential fatty acids, vitamins, and minerals (including potassium and magnesium).

The importance of even simple alterations in diet can be quite significant. In one study, for example, two medium-size carrots were eaten daily at breakfast by normal subjects. After 3 weeks, the following significant results were recorded: an 11 percent reduction in cholesterol levels; a 50 percent increase in fecal bile and fat excretion; and a 25 percent increase in stool weight.[135]

In another example of how simple food choices affect cholesterol levels, an evaluation of data from the National Health and Nutrition Examination Survey II disclosed that serum cholesterol levels are lowest among adults eating "ready-to-eat" cereal for breakfast.[136] Although individuals who consumed other breakfast foods had higher blood cholesterol levels, surprisingly, levels were highest among those who typically skipped breakfast. Due to the strong association of cholesterol levels to heart dis-

Table 14.5 Cholesterol Content of Selected Foods, in Milligrams (mg) per 3½-oz (100-g) Serving

Animal Food		*Plant Food*	
Type	*Cholesterol*	*Type*	*Cholesterol*
Egg, whole	550	All grains	0
Kidney, beef	375	All vegetables	0
Liver, beef	300	All nuts	0
Butter	250	All seeds	0
Oysters	200	All fruits	0
Cream cheese	120	All legumes	0
Lard	95	All vegetable oils	0
Beefsteak	70		
Lamb	70		
Pork	70		
Chicken	60		
Ice cream	45		

SOURCE: Pennington, J., *Food Values of Portions Commonly Used*, 14th ed., New York: Harper & Row, 1985.

ease, we may conclude from this study that breakfast should be consumed regularly to prevent heart disease. Furthermore, the study revealed that cereals, both hot and cold (and preferably from whole grains), may be the best food choices for breakfast.

In general, following the dietary guidelines discussed in Chapter 1 and the guidelines for designing a healthful diet in Chapter 11 will effectively lower a person's cholesterol levels and reduce the risk for cardiovascular disease. Since animal products are the primary sources of both saturated fats and cholesterol, the dietary intake of animal products must be limited in order to prevent or reverse atherosclerosis (see Table 14.5). Margarine (see page 42) and refined sugar should also be limited because of their role in contributing to the development of atherosclerosis.[137]

Instead of containing saturated fats and cholesterol, the diet should be composed of plant foods that provide essential fatty acids. There is some evidence that reduced levels of essential fatty acids contribute greatly to atherosclerosis.[138] Both omega-3 and omega-6 essential fatty acids lower cholesterol and triglyceride levels and decrease platelet aggregation.[139]

Another reason to reduce the intake of animal foods relates to evidence that the body handles plant proteins differently from how it handles animal proteins (see Chapter 3). While vegetable proteins have been shown to lower cholesterol levels, diets containing equivalent amounts of milk protein or other animal proteins actually raise cholesterol levels. To reduce

Table 14.6 Food Choices for Lowering Cholesterol

Eat Less of These	*Substitute with These*
Red meats, hamburgers, hot dogs, etc.	Fish and white meat of poultry
Eggs	Legumes
High-fat dairy products	Low-fat or nonfat dairy products
Butter, lard, and other saturated fats	Vegetable oils
Ice cream, pies, cake, cookies, etc.	Fruits
Refined cereals, white bread, etc.	Whole grains, whole-wheat bread
Fried foods, fatty snack foods	Vegetables, fresh salads
Salt and salty foods	Low-sodium light salt
Coffee and soft drinks	Herbal teas, fresh fruit and vegetable juices

cholesterol levels and the risk for atherosclerosis, animal products must be substantially reduced and plant foods must be substantially increased. A possible exception to the recommendation of reducing the intake of animal foods involves cold-water fish such as salmon, mackerel, and herring. These fish provide eicosapentaenoic acid (EPA), which has been shown in hundreds of studies to lower cholesterol and triglyceride levels. Table 14.6 presents a list of food choices for lowering cholesterol.

Importance of Antioxidants Antioxidants such as vitamin C, beta-carotene, selenium, and vitamin E exert protective effects against many of the processes responsible for the development of atherosclerosis, including the initial damage to the lining of the artery.[140] Diets rich in these protective factors are associated with a reduced risk for heart disease and strokes. This constitutes another strong case for increasing the consumption of plant foods rich in antioxidants.

Platelets and Atherosclerosis The importance of platelet activity in the development of atherosclerosis cannot be overemphasized. Once platelets aggregate, they release potent compounds that cause migration and proliferation of smooth muscle cells into the intima of the artery. Atherosclerosis can be prevented through inhibition of platelet function. Saturated fats increase platelet aggregation, while polyunsaturated fats—particularly linoleic acid, linolenic acid, and EPA—have the opposite effect. These effects are mediated through prostaglandin metabolism.

Many herbs and spices reduce platelet aggregation. Most notable among these are onions, garlic, ginger, and turmeric. These foods also reduce LDL cholesterol while raising HDL cholesterol.

Supporting the Structure of Artery Components A decline in the integrity of an artery's collagen matrix results in the depositing of cholesterol within the artery. Many researchers believe that if the collagen matrix of the artery remains strong, the atherosclerotic plaque will never develop. Many flavonoids, by increasing the integrity of collagen structures, may offer significant protection against atherosclerosis. Feeding flavonoid-rich extracts to animals has resulted in shrinkage of atherosclerotic plaques, as well as in decreased serum cholesterol levels (see page 91). Flavonoids appear to offer significant preventive effects. Nutrients important in maintaining the structure of artery components include vitamin C, vitamin B_6, copper, calcium, and magnesium.[141]

Other Recommendations

Quit smoking! Statistical evidence reveals a three- to fivefold increase in the risk of heart disease in smokers as compared to nonsmokers. The greater the number of cigarettes smoked and the longer the period of years spent smoking, the greater the risk of dying from a heart attack or stroke.

Exercise! Many studies have shown a direct relationship between physical activity and cholesterol levels. Physical exercise is also associated with a decreased risk of heart disease and stroke.

Hemorrhoids

In the United States, as well as in other industrialized countries, hemorrhoidal disease is extremely common. Although most individuals begin to develop hemorrhoids in their twenties, hemorrhoidal symptoms usually do not become evident until people reach their thirties.[142] Estimates indicate that 50 percent of persons over 50 years of age have symptomatic hemorrhoidal disease and that up to 33 percent of the total U.S. population have hemorrhoids to some degree.[143]

Dietary Considerations

Hemorrhoids are rarely seen in parts of the world where high-fiber, unrefined diets are consumed.[144] A low-fiber diet, high in refined foods, contributes greatly to the development of hemorrhoids.

Individuals consuming a low-fiber diet tend to strain more during bowel movements, since their smaller and harder stools are more difficult to pass. This straining increases the pressure in the abdomen, which obstructs venous return. The increased pressure increases pelvic congestion and may significantly weaken the veins, causing hemorrhoids to form.

A high-fiber diet is perhaps the most important component in a regimen to prevent or treat hemorrhoids. A diet rich in vegetables, fruits, legumes, and grains promotes regular bowel movements; and many fiber components attract water and form a gelatinous mass that keeps the feces soft, bulky, and easy to pass. The net effect of a high-fiber diet is significantly less straining during defecation.[145]

Natural bulking compounds can also be used to reduce fecal straining. These fibrous substances, particularly psyllium seed husks and guar gum, possess mild laxative action due to their ability to attract water and form a gelatinous mass. They are generally less irritating than wheat bran and other cellulose fiber products. Several double-blind clinical trials have demonstrated that supplementing the diet with bulk-forming fibers can significantly reduce the symptoms of hemorrhoids (bleeding, pain, pruritis, and prolapse) and can improve bowel habits.[146]

Other Recommendations

Topical therapy, in most circumstances, only provides temporary relief. Topical treatments involve the use of suppositories, ointments, and anorectal pads. Many over-the-counter products for hemorrhoids contain primarily natural ingredients, such as witch hazel (Hamamelis water), shark liver oil, cod liver oil, cocoa butter, Peruvian balsam, zinc oxide, live yeast cell derivatives, and allantoin.

Herpes Simplex

Herpes simplex virus (HSV) causes a recurrent viral infection of the skin or mucous membranes characterized by the appearance of single or multiple clusters of small blisters filled with a clear fluid on an inflamed base. It typically occurs about the mouth (herpes gingivostomatitis), lips (herpes labialis), genitals (herpes genitalis), and eye (herpes keratoconjunctivitis). After the initial infection, the virus becomes dormant in the nerve ganglia, and recurs following minor infections, trauma, stress (emotional, dietary, or environmental), and sun exposure.

The number of people with herpes infections is somewhat difficult to determine. Studies show that between 30 and 100 percent of the adults in the United States have had oral herpes, while genital herpes in found in a range of between 3 percent (among nuns) to 70 percent (among prostitutes).[147] Current estimates indicate that between 20 and 40 percent of the U.S. population have recurrent herpes infections.

Men seem more susceptible to recurrences. After resolution of the primary infection, HSV apparently becomes a dormant inhabitant within nerve ganglia. Recurrences develop at or near the site of primary infection and may be precipitated by many different stimuli: sunburn, sexual activity, menses, stress, food allergy, drugs, and certain foods. The risk of clinical herpes infection after sexual contact with an individual who has active lesions is estimated to be 75 percent. Since not everyone exposed to HSV develops clinical infection, however, it appears that host defense mechanisms are important in protecting against HSV infection.

Dietary Considerations

In general, the recommendations given in the Immune Function section (see pages 314–19), especially the advice to avoid refined carbohydrates and food allergens, are appropriate here as well. There are also some special dietary considerations. A lysine-rich/arginine-poor diet has become a popular treatment for herpes infections. This approach came from research showing that lysine has antiviral activity in vitro due to its antagonism to the metabolism of the amino acid arginine.[148] Possessing a greater amount of lysine than arginine is believed either to inhibit the synthesis of the arginine-rich proteins necessary for viral replication or to repress the activation of the virus's control genes.

Double-blind, placebo-controlled studies on the effectiveness of lysine supplementation with uncontrolled avoidance of arginine-rich foods have shown inconsistent results.[149] These results may be due to the lack of control over the amounts of arginine-rich foods consumed or to the severity of the cases (both placebo and treated groups had lesions for a remarkable 40 percent of the time in one negative study). In any event, better results can be achieved by limiting the intake of high-arginine/low-lysine foods, along with supplementation of 1,200 to 3,000 mg of lysine per day (see Table 14.7).

Other Recommendations

Licorice root contains a compound called glycyrrhetinic acid that inhibits both the growth and the cell-damaging effects of herpes simplex.[150] Regular consumption of licorice root tea should be encouraged in individuals prone to recurrent herpes infections.

High Blood Pressure

Each time the heart beats, it sends blood coursing through the arteries. The peak reading of the pressure exerted by this contraction is the systolic

Table 14.7 Arginine and Lysine Content of Selected Foods, in Milligrams (mg) per 3½-oz (100-g) Serving

Food	*Serving*	*Arginine*	*Lysine*
Almonds	70 nuts	2,730	580
Bacon	12 slices	2,100	2,000
Beans, green	¾ cup	80	80
Beans, lima	3.5 oz	1,170	1,470
Beans, mung	3.5 oz	1,320	1,930
Beans, red	⅓ cup	340	420
Beef, chuck	3.5 oz	1,600	2,200
Brazil nut	3.5 oz	2,250	470
Bread, whole-wheat	4 slices	510	290
Buckwheat	3.5 oz	1,200	460
Carob	3.5 oz	710	340
Cashews	40 nuts	1,950	740
Cheese, cheddar	3.5 oz	850	1,700
Chicken	3.5 oz	1,930	2,700
Chocolate	3.5 oz	4,500	2,000
Clams	½ cup	830	840
Coconut	3.5 oz	470	148
Crustaceans	3.5 oz	1,330	1,260
Eggs	2 large	840	820
Fish sticks	4–5 sticks	940	1,460
Halibut	3.5 oz	140	2,220
Hazelnut	3.5 oz	3,510	690
Lentil	3.5 oz	2,100	1,740
Linseed	3.5 oz	2,030	810
Liver, beef	3.5 oz	1,590	1,950
Milk, whole	3.5 oz	130	280
Millet	3.5 oz	410	260
Oatmeal, cooked	⅓ cup	130	70
Oysters	5–8 medium	310	280
Peanuts, w/o skins	3.5 oz	3,240	1,090
Peas, chick	3.5 oz	1,900	1,380
Peas, green	⅝ cup	420	220
Pecan	3.5 oz	2,030	810
Pork, lean	3.5 oz	1,510	1,850
Rice, brown	⅔ cup	120	100
Salmon	3.5 oz	1,530	2,350
Sardines	7 medium	1,190	1,850
Sesame	3.5 oz	2,590	580
Shrimp	3.5 oz	1,360	2,130
Soybeans, boiled	⅔ cup	620	620
Sunflower	3.5 oz	1,190	540
Tuna	⅝ can	1,530	2,530
Turkey	3.5 oz	1,700	2,450
Walnuts, English	27 whole	2,250	490
Yeast	3.5 oz	1,940	3,510

pressure. Between beats, the heart relaxes and blood pressure drops. The very lowest reading is referred to as the diastolic pressure. A normal blood pressure reading for adults is the following:

120 (systolic) / 80 (diastolic) mm Hg

Hypertension or high blood pressure is a major risk factor for a heart attack or stroke. The number of individuals with hypertension (a blood pressure reading of greater than 160/95) in the United States is estimated at 20 percent in the adult white population and 30 percent among Black adults. These figures nearly double if a blood-pressure reading of 140/90 mm Hg is considered the upper limit of normal.

Although physicians are primarily concerned with diastolic pressure (the second number in the blood-pressure reading), systolic pressure is also an important factor. Males with a normal diastolic pressure (less than 82 mm Hg) but an elevated systolic pressure (more than 158 mm Hg) have a twofold increase in cardiovascular death rate when compared to individuals with normal systolic pressures (less than 130 mm Hg).[151]

Most cases of hypertension can be brought under control through changes in diet and lifestyle.[152] Although well-designed long-term clinical studies have found that people with hypertension who do not take blood-pressure-lowering medicines actually fare much better than do those taking the prescription drugs, antihypertensive medications are among the most widely prescribed of all drugs.[153] Drug therapy usually involves using diuretics and/or beta-adrenergic-blocking drugs. These drugs can have many side effects.

Dietary Considerations

Although behavior patterns and stress play important roles, hypertension is most closely related to dietary factors. Hypertension is another of the many diseases or syndromes associated with the "Western" diet, and it is found almost entirely in developed countries.[154] People living in remote areas of China, the Solomon Islands, New Guinea, Panama, Brazil, and Africa show virtually no evidence of essential hypertension, nor do they experience a rise in blood pressure with advancing age.[155] Furthermore, when racially identical members of these societies migrate to less remote areas and adopt a more "civilized" diet, the incidence of hypertension increases dramatically.

Many dietary factors have been shown to be linked with high blood pressure, including the following:

Obesity
A high sodium-to-potassium ratio

A diet low in fiber and high in sugar
A diet high in saturated fats and low in essential fatty acids
A diet low in calcium and magnesium
A diet low in vitamin C

Several of these factors will be discussed here. The most important dietary recommendation is to increase the consumption of plant foods in the diet. When compared with nonvegetarians, vegetarians generally have lower blood-pressure levels and a lower incidence of hypertension and other cardiovascular diseases.[156] Dietary levels of sodium do not differ significantly between these two groups. However, a typical vegetarian's diet contains more potassium, complex carbohydrates, essential fatty acids, fiber, calcium, magnesium, and vitamin C, and less saturated fat and refined carbohydrate—all of which have a favorable influence on blood pressure.[157]

Obesity Numerous population and clinical studies have demonstrated repeatedly that obesity is a major factor in hypertension.[158] Weight reduction should be a primary therapeutic goal for decreasing hypertension in obese patients, and it may contribute to the management of moderately overweight hypertensives as well.

Sodium and Potassium The role of high sodium/low potassium intake in the development of high blood pressure is discussed in Chapter 3. In summary, excessive consumption of dietary sodium chloride (table salt), coupled with diminished dietary potassium, produces hypertension in susceptible individuals. It appears most often that sodium restriction alone does not improve blood-pressure control; it must be accompanied by a high potassium intake. Numerous studies have shown that a combination of sodium restriction and high potassium intake is of great therapeutic importance in treating high blood pressure.[159]

Sugar Sucrose (common table sugar) elevates blood pressure.[160] The most plausible explanation for this appears to be that sucrose increases adrenaline production, resulting in increased blood vessel constriction and increased sodium retention. In contrast to refined sugar, complex-carbohydrate, high-fiber foods actually lower blood pressure.

Calcium and Magnesium Population studies indicate that calcium and magnesium may offer some protection against the development of high blood pressure.[161] These data, along with several clinical studies demonstrating that calcium or magnesium supplementation has a blood-pressure-lowering effect, indicate that increasing a person's dietary calcium and magnesium intake (preferably from plant sources) may offer significant protective and therapeutic effects.[162]

Vitamin C An inverse relationship exists between serum vitamin C levels and blood pressure in hypertensive men; the lower the vitamin C level, the higher the blood pressure.[163] Whether this is due to better dietary habits or to a blood-pressure-lowering effect of vitamin C has yet to be determined. I believe that it is a combination of both.

Vitamin C is also important in helping the body eliminate heavy metals such as lead and cadmium. Chronic exposure to lead and cadmium from environmental sources, including drinking water and cigarette smoke, is associated with increased cardiovascular mortality. Elevated levels of lead in the blood have been found in a significant number of hypertensives.[164] Cadmium has also been shown to increase blood pressure. Studies have found blood cadmium levels to be three to four times higher in people with high blood pressure than in people with normal blood pressure.[165]

Cigarette smokers are known to have higher concentrations of lead and cadmium and lower concentrations of ascorbic acid than nonsmokers. This may be another reason why cigarette smoking is so strongly linked to high blood pressure.

Special Foods Special foods for people with high blood pressure include garlic, onions, nuts and seeds (or their oils, for their essential fatty acid content), green leafy vegetables (for their rich supply of calcium and magnesium), whole grains and legumes (for their fiber), and foods rich in vitamin C such as broccoli and citrus fruits.

Other Recommendations

Caffeine, alcohol, and tobacco use should be eliminated from the diet. Stress reduction techniques such as biofeedback, autogenics, meditation, yoga, hypnosis, and progressive muscle relaxation may offer some benefit in lowering blood pressure without the use of drugs. Regular aerobic exercise is extremely important for cardiovascular health.

Hives (Urticaria)

Hives or urticaria is a localized swelling of the skin that usually itches intensely. Hives are caused by the release of histamine within the skin. About 50 percent of patients with hives develop angioedema—a deeper, less-defined swelling that involves tissues beneath the skin as well as the skin itself.

Hives and angioedema are relatively common conditions: an estimated 15 to 20 percent of the general population have had hives at some time. Although persons in any age group may experience acute or chronic hives and/or angioedema, young adults (post-adolescence through the third decade of life) are most often affected.[166] Drugs are the leading cause of hives in adults. In children, hives are usually due to foods, food additives, or infections.[167]

Dietary Considerations

An elimination or low-antigenic diet is of utmost importance in treating most cases of hives, particularly in children. The diet should eliminate suspected allergens and all food additives. The strictest elimination diets allow only water, lamb, rice, pears, and vegetables. Foods most commonly associated with inducing urticaria (milk, eggs, chicken, fruits, nuts, and additives) should definitely be avoided.[168] Foods containing vasoactive amines should also be eliminated, even if no direct allergy to them is noted. The primary foods to eliminate are cured meats, alcoholic beverages, cheese, chocolate, citrus fruits, and shellfish.

The importance of eliminating food additives from the diet cannot be overstated. As discussed in Chapter 2, food additives such as tartrazine and benzoates stimulate production of a compound that increases the number of mast cells in the body.[169] Mast cells are involved in producing histamine and other allergic compounds. A person whose body has relatively many mast cells will typically be more prone to allergies. Examinations of patients with hives show that greater than 95 percent have an increase in mast cells.[170] Food additives appear to be a major factor in hives. Colorings (azo dyes), flavorings (salicylates, aspartame), preservatives (benzoates, nitrites, sorbic acid), antioxidants (hydroxytoluene, sulfite, gallate), and emulsifiers/stabilizers (polysorbates, vegetable gums) have all been shown to produce hives in sensitive individuals.[171]

Antibiotics in Foods Antibiotics, including penicillin and related compounds, are the most common cause of drug-induced hives. The rate of allergy to penicillin in the general population is thought to be at least 10 percent. Nearly 25 percent of these individuals display hives, angioedema, or severe allergic reactions upon ingestion of penicillin.[172] An important characteristic of penicillin is that it cannot be destroyed by boiling or steam distillation. This is a problem, since penicillin and related contaminants can exist undetected in foods.

The degree to which penicillin in our food supply contributes to urticarial reactions is unknown. However, urticaria and allergic symptoms have been traced to penicillin in milk, soft drinks, and frozen dinners.[173] In one study of 245 patients with chronic urticaria, 24 percent had positive skin tests and 12 percent had positive allergy tests for penicillin sensitivity.[174] Of the 42 patients sensitive to penicillin, 22 improved clinically on a dairy-product-free diet, while only 2 out of 40 patients with negative skin tests improved on the same diet. This study seems to provide indirect evidence of the importance of penicillin in the food supply as a cause of urticaria.

In an attempt to provide direct evidence, researchers gave penicillin-contaminated pork to penicillin-allergic volunteers; but no significant reactions were noted other than transient skin itchiness in two volunteers.[175] Penicillin in milk appears to be more allergenic than penicillin in meat.[176] Presumably this is because penicillin can be degraded into more allergenic compounds in the presence of carbohydrate and metals (as in milk) than in their absence (as in artificially contaminated meat).[177]

Other Recommendations

In one study involving 236 cases of chronic urticaria, psychological factors (such as stress) were reported to be the most frequent primary cause.[178] Stress appears to play an important role by increasing the person's susceptibility to allergies. In another study of 15 patients with chronic urticaria, relaxation therapy and hypnosis were shown to provide significant benefit.[179] Patients were given an audio tape and asked to use the relaxation techniques described on the tape at home. At a follow-up examination 5 to 14 months after the initial session, 6 patients were free of hives and 7 others reported improvement.

Hypoglycemia

Hypoglycemia or low blood sugar is not a disease per se but a symptom of faulty carbohydrate metabolism. Since glucose is the primary fuel for the brain, hypoglycemia usually affects mental function, and symptoms include such things as blurred vision, mental confusion, incoherent speech, bizarre behavior, convulsions, depression and other psychological disturbances, and irritability. One of the ways the body combats low blood-sugar levels is by increasing epinephrine (adrenaline) secretion by the adrenal gland. This can result in accompanying symptoms of headache, sweating, weakness, hunger, heart palpitations, and "inward trembling."

Dietary Considerations

The dietary factors discussed under Diabetes (see pages 286, 287) are appropriate here as well. Once again, the best diet for controlling blood-sugar levels is a diet rich in dietary fiber and complex carbohydrates; adequate in protein; and low in refined sugar, fat, and processed foods. Legumes and chromium-rich foods are particularly beneficial in stabilizing blood-sugar levels.

Other Recommendations

Since stress is often a contributing factor to hypoglycemia, it is important to practice stress reduction techniques such as exercise, relaxation, and meditation as part of your healthful lifestyle.

Immune Function

The immune system is among the most complex and fascinating systems of the human body. The immune system is composed of the lymphatic vessels and organs (thymus, spleen, tonsils, and lymph nodes), white blood cells (lymphocytes, neutrophils, basophils, eosinophils, monocytes, and so on), specialized cells residing in various tissue (macrophages, mast cells, and so on), and specialized serum factors. The immune system's prime functions are to protect the body against infection and against the development of cancer.

Dietary Considerations

The health of the body's immune system is largely determined by its state of stress and its nutritional status. Dietary factors that depress immune function include nutrient deficiency, sugar, and high cholesterol levels in the blood. Dietary factors that enhance immune function include all essential nutrients, antioxidants, flavonoids, and various other nutrients.

Consistent with good health, optimal immune function requires a healthful diet that has the following attributes: rich in whole, natural foods, such as fruits, vegetables, grains, beans, seeds, and nuts; low in fats and refined sugars; and supplied with adequate (but not excessive) amounts of protein. On top of this, for optimum immune function, an individual should consume 16 to 24 ounces of fresh fruit or vegetable juice per day, as well as five or six 8-ounce glasses of water per day (preferably pure); should take a good basic multivitamin–mineral supplement; should engage in a regular exercise program of at least 30 minutes or aerobic exercise and 5 to 10 minutes of passive stretching daily; should perform daily deep-breathing and relaxation exercises (meditation, prayer, and so on); should take time each day to play and enjoy family and friends; and should still get at least 6 to 8 hours of sleep daily.

Now let's look at some of the specific dietary factors that can play a role in immune function.

Nutrient Deficiency Undernourishment is generally regarded as the most frequent cause of immunodeficiency in the world. Although research relating nutritional status to immune function has historically concerned itself with severe states of malnutrition (namely, kwashiorkor and marasmas), attention is now shifting toward marginal deficiencies of single or multiple nutrients and toward overnutrition. Ample evidence supports the conclusion that any single nutrient deficiency can profoundly impair the immune system.

Nutrient deficiency is not limited to Third World countries. Nutrition surveys of the U.S. population have found that most Americans are deficient in at least one nutrient. Several studies have estimated that 19 to 66 percent of the elderly population in parts of North America consume two-thirds or less of the RDA for various nutrients.[180] The significance of these findings to the immune system is substantial, since virtually any nutrient deficiency impairs the immune system, putting the individual at greater risk for cancer and infections. Nutrients especially critical to healthy immune function include vitamin A, zinc, vitamin B_6, vitamin C, and selenium.

Obesity and Elevated Fats in the Blood Americans are typically overfed but undernourished. Unfortunately, the combination of nutritional inadequacies plus nutritional excesses greatly reduces immune function. Obesity is not only associated with such conditions as atherosclerosis, hypertension, diabetes mellitus, and joint disorders; it is also associated with decreased immune status, as evidenced by the decreased bacteria-killing activity of neutrophils and by the increased morbidity and mortality from infections and cancer.[181] Cholesterol and fat levels in the blood are usually elevated in obese individuals, and this may explain their impaired immune function. Increased blood levels of cholesterol, free fatty acids, triglycerides, and bile acids inhibit various immune functions, including the ability of white blood cells to produce antibodies and to migrate to areas of infections where they can engulf and destroy infectious organisms or cancer cells.[182] Optimal immune function therefore depends on maintaining healthful levels of cholesterol and other fats in the blood.

Sugar Ingesting 100 grams (roughly 3½ ounces) of a carbohydrate such as glucose, fructose, sucrose, honey, or pasteurized orange juice has been shown to reduce significantly the ability of white blood cells (neutrophils) to engulf and destroy bacteria.[183] In contrast, ingesting 100 grams of starch has no effect. These effects were found to become measurable within 30 minutes of ingestion and to last for more than 5 hours. Typically at least a 50 percent reduction in neutrophil activity occurred 2 hours after ingestion. Since neutrophils constitute 60 to 70 percent of the total circulating white blood cells, impairment of their activity leads to depressed immunity.

In addition, ingesting 75 grams of glucose has been shown to depress lymphocyte activity.[184] Other parameters of immune function are also undoubtedly affected by sugar consumption. It has been suggested that the ill effects of high glucose levels are a result of competition between blood glucose and vitamin C for membrane transport sites into the white blood cells.[185] This is based on evidence that vitamin C and glucose appear to have opposite effects on immune function, and both require insulin for membrane transport into many tissues.

Considering that the average American consumes 150 grams of sucrose (plus other refined simple sugars) each day, the inescapable conclusion is that most Americans have chronically depressed immune systems. Particularly during an infection or a chronic illness like cancer or AIDS, consumption of refined sugars is clearly harmful to immune function.

Carotenes As discussed in Chapter 4, beta-carotene has been shown to exert many beneficial effects on the immune system. Many of the immune-enhancing effects of carotenes (and other antioxidants) may be due to their ability to protect the thymus gland from damage. The thymus is the major gland of our immune system. It is composed of two soft pinkish-gray lobes that lie in a biblike fashion just beneath the thyroid gland and above the heart. The thymus gland shows maximum development immediately after birth. During the aging process, it undergoes a process of shrinkage or involution. The reason for this involution is that the thymus gland is extremely susceptible to free-radical and oxidative damage caused by stress, drugs, radiation, infection, and chronic illness. When the thymus gland becomes damaged, its ability to control the immune system is severely compromised.

The thymus is responsible for many immune system functions, including the production of T lymphocytes—a type of white blood cell. The thymus gland also releases such hormones as thymosin, thymopoeitin, and serum thymic factor, which regulate many immune functions. Low levels of these hormones in the blood are associated with depressed immunity and an increased susceptibility to infection. Typically, thymic hormone levels are very low in the elderly, in individuals prone to infection, in cancer and AIDS patients, and in individuals who are exposed to undue stress. Carotenes and other antioxidants may ensure optimal thymus gland activity by preventing damage to the thymus by free radicals and prooxidants.

The effects of carotenes on the immune system go well beyond protecting the thymus gland. Carotenes have been shown to enhance the function of several types of white blood cells and to increase the antiviral and anticancer properties of immune system mediators like interferon. Simply stated, carotene-rich foods and drinks seem to be able to boost immunity.

As mentioned in Chapter 4, considerable research is currently examining the relationship of vitamin A and carotenes to the incidence of epithelial cancer (cancer of the lungs, gastrointestinal tract, genitourinary tract, and skin). Studies have consistently demonstrated an inverse relationship between carotene intake and cancer incidence: the higher the intake of carotenes, the lower the incidence of cancer.

Although authorities generally agree that carotenes offer significant protection against many cancers, it is not known whether carotenes offer any therapeutic benefit with respect to existing cancers. Ample animal studies support the efficacy of carotenes—especially beta-carotene—in the prevention and treatment of cancer. Unfortunately, comparable studies in humans have not been performed.

Some human studies have been performed in relation to precancerous conditions, where oral beta-carotene has been shown to reverse the condition.[186] For example, beta-carotene has been shown to have "substantial" activity in reversing a precancerous condition of the mouth known as leukoplakia. *Leukoplakia* is a clinical term signifying a white plaquelike lesion occurring anywhere on the lips or oral cavity. It is generally a reaction to irritation, such as cigarette smoking or tobacco chewing. Leukoplakia almost invariably leads to cancer. In one study, 17 of 24 patients with leukoplakia responded to a relatively low dose of beta-carotene (30 mg/day) within a 3-month period.[187] These results are encouraging to cancer researchers because of beta-carotene's total lack of side effects.

Vitamin C Many claims have been made about the role of vitamin C (ascorbic acid) in enhancing the immune system, especially in regard to the prevention and treatment of the common cold. But despite numerous positive clinical and experimental studies, this effect for some reason remains hotly debated.[188] From a biochemical viewpoint, considerable evidence indicates that vitamin C plays a vital role in many immune mechanisms. Vitamin C has been shown to increase many different immune functions, including enhancing white blood cell function and activity and increasing interferon levels, antibody responses, antibody levels, secretion of thymic hormones, and integrity of ground substance.[189] Vitamin C has many biochemical effects similar to those produced by interferon, the body's natural antiviral and anticancer compound.

It is a good idea to eat foods rich in vitamin C when the immune system is under stress from an infection or cancer. The high concentration of vitamin C in white blood cells is rapidly depleted during infection, cancer, or stress. The cancer patient in particular needs adequate vitamin C. A cancer patient should supplement his or her diet with additional vitamin C (3 to 8 grams daily) and should consume high-vitamin-C-containing foods and juices—especially vegetable juices, because they are also rich sources of carotenes.

Antioxidants and Immune Function in Cancer and AIDS Antioxidants are critical in protecting the thymus gland from damage and in enhancing its function. Perhaps no one has greater need for the benefits of antioxidants than does the cancer or AIDS patient. In addition to dealing with the stress of these conditions, the patient's body must often deal with the side effects of current medical treatment. For example, in cancer therapy, chemotherapy and radiation expose both healthy cells and cancerous cells to free-radical damage. The result is great stress to antioxidant mechanisms and consequent depletion of valuable antioxidant enzymes and nutrients. Cancer patients thus need especially large quantities of antioxidant nutrients.[190] Likewise, individuals with AIDS or human immunodeficiency virus (HIV) have an increased need for antioxidant nutrients, because they are in a state of oxidative imbalance.[191] Specifically, AIDS patients have more pro-oxidants in their system than they have antioxidants. Furthermore, the development of AIDS in a symptom-free HIV-infected individual may depend on the cumulative effects of oxidative damage. If this is true, antioxidant therapy holds great promise as a means of delaying or precluding the onset of full-blown AIDS.

Supporting the cancer or AIDS patient with antioxidant nutrients such as coenzyme Q10, vitamin C, selenium, vitamin E, and sulfur compounds is gaining respect in orthodox research. In cancer patients, studies show that these nutrients can help reduce some of the side effects of chemotherapy drugs and radiation, thereby increasing their effectiveness.[192] Antioxidant therapy is also showing great promise in AIDS.[193]

Juicing fresh fruits and vegetables to provide important antioxidant compounds appears to be a good idea for patients. Furthermore, juicing can help deal with some nutritional problems that can develop as a result of the cancer. About two-thirds of all people with cancer develop a condition known as cachexia, characterized by a loss of appetite that results in decreased nutrient intake. This in turn leads to malnutrition, muscle wasting, and impaired immune function. Cachexia thus greatly reduces the patient's quality of life and contributes significantly to the development of further illness or even death. Juicing is used as part of the nutritional support program for cancer patients at several orthodox cancer treatment centers across the country, as well as in many alternative cancer treatments.

Particularly important for the cancer patient may be the inclusion of cabbage-family vegetables and garlic in the diet. The anticancer effects of the cruciferous or cabbage-family vegetables (cabbage, Brussels sprouts, broccoli, cauliflower, and so on) is discussed in Chapter 5. Even the American Cancer Society recommends regular consumption of these foods to prevent cancer. In addition to enhancing the detoxification of cancer-causing compounds, sulfur-containing compounds in cruciferous vegetables may have some therapeutic potential against cancer itself, as well. Specifically, in animal studies, these compounds are being shown to inhibit the progress of many types of tumors and cancers, including breast cancer. Cruciferous vegetables are also very good sources of carotenes and vitamin C. The cancer patient should try to consume 2 cups of cruciferous vegetables per day, in whole or juiced form.

Garlic possesses important immune-enhancing and anticancer properties. The famous Greek physician Hippocrates prescribed eating garlic as a treatment for cancers. Based on animal research and some human studies, this recommendation may have been extremely wise. Several garlic components have displayed significant immune-enhancing and anticancer effects.[194] Human studies showing garlic's immune-enhancing and anticancer effects are largely based on population studies. These studies suggest that an inverse relationship exists between cancer rates and garlic consumption: cancer rates are lowest where garlic consumption is greatest. For example, in China, a study comparing populations in different regions found that death from gastric cancers in regions with high garlic consumption was significantly less than in regions with lower garlic consumption.[195]

Since many of the therapeutic compounds in garlic have not been found in cooked, processed, and commercial garlic preparations, the plant's broad range of beneficial effects is best obtained from fresh, raw garlic. Consistently, the most potent garlic component is allicin—the component that is also responsible for garlic's strong odor. Juicing the garlic with chlorophyll-rich foods like parsley, celery, and kale may reduce the odor without compromising the positive effects of the raw garlic.

Other Recommendations

Numerous herbs have been shown to possess significant immune-enhancing properties. Perhaps the most popular herbs used to enhance the immune system in the United States are echinacea (*Echinacea augustifolia*) and goldenseal (*Hydrastis canadensis*). The medicinal use of these herbs is fully discussed in *The Healing Power of Herbs.* A complete discussion of the use of natural methods to address many common infectious conditions (including strep throat, sinus infections, and AIDS) is provided in *The Encyclopedia of Natural Medicine.*

Irritable Bowel Syndrome

Irritable bowel syndrome (IBS) is a very common condition in which the large intestine, or colon, fails to function properly. The problem is also known as nervous indigestion, spastic colitis, mucous colitis, and intestinal neurosis. IBS has numerous characteristic symptoms including various combinations of the following: abdominal pain and distension; more frequent bowel movements with pain; relief of pain with bowel movements; constipation; diarrhea; excessive production of mucus in the colon; symptoms of indigestion such as flatulence, nausea, or anorexia; and varying degrees of anxiety or depression. Estimates suggest that approximately 15 percent of the U.S. population have suffered from IBS.[196]

Dietary Considerations

Treating irritable bowel syndrome by increasing the intake of dietary fiber has a long history.[197] In general, consuming a diet rich in complex carbohydrates and dietary fiber is effective. Individuals usually respond better to fiber from sources other than wheat—particularly to water-soluble fiber like that found in vegetables, fruits, oat bran, guar gum, psyllium husks, and legumes (beans, peas, and their relatives). White table sugar or sucrose has a very detrimental effect on bowel function, particularly in patients with IBS. Its use should be severely restricted or, better yet, eliminated.[198]

Food allergies are another frequent cause of IBS. The majority of patients with IBS (approximately two-thirds) have at least one food intolerance, and some have multiple intolerances.[199] An elimination diet is perhaps the best method for determining food allergies in IBS. Many IBS patients have other symptoms suggestive of food allergy, such as heart palpitation, hyperventilation, fatigue, excessive sweating, and headaches.[200]

Other Recommendations

Ginger may offer some relief. Ginger is an excellent carminative (a substance that promotes the elimination of intestinal gas) and intestinal spasmolytic (a substance that relaxes and soothes the intestinal tract). As described in Chapter 10, a clue to ginger's success in eliminating gastrointestinal distress is offered by recent double-blind studies that demonstrated ginger's effectiveness in preventing the symptoms of motion sickness and of nausea and vomiting during pregnancy. To gain the maximum benefit from ginger, add some fresh ginger (about a ¼-inch slice) to fresh fruit or vegetable juice.

Kidney Stones

Kidney stones are extremely common in the United States. Each year, nearly 6 percent of the entire U.S. population develop a kidney stone. Over 10 percent of all males and 5 percent of all females experience the pain of a kidney stone during their lifetime. The rate of kidney stones has been steadily increasing, paralleling the rise in other chronic diseases associated with the so called "Western" diet.[201]

In the United States, most kidney stones are calcium-containing stones composed of calcium oxalate, calcium oxalate mixed with calcium phosphate, or (very rarely) calcium phosphate alone. The high rate of calcium-containing stones in affluent societies is directly associated with the following dietary patterns: low-fiber, highly refined carbohydrates; high alcohol; large amounts of animal protein; high-fat, high-calcium food; high salt; and high-vitamin-D-enriched food. Some of these factors are discussed more fully below.[202]

Dietary Considerations

Americans commonly eat more protein than their bodies require. When protein ingestion is too high, it leads to increased calcium excretion in the urine. America's high intake of protein is one of the main reasons we suffer from so many diet-related diseases, including those involving calcium metabolism like kidney stones and osteoporosis. Overconsumption of protein should be avoided, while fresh fruit and vegetable intake should be increased. Although vegetarians have a reduced risk for developing kidney stones, meat eaters who consume higher amounts of fresh fruits and vegetables have a lower incidence of kidney stones.[203] In addition the simple change from eating white bread to eating whole-wheat bread has lowered urinary calcium and reduced kidney stone formation in clinical studies.[204] The simple dietary adjustments of eating more fruits and vegetables, eating less sugar, and switching from white bread to whole-wheat bread would probably prevent kidney stone development or recurrence in many individuals.[205]

Excess body weight and faulty carbohydrate metabolism are high-risk factors for stone formation, since both lead to increased excretion of calcium in the urine. The common factor linking them may be the role that sugar (sucrose) plays. Following sugar ingestion, the level of urinary calcium rises. Refined carbohydrates should be restricted in the diet and largely or entirely replaced by complex carbohydrates such as whole grains, legumes, and vegetables.[206]

Magnesium and Vitamin B_6 Magnesium is of critical importance in the prevention of kidney stones.[207] Magnesium has been shown to increase the solubility of calcium oxalate and to inhibit the precipitation of both calcium phosphate and calcium oxalate. A low urinary magnesium-to-calcium ratio is an independent risk factor in stone formation. Supplemental magnesium alone has been shown to be effective in preventing recurrences of kidney stones. However, when magnesium is used in conjunction with vitamin B_6 (pyridoxine) an even greater effect is noted.[208] Authorities often recommended that foods with a high magnesium-to-calcium ratio and a high vitamin B_6 content be increased in the diet. Foods fulfilling these criteria include barley, bran, corn, buckwheat, rye, soy, oats, brown rice, avocado, banana, lima beans, and potato.

Avoiding Dairy Products Long-term overconsumption of milk or antacids is known to lead to the development of kidney stones. Recently, due to the increased incidence of osteoporosis, physicians and manufacturers of antacids have campaigned vigorously to convince women to use calcium carbonate antacids (Tums) as calcium supplements. This does not appear to be sound medical advice, because of the risk of developing kidney stones that attends overconsumption of antacids, especially in combination with high milk consumption.

Milk may not be suitable for people at risk for developing kidney stones, since most milk products are fortified with vitamin D. This vitamin increases the body's absorption of calcium, but it also increases the calcium concentration in the urine. Increasing the amount of urinary calcium greatly increases the risk of stone formation. Compounding this negative effect is the fact that consuming milk fortified with vitamin D lowers magnesium levels in the body.[209]

Juicing and Kidney Stones For all types of stones, increasing urine flow to dilute the urine is vital. Enough fluids (preferably from pure water and fresh fruit and vegetable juices) should be consumed to produce a daily urinary volume of at least 1½ quarts. As for specific juice recommendations, it is a good idea to avoid spinach-containing juices, since spinach is rich in both calcium and oxalate; but your diet should include other fresh juices. In fact, you should consume several juices regularly. For example, cranberry juice has been shown to reduce the amount of ionized calcium in the urine by over 50 percent in patients with recurrent kidney stones. Since high levels of urinary calcium greatly increase a person's risk of developing a kidney stone, cranberry juice may offer significant benefit—even though cranberries are fairly high in oxalate. Most cranberry juices on the market consist of one-third cranberry juice mixed with water and sugar. Fresh cranberry juice naturally sweetened with apple or grape juice is preferable.

Eating green leafy vegetables like kale, lettuce, and parsley is also of benefit, since they provide natural vitamin K_1. A natural compound in the urine that powerfully inhibits crystalline growth of calcium oxalate requires vitamin K for its synthesis. The presence of vitamin K in green leafy vegetables may be another reason why vegetarians have a lower incidence of kidney stones.

Finally, citrus juices may offer some protection because they provide citric acid. Decreased urinary citrate is found in 20 to 60 percent of patients with kidney stones.[210] This is extremely important, since citrate reduces urinary saturation of stone-forming calcium salts by forming complexes with calcium. If citrate levels are low, this inhibitory activity does not occur, and stone formation is likely to ensue. Citrate supplementation has been shown to be quite successful in preventing recurrent kidney stones. Potassium citrate and sodium citrate have been used to good effect in clinical studies.[211] Eating or juicing fresh citrus fruits may prove to be a more advantageous way to increase a person's intake of citrates.

Other Recommendations

Hair mineral analysis may be of value in patients with recurrent kidney stones, since many heavy metals (lead, mercury, aluminum, gold, uranium, and cadmium) are toxic to the kidney and may lead to stone formation.[212] Hair mineral analysis often (but not always) detects an increased body burden of cadmium and other heavy metals.

Multiple Sclerosis

Multiple sclerosis (MS) is a syndrome of progressive disturbances of the central nervous system (CNS) that occur early in life. Early symptoms of multiple sclerosis may include the following:

- Muscular symptoms – Feeling of heaviness, weakness, leg dragging, stiffness, tendency to drop things, clumsiness

- Sensory symptoms – Tingling, "pins-and-needles" sensation, numbness, dead feeling, bandlike tightness, electrical sensations
- Visual symptoms – Blurring, fogginess, haziness, eyeball pain, blindness, double vision
- Vestibular symptoms – Light-headedness, feeling of spinning, sensation of drunkenness, nausea, vomiting
- Genitourinary symptoms – Incontinence, loss of bladder sensation, loss of sexual function

Despite considerable research, many questions about MS remain. Mainstream medicine has become almost obsessed with finding a viral cause for this disease, although most current work suggests that it results from immune disturbances. In MS, the myelin sheath that surrounds nerves is destroyed. For this reason MS is classified as a "demyelinating" disease. Zones of demyelination (plaques) vary in size and location within the spinal cord. Symptoms correspond in a general way to the distribution of the plaques.

In about two-thirds of all cases, onset occurs between the ages of 20 and 40 (rarely is the onset after age 50); and women are affected slightly more often than men (60 percent female, 40 percent male). The cause of MS has yet to be definitively determined. Many causative factors have been proposed, including viruses, auto-immune factors, and diet.[213]

Dietary Considerations

Dr. Roy Swank, Professor of Neurology at the University of Oregon Medical School, has provided convincing evidence that a diet low in saturated fats, when maintained over a long period of time (one study lasted over 34 years), tends to halt the disease process.[214] Swank began successfully treating patients with his low-fat diet in 1948. Swank's recommended diet has the following features: a saturated fat intake of no more than 10 grams per day; a daily intake of 40 to 50 grams of polyunsaturated oils (margarine, shortening, and hydrogenated oils are not allowed); at least 1 teaspoon of cod liver oil daily; a normal allowance of protein; and the consumption of fish three or more times a week.[215]

Swank's diet was originally thought to help patients with MS by overcoming an essential fatty acid deficiency and by reducing the patients' intake of saturated fats. Currently, however, the beneficial effects are thought to be a result of three factors: decreasing platelet aggregation; decreasing the auto-immune response; and normalizing the decreased essential fatty acid levels found in the serum, red blood cells, platelets, and (perhaps most important) cerebrospinal fluid of patients with MS.

Linoleic acid, the essential fatty acid found in most vegetable oils, has been used as a treatment of MS. This therapy has been investigated in three double-blind trials.[216] Although the results of the studies were mixed (two showed an effect, and one did not), combined analysis indicates that patients supplementing their diets with linoleic acid had a less pronounced increase in disability, and reduced severity and duration of relapses, than did controls. These studies used sunflower seed oil at dosage of a little more than 1 tablespoon per day. Other vegetable oils that primarily contain linoleic acid include safflower oil and soy oil.

Better results would probably have been obtained in the double-blind studies if dietary saturated fatty acids had been restricted, if larger amounts of linoleic acid had been used (at least 2 tablespoons per day), and if the studies had been of longer duration (one study found that normalization of fatty acid levels required at least 2 years of supplementation). Even better results might be obtained by using flaxseed oil, as this oil contains both linoleic and alpha-linolenic acid (an omega-3 oil). Linolenic acid has a greater effect on platelets and is required for normal CNS composition.

There appears to be a strong rationale for supplementation with eicosapentaenoic acid (EPA) and DHA—the so-called "fish oils"—in the treatment of MS, although no direct clinical investigation of their effects has been done. EPA greatly inhibits platelet aggregation, and DHA is present in large concentration in lipids of the brain. This is consistent with Swank's protocol, which included liberal consumption of fish and supplementation with cod liver oil (a rich source of EPA and DHA). Supplements may be used to increase EPA and DHA, particularly in areas where cold-water fish are often unavailable.

Other Recommendations

Supplementing the dietary intake of vitamin E and selenium is definitely indicated, because of the increased lipid peroxidation seen in MS patients and because of the increased consumption of polyunsaturated fats, which increases vitamin E requirements. Pancreatic enzyme preparations and the protein-digesting enzyme of the pineapple, bromelain, have been demonstrated to be effective in treating auto-immune and immune complex diseases like MS.[217] In Germany, pancreatic enzyme preparations have produced good effects in reducing the severity and frequency of symptom flare-ups.[218]

Osteoarthritis

Osteoarthritis or degenerative joint disease is the most common form of arthritis. It is seen primarily, but not exclusively, in the elderly. Surveys have indicated that over 40 million Americans have osteoarthritis, including 80 percent of persons over the age of 50. In individuals under the age of 45, osteoarthritis is much more common in men; after age 45, however, it is 10 times more common in women than in men.[219]

The weight-bearing joints and the joints of the hands are the ones most often affected by the degenerative changes associated with osteoarthritis. Specifically, there is substantial cartilage destruction, followed by hardening and the formation of large bone spurs in the joint margins. Pain, deformity, and limitation of motion in the joint result. Inflammation is usually minimal.[220]

The onset of osteoarthritis can be very subtle; morning joint stiffness is often the first symptom. As the disease progresses, the patient feels pain on motion of the involved joint that is made worse by prolonged activity and relieved by rest. There are usually no signs of inflammation.[221]

Dietary Considerations

Perhaps the most important dietary recommendation for individuals suffering from osteoarthritis is that they achieve normal body weight. Being overweight means putting added stress on weight-bearing joints affected by osteoarthritis.

Both to prevent and to treat osteoarthritis with diet, the diet must be rich in whole natural foods—especially raw fruits and vegetables, because of their rich source of nutrients critical to joint health (particularly antioxidant factors like vitamin C, carotenes, and flavonoids). Especially beneficial are flavonoid-rich fruits like cherries, blueberries, and blackberries. Also important are sulfur-containing foods such as legumes, garlic, onions, Brussels sprouts, and cabbage; the sulfur content in fingernails of arthritis sufferers has been found to be lower than that of healthy controls.[222] Normalizing the sulfur content of the nails through colloidal sulfur treatments alleviated pain and swelling, according to clinical data from the 1930s.[223]

Childers, a horticulturist, popularized a diet for treating osteoarthritis that eliminated foods from the family Solanaceae (the nightshades) after finding that this simple dietary elimination cured his osteoarthritis.[224] Childers developed a theory that genetically susceptible individuals might develop arthritis (and various other complaints) from long-term low-level consumption of the alkaloids found in tomatoes, potatoes, eggplant, peppers, and tobacco. Presumably these alkaloids inhibit normal collagen repair in a joint or promote the inflammatory degeneration of the joint. Although its benefits remain to be proved, this diet may offer relief to some individuals and is certainly worth a try.

Individual Nutrients in Osteoarthritis A number of individual nutrients have been shown to be helpful to patients with osteoarthritis.[225] Most notable are niacinamide, the essential amino acid methionine, vitamin E, vitamin C, pantothenic acid, and vitamin B_6. All of these nutrients are required for the synthesis of normal collagen and the maintenance of joint structures. A deficiency of any one of these would allow accelerated joint degeneration.

Other Recommendations

Various physical therapy modalities (exercise, heat, cold, diathermy, ultrasound, and so on) performed by physical therapists, naturopathic physicians, and chiropractors are often very effective in improving joint mobility and reducing pain in sufferers of osteoarthritis. Physical therapy appears to be quite important, especially when administered regularly.

Osteoporosis

Osteoporosis, which literally means "porous bone," affects more than 20 million people in the United States. Normally there is a decline in bone mass after the age of 40 in both sexes. This bone loss is accelerated in patients with osteoporosis. Many factors can result in excessive bone loss, and different variants of osteoporosis exist. Postmenopausal osteoporosis is the most common form of osteoporosis.

Although the entire skeleton may be involved in postmenopausal osteoporosis, bone loss is usually greatest in the spine, hips, and ribs. Since these bones bear a great deal of weight, they become susceptible to pain, deformity, or fracture. At least 1.2 million fractures occur each year as a direct result of osteoporosis. The most catastrophic of fractures is the hip fracture, which is fatal in 12 to 20 percent of all cases and precipitates long-term nursing home care for half of those who survive. Nearly one-third of all women and one-sixth of all men will fracture their hips in their lifetime.

Osteoporosis involves both the mineral (inorganic) and the nonmineral (organic matrix, composed primarily of protein) components of bone. This is the first clue that there is more to osteoporosis than a lack of dietary calcium. In fact, lack of dietary calcium in the adult results in a separate condition known as osteomalacia or "softening of the bone." In osteomalacia there is only a deficiency of calcium in the bone, whereas in osteoporosis there is a lack of calcium and other minerals and a decrease in the nonmineral framework (organic matrix) of bone. Little attention has been given to the important role that this organic matrix plays in maintaining bone structure.

Calcium Metabolism and Hormonal Factors in Osteoporosis

Bone is dynamic living tissue that is constantly being broken down and rebuilt, even in adults. Normal bone metabolism depends on an intricate interplay of many nutritional and hormonal factors; the liver and kidney having a regulatory effect as well. Although over two dozen nutrients are necessary for optimal bone health, calcium and vitamin D are generally considered the most important factors. Hormones are also critical, however, as in women the incorporation of calcium into bone depends on the hormone estrogen. Approximately one in four postmenopausal women has osteoporosis.

Although many physicians recommend estrogen replacement for their postmenopausal women, authorities generally agree that the risk outweighs the benefit in most women who are at risk for osteoporosis. Instead of estrogen therapy, a greater emphasis should be placed on nutritional and lifestyle factors. In severe cases, improvement may result from the administration of estrogen, 1,5-(OH)2D3, or calcitonin (all of which are prescription medications).

Major Risk Factors for Osteoporosis in Women

The following factors have been identified as raising a woman's risk for osteoporosis:

Postmenopausal
White or Asian
Premature menopause
Positive family history
Short stature and small bones
Leanness
Low calcium intake
Inactivity
Nulliparity (never pregnant)
Gastric or small-bowel resection
Long-term glucocorticosteroid therapy
Long-term use of anticonvulsants
Hyperparathyroidism
Hyperthyroidism

Smoking
Heavy alcohol use

Dietary Considerations

Recently some doctors and financially interested companies have campaigned vigorously to get people to increase their dietary calcium. While this appears to be sound medical advice for many, osteoporosis is much more than a lack of dietary calcium. It is a complex condition involving hormonal, lifestyle, nutritional, and environmental factors. A comprehensive plan that addresses all of these factors offers the greatest protection against developing osteoporosis. In regard to calcium supplementation for women at high risk for osteoporosis, I recommend OsteoPrime, a bone-building supplement developed by Jonathan Wright, M.D., and Alan Gaby, M.D. OsteoPrime is made by Enzymatic Therapy and is available at health-food stores. Calcium citrate appears to be the best form of supplementary calcium.[226]

The primary goals of diet in the treatment and prevention of osteoporosis are to preserve adequate mineral mass, to prevent loss of the protein matrix and other structural components of bone, and to maintain optimal repair mechanisms for remodeling damaged areas of bone.

Many general dietary factors have been suggested as a cause of osteoporosis, including low calcium/high phosphorus intake, high-protein diet, high acid/ash diet, and trace mineral deficiencies.[227] To help slow down bone loss, foods high in calcium are often recommended. Besides dairy products, foods rich in calcium include kale, spinach, turnip greens, and other green leafy vegetables.

A vegetarian diet (whether lacto-ovo or vegan) is associated with a lower risk of osteoporosis.[228] Although bone mass in vegetarians does not differ significantly from bone mass in omnivores during the third, fourth, and fifth decades, significant differences are evident in the later decades. This indicates that the lower incidence of osteoporosis in vegetarians is due not to increased initial bone mass, but rather to decreased subsequent bone loss.

Several factors may be responsible for the slower rate of bone loss observed in vegetarians. Most important, probably, is a lower intake of protein. A high-protein diet or a diet high in phosphates is associated with increased excretion of calcium in the urine. Raising daily protein intake from 47 to 142 grams doubles the excretion of calcium in the urine.[229] A diet this high in protein is common in the United States and may be a significant factor in the increased number of people who suffer from osteoporosis in this country.

Another dietary factor that increases the loss of calcium from the body is refined sugar. Following sugar intake, urinary excretion of calcium increases.[230] Considering that the average American consumes every day 150 grams of sucrose, plus other refined simple sugars, and a glass of a carbonated beverage loaded with phosphates, in addition to the high-protein diet, it is little wonder that so many people suffer from osteoporosis in this country. When lifestyle factors are taken into account, it is easy to see why osteoporosis has become a major medical problem.

Green Leafy Vegetables Green leafy vegetables (kale, collard greens, parsley, lettuce, and so on) offer significant protection against osteoporosis. These foods are also a rich source of vitamins and minerals such as calcium, vitamin K_1, and boron. Vitamin K_1 is the form of vitamin K that is found in plants. As described in Chapter 3, one often overlooked function of vitamin K_1 is its role in converting inactive osteocalcin into its active form. Osteocalcin is the major noncollagen protein in bone. It serves to anchor calcium molecules and hold them in place within the bone.

A deficiency of vitamin K leads to impaired mineralization of the bone, due to inadequate osteocalcin levels. Very low blood levels of vitamin K_1 have been found in patients with fractures due to osteoporosis.[231] The severity of fracture strongly correlates with the level of circulating vitamin K: the lower the level of vitamin K, the greater the severity of the fracture. Since vitamin K is found in green leafy vegetables, it may be one of the key protective factors of a vegetarian diet against osteoporosis.

In addition to vitamin K_1, the high levels of such minerals as calcium and boron in green leafy vegetables may contribute to this protective effect. Boron is a trace mineral that has recently gained attention as a protective factor against osteoporosis.[232] Boron has been shown to have a positive effect on calcium and active estrogen levels in postmenopausal women—the group at highest risk for developing osteoporosis. In one study, supplementing the diet of postmenopausal women with 3 mg of boron per day reduced urinary calcium excretion by 44 percent and dramatically increased the level of the most biologically active estrogen. It appears that boron is required to activate certain hormones, including estrogen and vitamin D. Since fruits and vegetables are the main dietary sources of boron, diets low in these foods many be deficient in boron. Supplementation with boron is not necessary if the diet is rich in fruits and vegetables.

Other Recommendations

Physical fitness is actually the major determinant of bone density. Physical exercise consisting of 1 hour of moderate activity three times a week has been shown to prevent bone loss. In fact, this type of exercise can actually increase bone mass in postmenopausal women. Walking is probably the best exercise to start with. In contrast to exercise, immobilization doubles the rate of calcium excretion, increasing a person's likelihood of developing osteoporosis.

Coffee, alcohol, and smoking induce a negative calcium balance (more calcium is lost than absorbed) and are associated with an increased risk of developing osteoporosis. Obviously, these lifestyle factors must be eliminated.

Premenstrual Syndrome

Premenstrual syndrome (PMS), also called premenstrual tension, is a recurrent condition in women that is characterized by troublesome, yet often ill-defined, symptoms 7 to 14 days before menstruation. Typical symptoms include decreased energy, tension, irritability, depression, headache, altered sex drive, breast pain, backache, abdominal bloating, and swelling of the fingers and ankles. The syndrome affects about one-third of all women between 30 and 40 years of age, about 10 percent of whom may have a significantly debilitating form.[233]

Although there is a wide spectrum of symptoms, PMS patients exhibit common hormonal patterns when compared to symptom-free control groups. Perhaps the most common pattern is an elevation of plasma estrogen and a drop in plasma progesterone levels 5 to 10 days before the menses.

Dietary Considerations

Compared to symptom-free women, PMS patients consume 62 percent more refined carbohydrates, 275 percent more refined sugar, 79 percent more dairy products, 78 percent more sodium, 53 percent less iron, 77 percent less manganese, and 52 percent less zinc.[234] The first step in addressing PMS is to limit the consumption of refined sugar and to decrease or eliminate milk and dairy products. This will help eliminate some of the nutritional imbalances that eating these foods produces; it will also improve overall nutritional status.

Because many animals (beef and chicken especially) are fed growth-promoting hormones, they should be avoided as well. By decreasing their consumption of meat and dairy foods, women will turn to eating more plant foods to obtain necessary nutrition. As a result, they will decrease their intake of saturated fats and increase their intake of essential fatty acids. This consequence is critical, since many women with PMS have abnormalities in essential fatty acid metabolism.[235]

Furthermore, since vegetarian women are better able to clear estrogen metabolites from the body, deriving protein predominantly from plant foods is associated with more desirable ratios of estrogen to progesterone.[236] This is due to the differing types of bacterial flora associated with a vegetarian diet versus an omnivorous diet. Certain bacteria that are common in the omnivore's colon can synthesize estrogen and can liberate estrogen from bound forms in the colon. Since the primary route of excretion of estrogens is through the feces, an omnivorous diet is associated with increased absorption and reabsorption of estrogens from the intestines and may be a significant cause of the increased estrogen-to-progesterone ratio often seen in PMS. Another factor provided by a high intake of plant foods—especially legumes such as soybeans—is phytoestrogens. Phytoestrogens may help in PMS by antagonizing some of the effects of estrogens.

A diet rich in plant foods also increases the body's levels of magnesium and vitamin B_6, critical nutrients for PMS that have been shown to produce positive effects when supplemented to the diets of women with PMS.[237] Foods with high magnesium and vitamin B_6 levels should be increased in the diet. Items especially rich in these nutrients are whole grains and legumes.

Additional key dietary recommendations for the PMS sufferer include decreasing the intake of salt, alcohol, tobacco, and caffeine-containing foods and beverages such as coffee, tea, and chocolate.[238] Caffeine intake has been shown to produce a dose-dependent effect on the severity of symptoms: the more caffeine consumed, the greater the severity of the symptoms.[239]

Other Recommendations

Numerous studies have utilized vitamin B_6 at high doses (greater than 50 mg per day) in the treatment of PMS.[240] Most clinical studies have reported very good results from this. Although PMS has multiple causes, B_6 supplementation alone appears to benefit most patients.[241] However, following the preceding dietary recommendations and taking a high-potency multiple-vitamin and mineral supplement may provide better results than simply taking mega-doses of B_6.

Prostate Enlargement (BPH)

Nearly 60 percent of men between the ages of 40 and 59 years have an enlarged prostate gland—a condition that is known in the medical community as benign prostatic hyperplasia. Symptoms of BPH typically reflect obstruction of the bladder outlet: progressive urinary frequency, urgency, and nighttime awakening to empty the bladder; and hesitancy and intermittency of urination, with reduced force and caliber of urine. Left untreated, the condition eventually obstructs the bladder outlet, resulting in retention of urine in the blood.

Dietary Considerations

Diet appears to play a critical role in the development of BPH. Paramount to an effective plan of BPH prevention and treatment is adequate zinc intake and absorption. Zinc has been shown to reduce the size of the prostate—as determined by rectal examination, X ray, and endoscopy—and to reduce symptoms in the majority of patients.[242] The clinical efficacy of zinc is probably due to its critical involvement in many aspects of hormonal metabolism.[243]

Foods rich in zinc include nuts and seeds. These foods also provide an excellent source of essential fatty acids. Administering an essential fatty acid (EFA) complex containing linoleic, linolenic, and arachidonic acids has significantly improved urinary tract functioning in many BPH patients.[244] All 19 subjects in one uncontrolled study showed diminution of residual urine, and 12 of the 19 had no residual urine by the end of several weeks of treatment. These effects appear to be due to correction of an underlying essential fatty acid deficiency, since the prostatic and seminal lipid levels and ratios are often abnormal in BPH.[245] Based on this evidence alone, increasing the intake of nuts and seeds or supplementing the diet with an essential fatty acid complex appears indicated.

An old folk remedy for BPH is to eat ¼ to ½ cup of pumpkin seeds each day. This appears to be a very sound recommendation, given the high zinc and essential fatty acid content of pumpkin seeds. Flaxseed oil, sunflower oil, evening primrose oil, and soy oil are all appropriate vegetable oils to add to the diet to ensure that the essential fatty acid requirement is being met. One tablespoon per day is usually sufficient.

Cholesterol Breakdown products of cholesterol have been shown to accumulate in prostates that are affected with either BPH or cancer. These metabolites of cholesterol initiate degeneration of prostatic cells, which in turn can promote prostatic enlargement. Drugs that lower the body's cholesterol levels have been shown to have a favorable influence on BPH, preventing the accumulation of cholesterol in the prostatic cells and limiting subsequent formation of damaging cholesterol metabolites.[246] Every effort should be made to decrease serum cholesterol levels, since elevated cholesterol levels are implicated in so many diseases, including heart disease—the number one killer of Americans. (See the Heart Disease section on pages 300–305 for further discussion of how to lower cholesterol.)

Eating Organic Foods In any effort to treat or prevent BPH, the diet should be as free as possible from pesticides and other contaminants, since many of these compounds (such as dioxin, polyhalogenated biphenyls, hexachlorobenzene, and dibenzofurans) can ultimately lead to BPH.[247] Synthetic hormones fed to animals to fatten them up before slaughter have been shown to produce changes in rat prostates similar to BPH.[248]

It is quite possible that the tremendous increase in the occurrence of BPH in the last few decades is one reflection of the ever-increasing effect toxic chemicals have on our health. A diet rich in natural whole foods may offer some protection, due to the presence in these foods of many protective substances. In particular, minerals (calcium, magnesium, zinc, selenium, germanium, and so on), vitamins, plant pigments (flavonoids, carotenes, chlorophyll, and so on), fiber (especially gel-forming and mucilaginous types), and sulfur-containing compounds possess actions that help the body deal with toxic chemicals and heavy metals.

Other Recommendations

The liposterolic (fat and sterol) extract of saw palmetto (*Serenoa repens*) berries has been shown to greatly improve the signs and symptoms of an enlarged prostate in clinical studies.[249] The dosage is 160 mg of the extract (standardized to contain 85 to 95 percent fatty acids and sterols) twice daily.

Psoriasis

Psoriasis is an extremely common skin disorder. Its rate of occurrence in the United States is between 2 and 4 percent of the population. Psoriasis affects few Blacks and is rare in Native Americans and Blacks in tropical zones. The condition is caused by a pile-up of skin cells that have replicated too rapidly. The rate at which skin cells divide in psoriasis is roughly 1,000 times greater than that in normal skin. This is simply too fast for the cells to be shed, so they accumulate, resulting in the characteristic silvery scale of psoriasis.[250]

Dietary Considerations

A number of dietary factors appear to be responsible for psoriasis, including incomplete protein digestion, alcohol consumption, and excessive consumption of animal fats. Each of these factors will be discussed briefly below.

Protein Digestion and Bowel Toxemia A number of gut-derived toxins are implicated in the development of psoriasis.[251] For example, if protein digestion is incomplete or if intestinal absorption of amino acids is inadequate, bacteria can break the amino acids down into many toxic compounds. A group of toxic amino acids known as polyamines (for example, putrescine, spermidine, and cadaverine) have been shown to be increased in individuals with psoriasis.[252] These compounds contribute greatly to an excessive rate of cell proliferation. Lowered skin and urinary levels of polyamines are associated with clinical improvement in psoriasis.[253] The best way to prevent the excessive formation of polyamines is to maintain protein intake (especially from animal foods) at moderate levels while simultaneously increasing the intake of dietary fiber.

A diet low in dietary fiber is associated with increased levels of gut-derived toxins.[254] Dietary fiber is of critical importance in maintaining a healthy colon. Many fiber components can bind to bowel toxins, promoting their excretion in the feces. It is therefore essential that the diet of an individual with psoriasis be rich in plant foods.

Alcohol Alcohol consumption is known to worsen psoriasis considerably.[255] Alcohol's negative effects are a result of its increasing the absorption of toxins from the gut and impairing liver function. The connection between the liver and psoriasis involves one of the liver's basic tasks: filtering the blood. If the liver is overwhelmed by an increased number of gut-derived toxins, or if the liver's ability to filter these toxins decreases, the level of these compounds circulating in the blood will increase and the psoriasis will get much worse. Therefore, alcohol intake must be eliminated in individuals with psoriasis.

The Role of Fats in Psoriasis Dietary oils are extremely important in the management of psoriasis. Of particular benefit are omega-3 oils like flaxseed oil and fish oils like EPA. Several double-blind clinical studies have demonstrated that supplementing the diet with 10 to 12 grams of EPA produces significant improvement.[256] This amount is roughly equivalent to the amount of EPA in a 5-ounce serving of mackerel, salmon, or herring.

The improvement with EPA supplementation is largely due to EPA's inhibition of the production of inflammatory compounds. In the skin of individuals with psoriasis, the production of inflammatory leukotrienes from arachidonic acid (remember, this is found only in animal foods) is many times greater than normal. It is therefore necessary for these individuals to limit the intake of animal products, particularly animal fats and dairy products.

Psoriatic patients showed remarkable improvements while on a fasting and vegetarian treatment at a Swedish hospital where the effect of such diets on chronic inflammatory disease was being studied.[257] The improvement was probably due not only to the changes in the oil content, but also to decreased levels of gut-derived toxins and polyamines.

Other Recommendations

A special extract of milk thistle known as silymarin was discussed earlier in the Detoxification and Liver Support section (see page 285). Silymarin has been reported to be of value in the treatment of psoriasis, as well.[258] Presumably this is a result of its ability to improve liver function, inhibit inflammation, and reduce excessive cellular proliferation. The standard dosage of silymarin is 70 to 210 mg three times daily.

Rheumatoid Arthritis

Rheumatoid arthritis (RA) is a chronic inflammatory condition that affects the entire body but especially the synovial membranes of the joints. It is a classic example of an "auto-immune disease"—a condition in which the body's immune system attacks the body's own tissue.

In RA, the joints typically involved are the hands, feet, wrists, ankles, and knees. Somewhere between 1 and 3 percent of the population is affected; female patients outnumber males by almost 3:1; and the usual age of onset is 20 to 40 years, although rheumatoid arthritis may begin at any age.[259]

The onset of rheumatoid arthritis is usually gradual, but occasionally it is quite abrupt. Fatigue, low-grade fever, weakness, joint stiffness, and vague joint pain may precede the appearance of painful, swollen joints by several weeks. Several joints are usually involved in the onset, typically in a symmetrical fashion—for example, both hands, wrists, or ankles. In about one-third of persons with RA, initial involvement is confined to one or a few joints.[260]

Involved joints characteristically become quite warm, tender, and swollen. The skin over the joint takes on a ruddy purplish hue. As the disease progresses, joint deformities occur in the hands and feet. Terms used to describe these deformities include: *swan neck, boutonniere,* and *cockup toes.*[261]

There is abundant evidence that rheumatoid arthritis is an auto-immune reaction in which antibodies develop against components of joint tissues. Yet what triggers this reaction remains largely unknown. Speculation and investigation have centered on genetic susceptibility, abnormal bowel permeability, lifestyle and nutritional factors, food allergies, and microorganisms. Rheumatoid arthritis is a classic example of a multifactorial disease in which an interesting assortment of genetic and environmental factors seem to contribute to the disease process. For a full discussion of all of these factors, consult *The Encyclopedia of Natural Medicine.*

Dietary Considerations

Diet has been strongly implicated in many forms of arthritis for many years, in regard to both cause and cure. Various practitioners have recommended all sorts of specific diets for arthritis. In general—since rheumatoid arthritis is not found in societies that eat a more "primitive" diet, and since it is found at a relatively high rate in societies consuming the so-called "Western" diet—a diet rich in whole foods, vegetables, and fiber and low in sugar, meat, refined carbohydrate, and saturated fat seems to be indicated in preventing and possibly in treating rheumatoid arthritis. Strong scientific support exists for the roles that food allergies and dietary fats play in the inflammatory process.

Food Allergy Eliminating allergenic foods from the diet has been shown to offer significant benefit to some individuals with rheumatoid arthritis.[262] An elimination or low-allergenic diet, followed by systematic reintroduction, is often an effective way to isolate offending foods. Virtually any food is capable of aggravating RA, but the most common offending foods are wheat, corn, milk and other dairy products, beef, and nightshade-family foods (tomato, potato, eggplant, peppers, and tobacco).

Fasting, Juicing, and Vegetarian Diet Patients with rheumatoid arthritis have benefited from fasting; however, strict water fasting should only be done under direct medical supervision. Fasting presumably decreases the absorption of allergenic food components, although it may also affect the immune system.[263] A juice fast is safer and may actually yield better results.

A recent study highlights the effectiveness of juicing as part of a healthful diet and lifestyle in relieving rheumatoid arthritis.[264] In a 13-month study conducted in Norway at the Oslo Rheumatism Hospital, two groups of patients suffering from rheumatoid arthritis were studied to determine the effect of diet on their condition. One group followed a therapeutic diet (the treatment group), while members of the other group (control group) were allowed to eat as they wished. Both groups started the study by visiting a "health farm"—what we in America call a "spa"—for 4 weeks.

The treatment group began their therapeutic diet by fasting for 7 to 10 days and then began following a special diet. Dietary intake during the fast consisted of herbal teas, garlic, vegetable broth, decoction of potatoes and parsley, and the following juices: carrots, beets, and celery. No fruit juices were allowed.

After the fast the patients reintroduced a "new" food item every second day. If they noticed any increase in pain, stiffness, or joint swelling within 2 to 48 hours, this item was omitted from the diet for at least 7 days before being reintroduced a second time. If the food caused a worsening of symptoms on the second try, it was dropped permanently from the diet.

The results of the study indicated that short-term fasting followed by a vegetarian diet resulted in "a substantial reduction in disease activity" in many patients. The results indicated a therapeutic benefit beyond what might be expected from elimination of food allergies alone. The authors of the study suggested that the additional improvements were due to changes in dietary fatty acids.

The Role of Dietary Fats Vegetarian diets are often beneficial in the treatment of inflammatory conditions like rheumatoid arthritis, presumably because they decrease the availability of arachidonic acid for conversion into inflammatory prostaglandins and leukotrienes.

Another important way to decrease inflammatory response is to consume cold-water fish such as mackerel, herring, sardines, and salmon. These fish are rich sources of eicosapentaenoic acid (EPA), which competes with arachidonic acid for prostaglandin and leukotriene production. The net effect of consuming these fish or fish oil supplements is a significantly reduced inflammatory/allergic response. Several clinical studies have demonstrated the therapeutic effect of supplementing the diet with EPA (1.8 grams daily) or cod liver oil.[265] However, supplementation may not be necessary if at least one serving of one these cold-water fish is consumed daily. For vegetarians, flaxseed oil, canola oil, and evening primrose oil supplementation may provide similar benefit to EPA, although the research supporting this recommendation is not as solid.[266] Nonetheless, a vegetarian diet alone is clearly therapeutic for many rheumatoid arthritis sufferers.

Individual Nutrients A number of nutrients have been shown to be of benefit to people with rheumatoid arthritis. Most of these nutrients are involved in key antioxidant systems. This highlights the importance of a diet rich in nutrient-dense plant foods and fresh juices. Specific nutrients showing positive effects in rheumatoid arthritis include selenium, vitamin E, manganese, vitamin C, zinc, and pantothenic acid.[267] Consuming a diet rich in all classes of plant foods is the best way to ensure adequate levels of these nutrients in the body.

Special Foods The importance of flavonoids to joint structures was discussed earlier. Several bioflavonoids have demonstrated effects in experimental studies that indicate their potential value to individuals with rheumatoid arthritis (see Chapter 4 for a complete discussion). Good sources of the most beneficial flavonoids are cherries, berries, and citrus fruits.

Fresh pineapple may offer some benefit due to the presence of bromelain, a well-recognized anti-inflammatory enzyme. During flare-ups, fresh pineapple juice and fresh ginger may help because of their anti-inflammatory activity. Ginger exerts an anti-inflammatory action by inhibiting the manufacture of inflammatory compounds and by introducing an anti-inflammatory enzyme similar to bromelain. In one clinical study, seven patients with rheumatoid arthritis for whom conventional drugs had provided only temporary or partial relief were treated with ginger.[268] One patient took 50 grams per day of lightly cooked ginger while the remaining six took either 5 grams of fresh or 0.1 to 1 gram of powdered ginger daily. All patients reported substantial improvement, including pain relief, increased joint mobility, and decreased swelling and morning stiffness.[269]

Fresh ginger root is available at most grocery stores. Juicing fresh ginger along with fresh pineapple juice creates a delicious drink that offers significant benefit to sufferers of arthritis (see also the Osteoarthritis section on pages 326, 327).

Other Recommendations

Curcumin preparations available at health-food stores may be useful in countering inflammation. Standard physical therapy measures such as exercise, heat, cold, and massage—and the use of special physical therapy equipment such as diathermy, lasers, and paraffin baths—are also quite important in bringing relief.

Ulcer

The term *ulcer* usually refers to a peptic ulcer—any of a group of ulcerative disorders of the upper gastrointestinal tract. The major forms of peptic ulcer are the chronic duodenal ulcer and the gastric (stomach) ulcer. Although duodenal and gastric ulcerations occur at different locations, they appear to be the result of similar mechanisms. Specifically, their development is generally thought to be the result of damage by pepsin and stomach acids to the lining of the duodenum or stomach. Normally, enough protective factors are present to prevent the ulcer's formation; but when the integrity of these protective factors is decreased, ulceration occurs.

Although symptoms of a peptic ulcer may be absent or quite vague, peptic ulcers are usually associated with abdominal discomfort noted 45 to 60 minutes after meals or during the night. In the typical case, the pain is described as gnawing, burning, cramplike, or aching, or as "heartburn." Consuming antacids usually provides great relief.

The natural approach to peptic ulcers involves first identifying and then eliminating or reducing all factors that may contribute to the ulcers' development: food allergy, low-fiber diet, cigarette smoking, stress, and drugs such as aspirin and other nonsteroidal analgesics. Once the causative factors have been controlled or eliminated, the focus can be directed at healing the ulcers and promoting healthy tissue resistance.

NOTE: Patients with any symptoms of a peptic ulcer need competent medical care. Peptic ulcer complications such as hemorrhage, perforation, and obstruction constitute medical emergencies and require immediate hospitalization. Patients with peptic ulcers should be monitored by a physician, even if they are following the natural approaches discussed here.

Dietary Considerations

Strange as it may seem, clinical and experimental evidence points to food allergy as a prime causative factor in peptic ulcer.[270] The association between allergy and peptic ulcer has been investigated in several studies. In one study, 98 percent of patients with radiographic evidence of peptic ulcer had coexisting lower and upper respiratory tract allergic disease; and in another study, 25 of 43 allergic children had X-ray-diagnosed peptic ulcers.[271]

An elimination diet has been used with great success in treating and preventing recurrent ulcers. Food allergy is also consistent with the high recurrence rate of peptic ulcers. If food allergy is the cause, the ulcer will continue to recur until the food has been eliminated from the diet. Ironically, many people with peptic ulcers soothe themselves by consuming inordinate amounts of milk, a highly allergenic food.

Fiber A diet rich in fiber is associated with a reduced rate of peptic ulcers as compared with a low-fiber diet. The therapeutic use of a high-fiber diet in patients with recently healed duodenal ulcers has been shown to reduce the recurrence rate by half.[272] This is probably a result of fiber's ability to promote a healthy protective layer of mucin in the stomach and intestines.

Cabbage Juice As mentioned in Chapter 5, cabbage juice has been shown to be extremely effective in the treatment of peptic ulcers. Dr. Garnett Cheney from Stanford University's School of Medicine and other researchers in the 1950s clearly demonstrated that fresh cabbage juice is extremely effective in treating peptic ulcers—usually in less than 7 days. Further research has shown that the high glutamine content of the juice is probably responsible for the efficacy of cabbage in treating these ulcers. Here is one of Dr. Cheney's favorite juice recipe recommendations:

½ head or 2 cups of green cabbage

4 ribs of celery

2 carrots

Green cabbages are best, but red cabbages are also useful. Cut the cabbage into long wedges and feed these through the juicer, followed by the celery and then the carrots.

Other Recommendations

A special licorice extract known as "deglycyrrhizinated licorice" or DGL for short, is a remarkable antiulcer agent.[273] DGL's mode of action differs from that of medications currently used to treat peptic ulcers. Rather than inhibiting the release of acid, licorice stimulates the normal defense mechanisms that prevent ulcer formation. Numerous studies over the years have found DGL to be an effective antiulcer compound. In several head-to-head comparison studies, DGL has been shown to be more effective than Tagamet, Zantac, or antacids in both short-term treatment and maintenance therapy of peptic ulcers.[274] Moreover, while these drugs are associated with significant side effects, DGL is extremely safe and is available at only a fraction of the cost. The standard dose for DGL is two to four 380-mg tablets between or 20 minutes before meals. DGL should be continued for 8 to 16 weeks, depending on the response.

Varicose Veins

Varicose veins affect nearly 50 percent of middle-aged adults. The veins just under the skin of the legs are the veins most commonly affected, due to the tremendous strain that standing has on them. When an individual stands for long periods of time, the pressure exerted against the veins can increase up to 10 times. Hence, individuals with occupations that require long periods of standing are at greatest risk for developing varicose veins.

About four times more women are affected than men; obese individuals are at much greater risk; and the risk increases with age because of loss of tissue tone, loss of muscle mass, and weakening of the walls of the veins. Pregnancy may also lead to the development of varicose veins, since pregnancy increases venous pressure in the legs.[275]

In general, varicose veins do little harm if the vein in question is near the surface. These types of varicose veins are, however, cosmetically unappealing. Although significant symptoms are not common, the legs may feel heavy, tight, and tired. A more serious form of varicose veins involves obstruction and valve defects of the deeper veins of the leg.

Dietary Considerations

The relevant considerations here are similar to the findings with regard to hemorrhoids. Unlike in the United States and Great Britain, varicose veins are rarely seen in parts of the world where high-fiber, unrefined diets are consumed.[276] A low-fiber diet, high in refined foods, contributes to the development of varicose veins. Individuals who consume a low-fiber diet tend to strain more during bowel movements, since their smaller and harder stools are more difficult to pass. This straining increases the pressure in the abdomen, which obstructs the flow of blood up the legs. The increased pressure may, over time, significantly weaken the vein wall, leading to the formation of varicose veins (or hemorrhoids); or it may weaken the wall of the large intestine and produce diverticuli (small pockets) in the large intestine.[277]

A high-fiber diet is the most important element in treating and preventing varicose veins (and hemorrhoids). A diet rich in vegetables, fruits, legumes, and grains promotes easy bowel movements; and many fiber components attract water and form a gelatinous mass that keeps the feces soft, bulky, and easy to pass. The net effect of a high-fiber diet is significantly less straining during defecation.

Natural bulking compounds can also be used for this purpose. These substances, particularly psyllium seed husks, oat bran, and guar gum, exert a mild laxative action due to their ability to attract water and form a gelatinous mass. This keeps the feces soft and promotes peristalsis, significantly reducing straining during defecation. These types of fibers are generally less irritating than wheat bran and other cellulose fiber products.

Flavonoid-rich Foods Since increasing the integrity of the wall of the vein may also reduce the risk of developing varicose veins, flavonoid-rich berries such as cherries, blueberries, currants, and blackberries may be beneficial in preventing and treating varicose veins. Extracts of several of these berries are widely used as medications in Europe for various circulatory conditions, including varicose veins.[278]

The efficacy of these extracts is related to their ability to do four things: reduce capillary fragility; increase the integrity of the venous wall; inhibit the breakdown of the compounds that compose the ground substance; and increase the muscular tone of the vein. Consuming these berries or their extracts is indicated for individuals with varicose veins, as well as for individuals who wish to prevent them.

Bromelain and Other Fibrinolytic Compounds Individuals with varicose veins have a decreased ability to break down fibrin.[279] This is extremely important. When fibrin is deposited in the tissue near the varicose veins, the skin becomes hard and "lumpy" due to the presence of the fibrin and fat. In addition, a decreased ability to breakdown fibrin increases the risk of thrombus formation, which may result in thrombophlebitis, a heart attack, pulmonary embolism, or stroke.

Foods that increase the fibrinolytic activity of the blood are therefore indicated. Cayenne pepper, garlic, onion, and ginger all increase fibrin breakdown.[280] Liberal consumption of these spices in foods is recommended for individuals with varicose veins and other disorders of the cardiovascular system. Bromelain, from fresh pineapple, also promotes the breakdown of fibrin.[281]

Other Recommendations

Exercising and avoiding standing for long periods of time will reduce a person's risk of developing varicose veins. Walking, riding a bike, or jogging is particularly beneficial, since the contraction of leg muscles pushes pooled blood back into circulation.

Epilogue

What Is Naturopathic Medicine?

> *"Nature is doing her best each moment to make us well. She exists for no other end. Do not resist. With the least inclination to be well, we should not be sick."*
>
> —*Henry David Thoreau*

Naturopathy or "nature cure" is a method of healing that employs various natural means to empower an individual to achieve the highest level of health possible. Although the terms *naturopathy* and *naturopathic medicine* were not used until late in the nineteenth century, their philosophical roots go back thousands of years. Drawing on the healing wisdom of many cultures, including India (Ayurvedic), China (Taoist), and Greece (Hippocratic), naturopathic medicine is a system of medicine founded on six time-tested medical principles:

Principle 1. Nature possesses healing powers.

Naturopathic physicians believe that the body has considerable power to heal itself. The physician's role is to facilitate and enhance this process with the aid of natural, nontoxic therapies.

Principle 2. Identify and treat the cause.

The naturopathic physician is trained to seek the underlying causes of a disease rather than simply to suppress the symptoms. Symptoms are viewed as expressions of the body's attempt to heal itself, while the causes may have physical, mental/emotional, and spiritual sources.

Principle 3. First do no harm.

The naturopathic physician seeks to do no harm with medical treatment, by employing safe and effective natural therapies.

Principle 4. Treat the whole person.

Naturopathic physicians are trained to view an individual as being a whole composed of complex interactions of physical, mental/emotional, spiritual, social, and other factors.

Principle 5. The physician is a teacher.

The naturopathic physician is foremost a teacher, educating, empowering, and motivating the patient to assume more personal responsibility for his or her health by adopting a health-affirming attitude, lifestyle, and diet.

Principle 6. Prevention is the best cure.

Naturopathic physicians are preventive medicine specialists. Disease prevention is accomplished through education and altered life habits that support health.

Naturopathy: A Historical Perspective

Despite its philosophical links to many cultures, Western naturopathic medicine grew out of alternative healing systems of the eighteenth and nineteenth centuries. The European tradition of "taking the cure" at natural springs or spas had gained a foothold in America by the middle of the eighteenth century. The custom helped make Germany and the United States especially receptive to the ideas of naturopathy. Among the movement's earliest promoters were Father Sebastian Kneipp, a priest who credited his recovery from tuberculosis to bathing in the Danube, and Benedict Lust, a physician who trained at the water-cure clinic that Kneipp founded in Europe. Lust arrived in the United States in the 1890s and began using the term *naturopathy* to describe an eclectic compilation of doctrines of natural healing. In 1902, Lust opened the first naturopathic college of medicine in the United States, in New York City.

The early naturopaths attached great importance to a natural, healthful diet. So did many of their contemporaries. John Kellogg—a physician, Seventh-Day Adventist, and vegetarian—ran the Adventist Battle Creek Sanitarium, which utilized natural therapies; his brother, Will, built and ran a factory in Battle Creek, Michigan, to produce such health foods as shredded wheat and granola biscuits. Driven by personal convictions about the benefits of cereal fibers and by commercial interests, the Kellogg brothers (along with a former employee, C. W. Post) helped popularize naturopathic ideas about food.

Naturopathic medicine grew and flourished in the early part of the twentieth century. But in the mid-1930s, several factors enabled the medical profession to establish the foundation for its current virtual monopoly over health care:

1. Foundations, supported by the drug industry, began heavily subsidizing medical schools.
2. The medical profession finally stopped using "heroic" therapies (blood letting and mercury dosing) and was able to replace these with new therapies that were more effective for treating symptoms and much less toxic.
3. The medical profession became more politically astute and was able to convince both the public and politicians of the apparent superiority of its system, leading to legislation that severely restricted the viability of other healthcare systems.

Naturopathy has experienced a tremendous resurgence in the last two decades. This is largely due to increased public awareness of the role of diet and lifestyle in the cause of chronic disease, and the failure of modern medicine to deal effectively with these disorders.

Naturopathic Medical Schools

Currently, the Bastyr College of Natural Health Sciences in Seattle, founded in 1978, is the only fully accredited school that trains naturopathic physicians, although the National College of Naturopathic Medicine, in Portland, Oregon, founded in 1956, is currently a candidate for accreditation. (Accreditation is done by the Council of Naturopathic Medical Education and by regional accrediting agencies of the U.S. Department of Education.) Both colleges offer a 4-year doctoral program leading to the Doctor of Naturopathic Medicine (N.D.) degree. Preadmission requirements at both schools are a conventional undergraduate premedical program designed to prepare entering students for 4 years of training in basic medical and clinical science as well as in naturopathic treatments. For more information, write the following addresses (or telephone):

Bastyr College of Natural Health Sciences
144 N.E. 54th St.
Seattle, WA 98105
(206) 523-9585

National College of Naturopathic Medicine
11231 S.E. Market St.
Portland, OR 97216
(503) 255-4860

Professional Licensure

The American Association of Naturopathic Physicians (AANP) is the professional organization of licensed naturopathic physicians. It is seeking to expand licensure of naturopaths in individual states and provinces. Although naturopaths practice in virtually every state and Canadian province, currently only Alaska, Alberta, Arizona, British Columbia, Connecticut, District of Columbia, Hawaii, Manitoba, Montana, Ontario, Oregon, Saskatchewan, and Washington offer licensure to naturopaths. The organization is also seeking to differentiate the professionally trained naturopath from the unscrupulous individual claiming to be a naturopath on the basis of having received a "mail-order" degree. For more information and for a referral service, write to the following address (or telephone):

American Association of Naturopathic Physicians
P.O. Box 20386
Seattle, WA 98102
(206) 323-7610

What a Naturopath Is Trained to Do

The modern naturopathic physician provides all phases of primary health care. This means that he or she is trained to be the doctor first seen by the patient for general (nonemergency) health care. In addition to providing recommendations on lifestyle, diet, and exercise, naturopathic physicians may use various healing techniques. Some naturopathic physicians emphasize one particular healing technique, while others are more eclectic and use a number of techniques. Still other naturopaths specialize in a particular medical field, such as pediatrics, natural childbirth, or physical medicine.

Naturopathy is inclusive, incorporating various healing techniques. The current scope of treatments that naturopathic physicians receive training in include clinical nutrition, botanical or herbal medicine, homeopathy, Oriental medicine and acupuncture, hydrotherapy, physical medicine (including massage and therapeutic manipulation), counseling and other psychotherapies, and minor surgery.

Clinical Nutrition

Clinical nutrition, or the use of diet as a therapy, serves as the foundation of naturopathic medicine. An ever-increasing body of knowledge supports the use of whole foods and nutritional supplements to maintain health and treat disease.

Botanical Medicine

Plants have been used as medicines since antiquity. Naturopathic physicians are professionally trained herbalists and know both the historical uses of plants and modern pharmacological mechanisms.

Homeopathy

The term *homeopathy* is derived from the Greek words *homeos,* meaning similar, and *pathos,* meaning disease. Homeopathy is a system of medicine that treats a disease with a dilute, potentized agent or drug that, when given to a healthy individual, produces the same symptoms the disease does. The fundamental principle here is that like cures like. Homeopathic medicines are derived from a wide range of plant, mineral, and chemical substances.

Oriental Medicine and Acupuncture

Acupuncture is an ancient Chinese system of medicine involving the stimulation of specific points on the body to enhance the flow of vital energy (*Chi*) along pathways called *meridians.* Acupuncture points can be stimulated by the insertion and withdrawal of needles, by the application of heat (moxibustion), by massage, by laser, by electrical means, or by a combination of these methods.

Hydrotherapy

Hydrotherapy may be defined as the use of water in any of its forms (hot, cold, ice, steam, and so on) and methods of application (sitz bath, douche, spa and hot tub, whirlpool, sauna, shower, immersion bath, pack, poultice, foot bath, fomentation, wrap, colonic irrigations, and so on) to help maintain health or treat disease. It is an ancient method of treatment. Hydrotherapy has been used to treat disease and injury by many different cultures, including the Egyptians, Assyrians, Persians, Greeks, Hebrews, Hindus, and Chinese.

Physical Medicine

Physical medicine refers to the use of physical measures in the treatment of an individual. This includes the use of physiotherapy equipment such as ultrasound, diathermy, and other electromagnetic energy agents; therapeutic exercise; massage; joint mobilization (manipulative) and immobilization techniques; and hydrotherapy.

Counseling and Lifestyle Modification

Counseling and lifestyle modification techniques are essential to the naturopathic physician. A naturopath is formally trained in the following counseling areas:

- Interviewing and responding skills, active listening, assessing body language, and other contact skills necessary for the therapeutic relationship
- Recognizing and understanding prevalent psychological issues, including developmental problems, abnormal behavior, addictions, stress, and sexuality
- Various treatment measures, including hypnosis and guided imagery, counseling techniques, correction of underlying organic factors, and family therapy

What to Expect when You Visit a Naturopath

A typical first office visit with a naturopathic doctor takes 1 hour. Since naturopathic physicians consider teaching the patient how to live healthfully to be one of their primary goals, the time devoted to discussing and explaining principles of health maintenance is one aspect that sets naturopaths apart from orthodox physicians, who often seem to be rushing from one patient to the next.

The relationship begins with a thorough medical history and interview process designed to view all aspects of a patient's lifestyle. If necessary, the physician will perform standard diagnostic procedures, including physical exam and blood and urine analysis. Once a good understanding of the patient's health and disease status is established (and diagnosing a disease is only one part of this process), the doctor and patient work together to establish a treatment and health-promoting program.

The Future of Naturopathic Medicine

To the uninformed, naturopathic medicine—and indeed the entire concept of natural medicine—appears to be a passing fad. To the informed, naturopathic medicine is quite clearly at the forefront of future health care.

One great fallacy promoted by the U.S. medical establishment is that no firm scientific evidence supports the use of many natural therapies. This assumption is simply untrue. In fact, during the last 10 to 20 years, an explosion of information supporting the use of natural medicines has occurred in the scientific literature.

Science and medicine now possess the technology and understanding needed to appreciate many aspects of natural medicine. It is becoming increasingly common for medical organizations that in the past have spoken out strongly against naturopathic medicine to endorse such naturopathic techniques as lifestyle modification, stress reduction, exercise, and dietary measures such as consuming a high-fiber diet rich in plant foods.

This illustrates the paradigm shift that is now occurring in medicine. What was once scoffed at is now becoming generally accepted as constituting an effective alternative. In fact, in most instances the naturopathic alternative offers significant benefit over standard medical practices. In the future, many of the concepts, philosophies, and practices of naturopathy will undoubtedly be vindicated. The future looks very bright for naturopathic medicine.

Appendix

Tables of Nutritive Values of Various Food Groups

Table A.1 Nutritive Value of Edible Part of Selected Vegetables

									Minerals (Macro)					Minerals (Micro)		
Food Item Name	*Approximate Measure*	*Weight (g)*	*Moisture (%)*	*Food Energy Calories (kcal)*	*Protein (g)*	*Fats (g)*	*Carbohydrates (g)*	*Fiber (g)*	*Calcium (mg)*	*Phosphorus (mg)*	*Sodium (mg)*	*Magnesium (mg)*	*Potassium (mg)*	*Iron (mg)*	*Zinc (mg)*	*Copper (mg)*
Artichokes																
Globe or French, boiled, drained	1 lg	100	90.2	38.0	3.4	.1	5.8	1.9	67.0	67.0	30.0	27.2	301.0	.90	.35	(.03)
Asparagus																
spears, raw	5 spears	100	91.7	26.0	2.5	.2	5.0	.7	22.0	62.0	2.0	20.0	278.0	1.00	.70	.04
fresh, cooked, drained	5 spears	100	93.6	20.0	2.2	.2	3.6	.7	21.0	50.0	1.0	(10.3)	183.0	.60	(.31)	(.22)
Beet Greens																
raw	1 cup	33	90.9	7.9	.7	.1	1.5	.4	39.3	13.2	42.9	35.0	188.1	1.09	.01	—
boiled, drained	1 cup	200	93.6	36.0	3.4	.4	6.6	2.2	198.0	50.0	152.0	—	664.0	3.80	—	—
Beets																
raw	1 cup	170	87.3	73.1	2.7	.2	16.8	1.4	27.2	56.1	102.0	42.5	569.5	1.19	.20	.03
fresh, boiled, drained	1 cup	200	90.9	64.0	2.2	.2	14.4	1.6	28.0	46.0	86.0	—	416.0	1.00	.25	—
Bell (Sweet) Peppers																
green, raw	1 med	40	93.4	8.8	.5	.1	1.9	.6	3.6	8.8	5.2	7.2	85.2	.28	.01	.02
green, boiled, drained	1 oz	28	94.7	5.0	.3	.1	1.1	.4	2.5	4.5	2.5	(2.8)	41.7	.14	(.06)	(.02)
red, raw	1 avg	90	90.7	27.9	1.3	.3	6.4	1.5	11.7	27.0	5.4	11.7	108.0	.54	—	—
Broccoli																
spears, raw	1 cup	155	89.1	49.6	5.6	.5	9.1	2.3	159.7	120.9	23.3	28.7	592.1	1.71	1.01	1.24
spears, cooked	1 cup	150	91.3	39.0	4.7	.5	6.8	2.4	132.0	93.0	15.0	—	400.5	1.20	.23	—
Brussels Sprouts																
raw	1 med	10	85.2	4.5	.5	Trace	.8	.2	3.6	8.0	1.4	2.9	39.0	.15	—	—
cooked	1 cup	150	88.2	54.0	6.3	.6	9.6	2.4	48.0	108.0	15.0	—	409.5	1.65	.54	—

	Fat-Soluble Vitamins		Water-Soluble Vitamins						
Food Item Name	*Vitamin A (IU)*	*Vitamin E (Alpha Tocopherol) (mg)*	*Vitamin C (mg)*	*Thiamine (mg)*	*Riboflavin (mg)*	*Niacin (mg)*	*Pantothenic Acid (mg)*	*Vitamin B_6 (Pyridoxine) (mg)*	*Folacin (Folic Acid) (mcg)*
Artichokes									
Globe or French, boiled, drained	90.0	—	8.40	.07	.03	.93	.21	.07	32.00
Asparagus									
spears, raw	900.0	—	33.00	.18	.20	1.50	.62	.15	109.0
fresh, cooked, drained	900.0	(2.50)	26.00	.16	.18	1.40	(.14)	(.04)	(30.06)
Beet Greens									
raw	2013.0	0.57	9.90	.03	.07	.13	.08	.03	—
boiled, drained	10200.0	—	30.00	.14	.30	.60	—	—	—
Beets									
raw	34.0	—	17.00	.05	.09	.68	.26	.09	22.95
fresh, boiled, drained	40.0	—	12.00	.06	.08	.60	—	—	156.00
Bell (Sweet) Peppers									
green raw	168.0	(.32)	51.20	.032	.03	.20	.09	.10	7.60
green, boiled, drained	117.6	(.23)	26.88	.017	.02	.14	(.05)	(.04)	(3.11)
red, raw	4005.0	—	183.60	.072	.07	.45	.24	—	—
Broccoli									
spears, raw	3875.0	2.00	175.15	.26	.36	1.4	1.55	.33	201.50
spears, cooked	3750.0	—	135.00	.14	.30	1.20	—	—	84.00
Brussels Sprouts									
raw	55.0	—	10.20	.01	.02	.09	.07	.02	4.90
cooked	780.0	—	130.50	.12	.21	1.20	—	—	54.00

Table A.1 *(continued)*

Food Item Name	Approximate Measure	Weight (g)	Moisture (%)	Food Energy Calories (kcal)	Protein (g)	Fats (g)	Carbohydrates (g)	Fiber (g)	Minerals (Macro) Calcium (mg)	Phosphorus (mg)	Sodium (mg)	Magnesium (mg)	Potassium (mg)	Minerals (Micro) Iron (mg)	Zinc (mg)	Copper (mg)
Cabbage																
common, raw	1 cup	70	92.4	16.8	1.0	.1	3.8	.6	34.3	20.3	14.0	9.1	163.1	.28	.28	.04
common, shredded, cooked in small amount of water	1 cup	145	93.9	29.0	1.6	.3	6.2	1.2	63.8	29.0	20.3	—	236.4	.44	.58	—
red, raw	1 cup	100	90.2	31.0	2.0	.2	6.9	1.0	42.0	35.0	26.0	17.0	268.0	.80	.34	.10
Cabbage, Chinese (Bok Choy)																
raw	1 cup	44	95.0	6.2	.5	0	1.3	.3	18.9	17.6	10.1	6.2	171.3	.26	.28	—
Carrots																
raw	1 lg	100	59.0	42.0	1.2	.2	9.7	1.0	37.0	36.0	47.0	18.5	341.0	.70	.40	.01
boiled, drained	1 cup	150	91.2	46.5	1.4	.3	10.7	1.5	49.5	46.5	49.5	9.3	333.0	.90	.45	(.12)
Cauliflower																
raw	1 cup	100	91.0	27.0	2.7	.2	5.2	1.0	25.0	56.0	13.0	24.0	295.0	1.10	.34	.14
boiled, drained	1 cup	120	92.8	26.4	2.8	.2	4.9	1.2	25.2	50.4	10.8	(10.7)	247.2	.84	.40	(.04)
Celery																
raw	4 ribs	100	94.1	17.0	.9	.1	3.9	.6	39.0	28.0	126.0	8.7	341.0	.30	.07	.01
boiled, drained	1 cup	125	95.3	17.5	1.0	.1	3.9	.8	38.8	27.5	110.0	3.9	298.8	.25	(.13)	.13
Chives																
raw	1 tbls	10	91.3	2.8	.2	Trace	.6	.1	6.9	4.4	—	2.4	25.0	.17	—	—
Collards																
leaves w/stems, cooked in small amount of water	1 cup	200	90.8	58.0	5.4	1.2	9.8	1.6	304.0	78.0	50.0	—	468.0	1.20	.05	(.08)

	Fat-Soluble Vitamins		*Water-Soluble Vitamins*						
Food Item Name	*Vitamin A (IU)*	*Vitamin E (Alpha Tocopherol) (mg)*	*Vitamin C (mg)*	*Thiamine (mg)*	*Riboflavin (mg)*	*Niacin (mg)*	*Pantothenic Acid (mg)*	*Vitamin B_6 (Pyridoxine) (mg)*	*Folacin (Folic Acid) (mcg)*
Cabbage									
common, raw	91.0	.04	32.90	.04	.04	.21	.14	.11	46.20
common, shredded, cooked in small amount of water	188.5	—	47.85	.06	.06	.44	—	—	26.10
red, raw	40.0	.22	61.00	.09	.06	.40	.32	.20	34.00
Cabbage, Chinese (Bok Choy)									
raw	66.0	—	11.00	.02	.02	.26	—	—	36.52
Carrots									
raw	11000.0	.45	0	.06	.05	.60	.28	.15	32.00
boiled, drained	15750.0	.17	9.00	.08	.08	.75	(.29)	(.15)	36.00
Cauliflower									
raw	60.0	(.22)	78.00	.11	.10	.70	1.00	.21	55.00
boiled, drained	72.0	(.14)	66.00	.11	.10	.72	(.52)	(.16)	40.80
Celery									
raw	240.0	.46	9.00	.03	.03	.30	.43	.06	12.00
boiled, drained	287.5	.48	7.50	.03	.04	.38	(.37)	(.75)	(7.56)
Chives									
raw	580.0	—	5.60	.01	.01	.05	—	.02	—
Collards									
leaves w/stems, cooked in small amount of water	10800.0	—	92.00	.28	.40	2.40	—	—	—

Table A.1 (*continued*)

										Minerals (Macro)					Minerals (Micro)		
Food Item Name	*Approximate Measure*	*Weight (g)*	*Moisture (%)*	*Food Energy Calories (kcal)*	*Protein (g)*	*Fats (g)*	*Carbohydrates (g)*	*Fiber (g)*	*Calcium (mg)*	*Phosphorus (mg)*	*Sodium (mg)*	*Magnesium (mg)*	*Potassium (mg)*	*Iron (mg)*	*Zinc (mg)*	*Copper (mg)*
Cucumbers																
raw, not pared	1 med	100	95.1	15.0	.9	.1	3.4	.6	25.0	27.0	6.0	12.0	160.0	1.10	.12	.01
raw, pared	1 med	100	95.7	14.0	.6	.1	3.2	.3	17.0	18.0	6.0	10.0	160.0	.30	—	—
Dandelions																
raw	1 cup	142	85.6	63.9	3.8	1.0	13.1	2.3	265.5	93.7	107.9	51.1	563.7	4.40	.62	.21
boiled, drained	1 cup	200	89.8	66.0	4.0	1.2	12.8	2.6	280.0	84.0	88.0	—	464.0	3.60	.80	—
Eggplant																
raw	½ cup	100	92.4	25.0	1.1	.2	5.6	.9	12.0	26.0	2.0	82.0	214.0	.70	—	.01
boiled, drained	1 cup	200	94.3	38.0	2.2	.4	8.2	1.8	22.0	42.0	2.0	—	300.0	1.20	.24	—
Fennel																
common, leaves, raw	1 cup	60	90.0	16.8	1.7	.2	3.1	.3	60.0	30.6	—	—	238.2	1.62	—	—
Garlic																
clove, raw	1 avg	3	61.3	4.1	.2	0	.9	0	.9	6.1	.6	.7	15.9	.05	.02	.01
Jerusalem Artichokes																
raw	3½ oz	100	79.8	41.0	2.3	.1	16.7	.8	14.0	78.0	—	11.0	—	3.40	.06	—
Kale																
boiled, drained, leaves w/stems	1 cup	110	91.2	30.8	3.5	.8	4.4	1.2	147.4	50.6	47.3	—	243.1	1.32	.30	—
Onions																
young green, raw, bulb & entire top	1 med	20	89.4	7.2	.3	0	1.6	.2	10.2	7.8	1.0	(2.2)	46.2	.20	.06	.01

	Fat-Soluble Vitamins		Water-Soluble Vitamins						
Food Item Name	*Vitamin A (IU)*	*Vitamin E (Alpha Tocopherol) (mg)*	*Vitamin C (mg)*	*Thiamine (mg)*	*Riboflavin (mg)*	*Niacin (mg)*	*Pantothenic Acid (mg)*	*Vitamin B_6 (Pyridoxine) (mg)*	*Folacin (Folic Acid) (mcg)*
Cucumbers									
raw, not pared	250.0	Trace	11.00	.03	.04	.20	.25	.04	(16.05)
raw, pared	—	—	11.00	.03	.04	.20	—	.05	15.00
Dandelions									
raw	19880.0	—	49.70	.27	.37	1.14	—	—	—
boiled, drained	23400.0	—	36.00	.26	.32	—	—	—	—
Eggplant									
raw	10.0	—	5.00	.05	.05	.60	.22	.08	—
boiled, drained	20.0	—	6.00	.10	.08	1.00	—	—	32.00
Fennel									
common, leaves, raw	2100.0	—	18.60	—	—	—	.15	.06	—
Garlic									
clove, raw	—	—	.45	.01	Trace	.02	—	—	—
Jerusalem Artichokes									
raw	20.0	—	4.00	.20	.06	1.30	.07	0	—
Kale									
boiled, drained, leaves w/stems	8140.0	—	68.20	—	—	—	—	—	—
Onions									
young green, raw, bulb & entire top	400.0	Trace	6.40	.01	.01	.08	.03	(.02)	(8.04)

Table A.1 *(continued)*

Food Item Name	Approximate Measure	Weight (g)	Moisture (%)	Food Energy Calories (kcal)	Protein (g)	Fats (g)	Carbohydrates (g)	Fiber (g)	Minerals (Macro) Calcium (mg)	Phosphorus (mg)	Sodium (mg)	Magnesium (mg)	Potassium (mg)	Minerals (Micro) Iron (mg)	Zinc (mg)	Copper (mg)
young green, raw, tops only (green portion)	1 cup	100	91.8	27.0	1.6	.4	5.5	1.3	56.0	39.0	5.0	24.0	231.0	2.20	—	—
mature (dry), yellow, raw	1 med	110	89.1	41.8	1.5	.1	9.6	.7	29.7	39.6	11.0	13.2	172.7	.55	.33	.11
mature (dry), yellow, boiled, drained	1 cup	210	91.8	60.9	2.5	.2	13.7	1.2	50.4	60.9	14.7	—	231.0	.84	—	—
Parsley																
raw	1 tbls	4	85.1	1.8	.1	0	.3	.1	8.1	2.5	1.8	1.6	29.1	.25	.04	0
dried	1 tsp	1	9.0	2.8	.2	0	.5	.1	14.7	3.5	4.5	2.5	38.1	.98	.05	.01
Parsnips																
raw	1 lg	200	79.1	152.0	3.4	1.0	35.0	4.0	100.0	154.0	24.0	91.2	1082.0	1.40	(.22)	.20
boiled, drained	1 cup	200	82.2	132.0	3.0	1.0	29.8	4.0	90.0	124.0	16.0	25.2	758.0	1.20	(.22)	(.26)
Potatoes																
raw	1 avg	100	79.8	76.0	2.1	.1	17.1	.5	7.0	53.0	3.0	14.0	407.0	.60	.30	.05
baked in skin	1 med	100	75.1	93.0	2.6	.1	21.1	.6	9.0	65.0	4.0	(28.8)	503.0	.70	(.31)	(.18)
boiled in skin	1 med	100	79.8	76.0	2.1	.1	17.1	.5	7.0	53.0	3.0	—	407.0	.60	.30	—
boiled, pared before cooking	1 med	100	82.8	65.0	1.9	.1	14.5	.5	6.0	42.0	2.0	(15.3)	285.0	.50	.30	(.12)
mashed, milk added	1 cup	200	82.8	130.0	4.2	1.4	26.0	.8	48.0	98.0	602.0	—	522.0	.80	.60	—
fried from raw	1 cup	170	46.9	455.6	6.8	24.1	55.4	1.7	25.5	171.7	379.1	—	1317.5	1.87	.23	—
french fried in cottonseed oil	1 piece	5	44.7	13.7	.2	.7	1.8	.1	.8	5.6	.3	—	42.7	.07	—	—

	Fat-Soluble Vitamins		Water-Soluble Vitamins						
Food Item Name	*Vitamin A (IU)*	*Vitamin E (Alpha Tocopherol) (mg)*	*Vitamin C (mg)*	*Thiamine (mg)*	*Riboflavin (mg)*	*Niacin (mg)*	*Pantothenic Acid (mg)*	*Vitamin B_6 (Pyridoxine) (mg)*	*Folacin (Folic Acid) (mcg)*
young green, raw, tops only (green portion)	4000.0	—	51.00	.07	.10	.60	—	—	80.00
mature (dry), yellow, raw	44.0	.24	11.00	.03	.04	.22	.14	.14	27.50
mature (dry), yellow, boiled, drained	84.0	—	14.70	.06	.06	.42	—	—	27.30
Parsley									
raw	340.0	(.07)	6.88	Trace	.01	.05	.01	.01	4.64
dried	233.4	(2.13)	1.22	Trace	.01	.08	(.68)	.01	(61.20)
Parsnips									
raw	60.0	(2.08)	32.00	.16	.18	.40	1.20	.18	(134.22)
boiled, drained	60.0	—	20.00	.14	.16	.20	—	—	—
Potatoes									
raw	40.0	.05	20.00	.100	.04	1.50	.38	.25	19.00
baked in skin	Trace	.03	20.00	.100	.04	1.70	(.22)	(.17)	(10.11)
boiled in skin	—	.04	16.00	.090	.04	1.50	—	—	—
boiled, pared before cooking	Trace	.04	16.00	.090	.03	1.20	(.21)	(.19)	(10.09)
mashed, milk added	40.0	—	20.00	.160	.10	2.00	—	—	20.00
fried from raw	—	—	32.30	.20	.12	4.76	—	—	—
french fried in cottonseed oil	—	—	1.05	.01	Trace	.16	—	—	1.10

Table A.1 *(continued)*

									Minerals (Macro)					Minerals (Micro)		
Food Item Name	Approximate Measure	Weight (g)	Moisture (%)	Food Energy Calories (kcal)	Protein (g)	Fats (g)	Carbohydrates (g)	Fiber (g)	Calcium (mg)	Phosphorus (mg)	Sodium (mg)	Magnesium (mg)	Potassium (mg)	Iron (mg)	Zinc (mg)	Copper (mg)
Pumpkin																
raw	1 oz	28	—	4.2	.2	Trace	.9	.14	11.0	5.3	.3	—	86.3	.11	.06	.03
canned	1 cup	243	90.2	80.2	2.4	.7	19.2	3.2	60.8	89.9	12.2	63.2	537.0	.97	.37	.27
Radishes																
raw, common	1 sm	10	94.5	1.7	.1	0	.4	.1	3.0	3.1	1.8	1.5	32.2	.10	0	.01
raw, oriental	1 cup	95	94.1	18.1	.9	.1	4.0	.7	33.3	24.7	—	—	171.0	.57	—	—
Rutabagas																
raw	1 oz	28	87.0	12.9	.3	0	3.0	.3	18.5	10.9	1.4	4.2	66.9	.11	—	—
boiled, drained	1 cup	200	90.2	70.0	1.8	.2	16.4	2.2	118.0	62.0	8.0	—	334.0	.60	—	—
Spinach																
raw	1 cup	100	90.7	26.0	3.2	.3	4.3	.6	93.0	51.0	71.0	88.0	470.0	3.10	.80	.20
boiled, drained	1 cup	180	92.0	41.4	5.4	.5	6.5	1.1	167.4	68.4	90.0	(106.2)	583.2	3.96	1.26	(.45)
Squash, Summer																
all varieties, raw	1 cup	200	94.0	38.0	2.2	.2	8.4	1.2	56.0	58.0	2.0	32.0	404.0	.80	.36	—
all varieties, boiled, drained	1 cup	210	95.5	29.4	1.9	.2	6.5	1.3	52.5	52.5	2.1	(25.2)	296.1	.84	(.34)	(.11)
Squash, Winter																
all varieties, raw	1 cup	200	85.1	100.0	2.8	.6	24.8	2.8	44.0	76.0	2.0	34.0	738.0	1.20	—	—
all varieties, baked	1 cup	205	81.4	129.2	3.7	.8	31.6	3.7	57.4	98.4	2.1	—	945.1	1.64	—	—
all varieties, boiled, mashed	1 cup	205	88.8	77.9	2.3	.6	18.9	2.9	41.0	65.6	2.1	(28.7)	528.9	1.03	.35	(.10)

Food Item Name	Fat-Soluble Vitamins: Vitamin A (IU)	Fat-Soluble Vitamins: Vitamin E (Alpha Tocopherol) (mg)	Water-Soluble Vitamins: Vitamin C (mg)	Thiamine (mg)	Riboflavin (mg)	Niacin (mg)	Pantothenic Acid (mg)	Vitamin B_6 (Pyridoxine) (mg)	Folacin (Folic Acid) (mcg)
Pumpkin									
raw	700.0	Trace	1.49	.01	.01	.01	.11	.02	3.87
canned	66540.7	—	12.15	.07	.12	.97	(.97)	(.10)	36.45
Radishes									
raw, common	1.0	0	2.60	Trace	Trace	.03	.02	.01	2.40
raw, oriental	9.5	—	30.40	.03	.02	.38	—	—	—
Rutabagas									
raw	162.4	—	12.04	.02	.02	.31	.05	.03	—
boiled, drained	1100.0	—	52.00	.12	.12	1.60	—	—	42.00
Spinach									
raw	8100.0	—	51.00	.10	.20	.60	.30	.28	193.00
boiled, drained	14580.0	(3.62)	50.40	.13	.25	.90	(.40)	(.32)	163.80
Squash, Summer									
all varieties, raw	820.0	—	44.00	.10	.18	2.00	.72	.16	62.00
all varieties, boiled, drained	819.0	—	21.00	.11	.17	1.68	(.23)	(.12)	35.70
Squash, Winter									
all varieties, raw	7400.0	—	26.00	.10	.22	1.20	.80	.31	34.00
all varieties, baked	8405.0	—	26.65	.10	.26	1.44	—	—	—
all varieties, boiled, mashed	7175.0	—	16.40	.08	.20	.82	(.45)	(.23)	—

Table A.1 *(continued)*

Food Item Name	Approximate Measure	Weight (g)	Moisture (%)	Food Energy Calories (kcal)	Protein (g)	Fats (g)	Carbohydrates (g)	Fiber (g)	Minerals (Macro) Calcium (mg)	Phosphorus (mg)	Sodium (mg)	Magnesium (mg)	Potassium (mg)	Minerals (Micro) Iron (mg)	Zinc (mg)	Copper (mg)
Sweet Potato																
all varieties, raw	1 sm	100	70.6	114.0	1.8	.4	26.3	.7	32.0	47.0	10.0	31.0	243.0	.70	.08	.15
baked in skin	1 sm	100	63.7	141.0	2.1	.5	32.5	.9	40.0	58.0	12.0	—	300.0	.90	—	—
boiled in skin	1 sm	100	70.6	114.0	1.7	.4	26.3	.7	32.0	47.0	10.0	(12.0)	243.0	.70	—	(.16)
Swiss Chard																
raw	1 cup	166	91.1	41.5	4.0	.5	7.6	1.3	146.1	64.7	244.0	107.9	913.0	5.31	—	—
boiled, drained	1 cup	166	93.7	29.9	3.0	.3	5.5	1.2	121.2	39.8	142.8	—	532.9	2.99	—	—
Tomatoes																
green, raw	1 sm	100	93.0	24.0	1.0	.2	5.1	.5	13.0	27.0	3.0	14.0	244.0	.50	—	—
ripe, raw	1 sm	100	93.5	22.0	1.0	.2	4.7	.5	13.0	27.0	3.0	17.7	244.0	.50	.20	.01
ripe, boiled	1 cup	240	92.4	62.4	2.4	.5	13.2	1.4	36.0	76.8	9.6	—	688.8	1.44	.48	—
Turnip Greens																
raw	1 cup	200	90.3	56.0	5.8	.6	10.0	1.6	492.0	116.0	20.0	116.0	880.0	3.60	3.82	.70
boiled in small amount of water, drained	1 cup	150	93.2	30.0	3.3	.3	5.4	1.1	276.0	55.5	(11.0)	(15.3)	(116.9)	1.65	.62	.23
Turnips																
raw	1 cup	132	91.5	39.6	1.5	.3	8.7	1.2	51.5	39.6	64.7	12.5	353.8	.66	.49	.21
boiled, drained	1 cup	150	93.6	34.5	1.2	.3	7.4	1.4	52.5	36.0	51.0	—	282.0	.60	.42	.12
Watercress																
leaves & stems, raw	1 piece	1	93.3	.2	0	0	0	Trace	1.5	.5	.5	.2	2.8	.02	Trace	0

	Fat-Soluble Vitamins		*Water-Soluble Vitamins*						
Food Item Name	*Vitamin A (IU)*	*Vitamin E (Alpha Tocopherol) (mg)*	*Vitamin C (mg)*	*Thiamine (mg)*	*Riboflavin (mg)*	*Niacin (mg)*	*Pantothenic Acid (mg)*	*Vitamin B_6 (Pyridoxine) (mg)*	*Folacin (Folic Acid) (mcg)*
Sweet Potato									
all varieties, raw	8800.0	4.00	21.00	.10	.06	.60	.82	.22	12.00
baked in skin	8100.0	—	22.00	.09	.07	.70	—	—	18.00
boiled in skin	7900.0	4.00	17.00	.09	.06	.60	(.65)	(.12)	18.00
Swiss Chard									
raw	10790.0	—	53.12	.100	.28	.83	.29	—	—
boiled, drained	8964.0	—	26.56	.076	.18	.66	—	—	—
Tomatoes									
green, raw	270.0	—	20.00	.06	.04	.50	—	—	—
ripe, raw	900.0	.40	23.00	.06	.04	.70	.33	.10	39.00
ripe, boiled	2400.0	—	57.60	.17	.12	1.92	—	—	—
Turnip Greens									
raw	15200.0	4.48	278.00	.42	.78	1.60	.76	.53	190.00
boiled in small amount of water, drained	9450.0	(1.50)	103.50	.23	.36	.90	(.47)	(.23)	(165.32)
Turnips									
raw	0	0	47.52	.05	.09	.79	.26	.12	26.40
boiled, drained	0	0	33.00	.06	.08	.45	(.23)	(.10)	19.50
Watercress									
leaves & stems, raw	49.0	(.01)	.79	0	.00	.01	Trace	Trace	—

SOURCE: Ensminger, A. H.; Ensminger, M. E.; Konland, G. E.; and Robson, J. R. K., *Foods and Nutrition Encyclopedia*. (Clovis, Calif.: Pegus Press, 1983).

Table A.2 Nutritive Value of Edible Part of Selected Fruits

Food Item Name	*Approximate Measure*	*Weight (g)*	*Moisture (%)*	*Food Energy Calories (kcal)*	*Protein (g)*	*Fats (g)*	*Carbohydrates (g)*	*Fiber (g)*	*Minerals (Macro)* Calcium (mg)	Phosphorus (mg)	Sodium (mg)	Magnesium (mg)	Potassium (mg)	*Minerals (Micro)* Iron (mg)	Zinc (mg)	Copper (mg)
Apples																
raw, fresh, unpared	1 med	150	84.8	84.0	.3	.9	21.2	1.5	4.5	9.0	1.5	7.2	208.5	.15	.08	.06
raw, fresh, pared	1 med	145	85.3	76.9	.3	.4	20.2	.9	2.9	8.7	1.5	4.6	176.9	.15	.07	.05
baked, unpared	1 med	150	—	187.5	.3	.9	—	—	9.0	15.0	1.5	—	165.0	.45	—	—
Apricots																
raw	1 med	38	85.3	19.4	.4	.1	4.9	.2	3.0	5.7	.4	3.5	121.2	.19	.05	.03
Avocados																
all varieties, raw, halved, fruit served w/skin	1 avg	250	74.0	417.5	5.3	41.0	15.8	4.0	25.0	105.0	10.0	112.5	1510.0	1.50	0	1.00
Bananas																
common, yellow	1 avg	100	68.8	110.0	1.2	.2	29.0	.4	7.0	28.0	—	—	—	.50	.19	—
Blackberries																
raw	1 cup	144	84.5	83.5	1.7	1.3	18.6	5.9	20.2	27.4	1.4	28.5	305.3	.58	0	.16
Blueberries																
raw	1 cup	140	83.2	86.8	1.0	.7	21.4	2.1	21.0	18.2	1.4	8.4	113.4	1.40	.16	.15
Cantaloupe																
raw	1 whole	770	91.2	231.0	4.6	.8	57.8	2.3	107.8	123.2	92.4	64.7	1932.7	3.08	1.08	.11
Cherries																
sweet, raw	1 cup	200	80.4	140.0	2.6	.6	34.8	.8	20.0	26.0	4.0	32.4	500.0	.40	0	.27
sour red, raw	1 cup	200	83.7	116.0	2.4	.6	28.6	.4	12.0	22.0	4.0	23.0	382.0	.80	0	.18

	Fat-Soluble Vitamins		Water-Soluble Vitamins						
Food Item Name	Vitamin A (IU)	Vitamin E (Alpha Tocopherol) (mg)	Vitamin C (mg)	Thiamine (mg)	Riboflavin (mg)	Niacin (mg)	Pantothenic Acid (mg)	Vitamin B_6 (Pyridoxine) (mg)	Folacin (Folic Acid) (mcg)
Apples									
raw, fresh, unpared	135.0	.47	10.50	.05	.03	.15	.16	.05	12.00
raw, fresh, pared	58.0	—	5.80	.04	.03	.15	.15	.04	11.60
baked, unpared	139.5	—	4.50	.05	.03	.20	—	—	—
Apricots									
raw	1026.0	—	3.80	.01	.01	.23	.09	.03	1.25
Avocados									
all varieties, raw, halved, fruit served w/skin	725.0	—	35.00	.28	.50	4.00	2.68	1.05	127.50
Bananas									
common, yellow	65.0	—	15.00	.04	.04	.70	—	—	—
Blackberries									
raw	288.0	5.00	30.24	.04	.06	.58	.35	.07	19.73
Blueberries									
raw	140.0	—	19.60	.04	.08	.70	.22	.09	8.40
Cantaloupe									
raw	26180.0	1.08	254.10	.40	.26	4.62	1.93	.42	231.00
Cherries									
sweet, raw	220.0	—	20.00	.10	.12	.80	.52	.06	16.00
sour red, raw	2000.0	—	20.00	.10	.12	.80	.29	.13	16.00

Table A.2 *(continued)*

Food Item Name	Approximate Measure	Weight (g)	Moisture (%)	Food Energy Calories (kcal)	Protein (g)	Fats (g)	Carbohydrates (g)	Fiber (g)	Minerals (Macro) Calcium (mg)	Phosphorus (mg)	Sodium (mg)	Magnesium (mg)	Potassium (mg)	Minerals (Micro) Iron (mg)	Zinc (mg)	Copper (mg)
Cranberries																
raw	1 cup	100	87.9	46.0	.4	.7	10.8	1.4	7.0	6.0	2.0	4.5	67.0	.20	0	.06
Currants																
Black European, raw	1 cup	132	84.2	71.3	2.2	.1	17.3	3.2	79.2	52.8	4.0	22.6	491.0	1.45	—	(.17)
red & white, raw	1 cup	133	85.7	66.5	1.9	.3	16.1	4.5	42.6	30.6	2.7	20.0	341.8	1.33	—	.15
Dates																
domestic, natural, dry	1 cup	178	23.8	482.4	3.5	.9	128.5	4.1	58.7	64.1	1.8	60.5	1185.5	1.85	.52	.50
Figs																
raw	1 med	41	77.5	32.8	.5	.1	8.3	.5	14.4	5.7	.4	8.2	95.1	.16	0	.03
Grapefruit																
pink-red-white, all varieties	1 whole	482	88.4	197.6	2.4	.5	51.1	1.0	77.1	77.1	4.8	57.8	650.7	1.93	.48	.20
Grapes																
American type, slip skin, raw	1 cup	153	81.6	105.6	2.0	1.5	24.0	.9	24.5	18.4	4.6	19.9	241.7	.61	.06	.05
European type, adherent skin, raw	1 cup	153	81.4	102.5	.9	.5	26.5	.8	18.4	30.6	4.6	9.2	264.7	.61	.06	1.45
Lemons																
pulp w/peel, raw	1 sm	100	87.4	20.0	1.2	.3	10.7	(5.1)	61.0	15.0	3.0	(11.9)	145.0	.70	(.11)	(.26)
pulp w/o peel, raw	1 med	100	90.1	27.0	1.1	.3	8.2	.4	26.0	16.0	2.0	9.0	138.0	.60	—	.26
Limes																
acid type, raw	1 med	100	89.3	28.0	.8	.2	9.5	.5	33.0	18.0	2.0	—	102.0	.60	—	—

	Fat-Soluble Vitamins		*Water-Soluble Vitamins*						
Food Item Name	*Vitamin A (IU)*	*Vitamin E (Alpha Tocopherol) (mg)*	*Vitamin C (mg)*	*Thiamine (mg)*	*Riboflavin (mg)*	*Niacin (mg)*	*Pantothenic Acid (mg)*	*Vitamin B_6 (Pyridoxine) (mg)*	*Folacin (Folic Acid) (mcg)*
Cranberries									
raw	40.0	—	11.00	.03	.02	.10	.22	.04	2.00
Currants									
Black European, raw	303.6	1.32	264.00	.07	.07	.40	.53	.09	—
red & white, raw	159.6	(.17)	54.53	.05	.07	.13	.09	.05	—
Dates									
domestic, natural, dry	89.0	—	0	.16	.18	3.92	1.39	.35	25.45
Figs									
raw	32.8	—	.82	.03	.02	.16	.12	.05	5.74
Grapefruit									
pink-red-white, all varieties	385.6	1.21	183.16	.19	.10	.96	1.36	.16	53.02
Grapes									
American type, slip skin, raw	153.0	—	6.12	.14	.09	.46	.12	.19	10.71
European type, adherent skin, raw	153.0	1.07	6.12	.14	.09	.46	.12	.19	10.71
Lemons									
pulp w/peel, raw	30.0	—	77.00	.05	.04	.20	(.22)	(.12)	12.00
pulp w/o peel, raw	20.0	—	53.00	.04	.02	.10	.19	.08	—
Limes									
acid type, raw	10.0	—	37.00	.03	.02	.20	.22	—	4.00

Table A.2 *(continued)*

Food Item Name	Approximate Measure	Weight (g)	Moisture (%)	Food Energy Calories (kcal)	Protein (g)	Fats (g)	Carbohydrates (g)	Fiber (g)	Minerals (Macro) Calcium (mg)	Phosphorus (mg)	Sodium (mg)	Magnesium (mg)	Potassium (mg)	Minerals (Micro) Iron (mg)	Zinc (mg)	Copper (mg)
Loganberries																
raw	1 cup	150	83.0	93.0	1.5	.9	22.4	4.5	52.5	25.5	1.5	37.5	255.0	1.80	—	(.21)
Mangos																
raw	1 whole	200	81.7	132.0	1.4	.8	33.6	1.8	20.0	26.0	14.0	17.6	378.0	.80	0	.23
Oranges																
all varieties, w/o peel, raw	1 sm	100	86.0	49.0	.9	.2	12.2	.5	41.0	20.0	1.0	6.7	200.0	.40	.20	Trace
Peaches																
raw	1 med	100	89.1	38.0	.6	.1	9.7	.6	9.0	19.0	1.0	6.6	202.0	.50	.20	.07
Pears																
raw, w/skin	1 avg	200	83.2	122.0	1.4	.8	30.6	2.8	16.0	22.0	4.0	14.0	260.0	.60	.16	.23
raw, peeled	1 med	182	—	66.4	.5	Trace	17.1	5.1	13.1	27.1	5.3	8.7	184.5	.40	.15	.18
Pineapple																
raw	1 cup	132	85.3	76.6	.4	.3	18.1	.5	22.4	10.6	1.3	17.2	192.7	.66	.28	.19
Plantain (Baking Banana)																
green, raw	1 sm	100	66.4	119.0	1.1	.4	31.2	.4	7.0	30.0	5.0	—	385.0	.70	1.5	—
Plums																
Japanese hybrid, 2⅛" diameter, raw	1 avg	70	86.6	33.6	.4	.1	8.6	.4	8.4	12.6	.7	6.3	119.0	.35	.06	—
prune type, raw	1 med	50	78.7	37.5	.4	.1	9.9	.2	6.0	9.0	.5	4.5	85.0	.25	—	—

Food Item Name	*Fat-Soluble Vitamins* Vitamin A (IU)	Vitamin E (Alpha Tocopherol) (mg)	*Water-Soluble Vitamins* Vitamin C (mg)	Thiamine (mg)	Riboflavin (mg)	Niacin (mg)	Pantothenic Acid (mg)	Vitamin B_6 (Pyridoxine) (mg)	Folacin (Folic Acid) (mcg)
Loganberries									
raw	300.0	(.44)	36.00	.04	.06	.60	(.35)	(.09)	—
Mangos									
raw	9600.0	—	70.00	.10	.10	2.20	.32	—	—
Oranges									
all varieties, w/o peel, raw	200.0	.23	50.00	.10	.04	.40	.25	.06	46.00
Peaches									
raw	1330.0	—	7.00	.02	.05	1.00	.17	.02	8.00
Pears									
raw, w/skin	40.0	—	8.00	.04	.08	.20	.14	.03	28.00
raw, peeled	30.8	Trace	5.86	.05	.05	.35	.13	.04	25.48
Pineapple									
raw	92.4	—	22.44	.12	.04	.26	.21	.12	14.52
Plantain (Baking Banana)									
green, raw	605.0	—	14.00	.06	.04	.60	.37	—	16.00
Plums									
Japanese hybrid, 2⅛" diameter, raw	175.0	—	4.20	.02	.02	.35	.13	.04	4.20
prune type, raw	150.0	—	2.00	.02	.02	.25	.09	.04	3.00

Table A.2 *(continued)*

Food Item Name	Approximate Measure	Weight (g)	Moisture (%)	Food Energy Calories (kcal)	Protein (g)	Fats (g)	Carbohydrates (g)	Fiber (g)	Minerals (Macro) Calcium (mg)	Phosphorus (mg)	Sodium (mg)	Magnesium (mg)	Potassium (mg)	Minerals (Micro) Iron (mg)	Zinc (mg)	Copper (mg)
Prunes																
dried, softenized, uncooked	1 lg	10	32.4	23.9	.3	.1	6.3	.2	5.1	7.9	.4	4.5	75.4	.25	.05	.04
dried, softenized, cooked w/o sugar	1 cup	270	66.4	321.3	2.7	.8	84.8	2.2	64.8	99.9	10.8	54.0	882.9	4.86	.89	.68
dehydrated, uncooked	1 lg	10	2.5	34.4	.3	.1	9.1	.2	9.0	10.7	1.1	—	94.0	.44	—	—
Raisins																
California, Thompson seedless	1 tbls	10	17.0	28.9	.3	0	7.7	.1	8.6	10.2	1.7	3.5	67.8	.21	.02	.04
Raspberries																
black, raw	1 cup	123	80.8	89.8	1.8	1.7	19.3	6.3	36.9	27.1	1.2	36.9	244.8	1.11	.56	.16
red, raw	1 cup	132	84.2	75.2	1.6	.7	18.0	4.0	29.0	29.0	1.3	26.4	221.8	1.19	0	.08
Strawberries																
raw	1 cup	150	89.9	55.5	1.1	.8	12.6	2.0	31.5	31.5	1.5	18.0	246.0	1.50	0	.04
Tangelos																
raw	1 med	170	89.4	39.0	.5	.1	9.2	—	27.2	20.4	1.7	19.0	295.8	.17	0	.06
Tangerines																
Dancy, raw	1 med	116	87.0	53.4	.9	.2	13.5	.6	19.7	11.6	2.3	14.3	187.9	.46	.17	.03
Watermelon																
raw	1 cup	200	92.6	52.0	1.0	.4	12.8	.6	14.0	20.0	2.0	20.4	200.0	1.00	.18	.03

	Fat-Soluble Vitamins		Water-Soluble Vitamins						
Food Item Name	*Vitamin A (IU)*	*Vitamin E (Alpha Tocopherol) (mg)*	*Vitamin C (mg)*	*Thiamine (mg)*	*Riboflavin (mg)*	*Niacin (mg)*	*Pantothenic Acid (mg)*	*Vitamin B_6 (Pyridoxine) (mg)*	*Folacin (Folic Acid) (mcg)*
Prunes									
dried, softenized, uncooked	199.4	—	.33	.01	.02	.19	.05	.03	.40
dried, softenized, cooked w/o sugar	2025.0	—	2.70	.08	.19	1.89	(.62)	(.41)	Trace
dehydrated, uncooked	217.0	—	.40	.01	.02	.21	—	—	—
Raisins									
California, Thompson seedless	2.0	—	.09	.01	Trace	.06	.01	.02	.40
Raspberries									
black, raw	—	—	22.14	.04	.11	1.11	.30	.07	6.15
red, raw	171.6	(.41)	33.00	.04	.12	1.19	.32	.08	6.60
Strawberries									
raw	90.0	.20	88.50	.05	.11	.90	.51	.08	24.00
Tangelos									
raw	—	—	26.00	—	—	—	—	.09	23.80
Tangerines									
Dancy, raw	487.2	—	35.96	.07	.02	.12	.23	.08	24.36
Watermelon									
raw	1180.0	—	14.00	.06	.06	.40	.60	.14	16.00

SOURCE: Ensminger, A. H.; Ensminger, M. E.; Konland, G. E.; and Robson, J. R. K., *Foods and Nutrition Encyclopedia*. (Clovis, Calif.: Pegus Press, 1983).

Table A.3 Nutritive Value of Selected Grains and Grain Products

									Minerals (Macro)					Minerals (Micro)		
Food Item Name	*Approximate Measure*	*Weight (g)*	*Moisture (%)*	*Food Energy Calories (kcal)*	*Protein (g)*	*Fats (g)*	*Carbohydrates (g)*	*Fiber (g)*	*Calcium (mg)*	*Phosphorus (mg)*	*Sodium (mg)*	*Magnesium (mg)*	*Potassium (mg)*	*Iron (mg)*	*Zinc (mg)*	*Copper (mg)*
Cereals																
Amaranth																
whole grain	1 oz	28	12.3	100.2	3.6	2.0	18.2	1.9	69.2	140.0	—	—	—	.95	.75	—
toasted	1 oz	28	4.3	108.1	3.8	2.3	19.9	2.8	81.8	144.8	—	—	—	.45	—	—
Barley, Pearled																
light, boiled	½ cup	100	—	120.0	2.8	.6	27.5	.2	3.2	71.0	1.0	7.3	40.0	.30	.07	.05
Buckwheat																
whole grain	1 cup	100	11.0	360.0	11.7	2.4	72.9	9.9	114.0	282.0	—	252.6	448.0	3.10	—	.82
Corn, Sweet																
raw, white & yellow	1 med ear	140	72.7	134.4	4.9	1.4	30.9	1.0	4.2	155.4	(1.4)	67.2	392.0	.98	.70	.08
fresh, white & yellow, cooked on cob	1 med	140	74.1	127.4	4.6	1.4	29.4	1.0	4.2	124.6	(2.5)	(63.3)	274.4	.84	.56	(.20)
fresh, white & yellow, cut off cob before cooking	1 cup	165	76.5	137.0	5.3	1.7	31.0	1.2	5.0	146.9	—	—	272.3	.99	.83	—
Cornmeal																
degermed, unenriched, cooked	1 cup	238	87.7	119.0	2.6	.5	25.5	.2	2.4	33.3	—	16.7	38.1	.48	.24	—
degermed, enriched, cooked	1 cup	238	87.7	119.0	2.6	.5	25.5	.2	2.4	33.3	—	16.7	38.1	.95	.24	—
Grits																
corn, degermed, unenriched, cooked	1 cup	242	87.1	121.0	2.9	.2	26.6	.2	2.4	24.2	—	7.3	26.6	.24	—	—

	Fat-Soluble Vitamins		Water-Soluble Vitamins						
Food Item Name	*Vitamin A (IU)*	*Vitamin E (Alpha Tocopherol) (mg)*	*Vitamin C (mg)*	*Thiamine (mg)*	*Riboflavin (mg)*	*Niacin (mg)*	*Pantothenic Acid (mg)*	*Vitamin B_6 (Pyridoxine) (mg)*	*Folacin (Folic Acid) (mcg)*
Cereals									
Amaranth									
whole grain	0	—	.84	.04	.09	.28	—	—	—
toasted	—	—	—	0	.09	.31	—	—	—
Barley, Pearled									
light, boiled	0	Trace	—	—	—	—	—	—	—
Buckwheat									
whole grain	0	—	0	.60	—	4.40	—	—	—
Corn, Sweet									
raw, white & yellow	560.0	.08	16.80	.21	.17	2.38	.76	.66	46.20
fresh, white & yellow, cooked on cob	560.0	(.73)	12.60	.17	.14	1.96	(.55)	(.24)	(46.35)
fresh, white & yellow, cut off cob before cooking	660.0	—	11.55	.18	.17	2.15	—	—	54.45
Cornmeal									
degermed, unenriched, cooked	142.8	1.52	0	.05	.02	.24	1.64	—	21.42
degermed, enriched, cooked	142.8	1.52	0	.14	.10	1.19	1.64	—	21.42
Grits									
corn, degermed, unenriched, cooked	145.2	.75	0	.05	.02	.48	—	—	—

Table A.3 *(continued)*

Food Item Name	Approximate Measure	Weight (g)	Moisture (%)	Food Energy Calories (kcal)	Protein (g)	Fats (g)	Carbohydrates (g)	Fiber (g)	Minerals (Macro) Calcium (mg)	Phosphorus (mg)	Sodium (mg)	Magnesium (mg)	Potassium (mg)	Minerals (Micro) Iron (mg)	Zinc (mg)	Copper (mg)
corn, degermed, enriched, cooked	1 cup	242	87.1	121.0	2.9	.2	26.6	.2	2.4	24.2	—	7.3	26.6	.73	—	—
hominy, enriched, dry	1 cup	156	10.7	558.5	13.3	1.4	123.4	.8	3.1	121.7	1.6	31.2	166.9	4.46	0	.06
Millet																
whole grain	1 cup	230	10.8	795.8	20.5	8.5	172.3	3.9	48.3	641.7	—	—	—	8.51	—	—
Quinoa																
whole grain	3½ oz	100	11.0	351.0	12.3	6.1	67.7	4.6	112.0	286.0	—	—	—	7.50	—	—
Rice																
bran	1 oz	28	9.7	77.3	3.7	4.4	14.2	.4	21.3	388.1	—	—	418.6	5.43	—	—
brown, cooked	1 cup	150	70.3	178.5	3.8	1.2	38.3	.5	18.0	109.5	423.0	43.5	105.0	.75	.90	—
polished	1 cup	105	9.8	278.3	12.7	13.4	60.6	2.5	72.5	1161.3	—	—	749.7	16.91	.37	—
white, enriched (all varieties), cooked	1 cup	150	72.6	160.5	3.0	.3	36.3	.2	15.0	42.0	561.0	12.0	42.0	1.35	.60	—
Rye																
whole grain	1 cup	185	12.1	669.7	22.4	4.1	135.8	3.7	70.3	695.6	1.9	246.6	864.0	6.85	6.01	.47
Wheat																
whole grain, cooked	1 cup	42	87.7	18.9	.8	.1	3.9	.12	2.9	21.8	89.0	—	20.2	.21	.21	—
bran, unprocessed	1 tbls	9	14.0	31.8	1.4	.4	5.6	.8	10.7	114.8	.8	53.8	100.9	1.34	.88	(.11)
germ, unprocessed	1 tbls	9	14.0	35.2	2.4	1.0	4.2	.2	6.5	100.6	.3	30.6	74.4	.85	1.29	.07
germ, toasted	1 tbls	6	4.2	23.5	1.5	.7	3.0	.1	2.8	65.0	.1	21.9	56.8	.53	.92	.08
Wild Rice																
raw	1 cup	112	8.5	395.4	15.8	.8	84.3	1.1	21.3	379.7	7.8	144.5	246.4	4.70	—	—

	Fat-Soluble Vitamins		Water-Soluble Vitamins						
Food Item Name	*Vitamin A (IU)*	*Vitamin E (Alpha Tocopherol) (mg)*	*Vitamin C (mg)*	*Thiamine (mg)*	*Riboflavin (mg)*	*Niacin (mg)*	*Pantothenic Acid (mg)*	*Vitamin B_6 (Pyridoxine) (mg)*	*Folacin (Folic Acid) (mcg)*
corn, degermed, enriched, cooked	145.2	.75	0	.04	.03	.40	—	—	—
hominy, enriched, dry	0	—	0	.69	.41	5.49	0	.19	18.72
Millet									
whole grain	38.4	—	—	.76	.32	4.14	—	—	—
Quinoa									
whole grain	0	—	3.00	.36	.42	1.40	—	—	—
Rice									
bran	0	—	0	.63	.07	8.34	.78	.70	10.92
brown, cooked	0	.23	0	.14	.03	2.10	2.28	.93	—
polished	0	—	0	1.93	.19	29.61	3.50	2.10	201.60
white, enriched (all varieties), cooked	0	.27	0	.17	.11	1.50	1.13	.06	24.00
Rye									
whole grain	0	3.05	0	.80	.41	2.96	—	—	—
Wheat									
whole grain, cooked	0	—	0	.03	.01	.25	.58	.22	2.72
bran, unprocessed	0	.15	0	.07	.03	1.89	.27	.12	23.22
germ, unprocessed	0	(1.22)	0	.18	.06	.38	.11	—	29.52
germ, toasted	6.6	—	.60	.10	.06	.32	.07	.07	25.20
Wild Rice									
raw	0	—	0	.50	.71	6.94	1.14	—	—

Table A.3 *(continued)*

Food Item Name	*Approximate Measure*	*Weight (g)*	*Moisture (%)*	*Food Energy Calories (kcal)*	*Protein (g)*	*Fats (g)*	*Carbohydrates (g)*	*Fiber (g)*	*Minerals (Macro)* *Calcium (mg)*	*Phosphorus (mg)*	*Sodium (mg)*	*Magnesium (mg)*	*Potassium (mg)*	*Minerals (Micro)* *Iron (mg)*	*Zinc (mg)*	*Copper (mg)*
Breakfast Cereals																
Oats																
rolled (oatmeal), cooked	1 cup	236	86.5	112.7	4.7	2.4	22.9	.5	21.2	134.5	514.5	49.6	144.0	1.42	1.18	—
Rice																
cream of, cooked	1 oz	28	87.5	14.0	.2	Trace	3.1	Trace	.6	3.6	49.3	2.2	Trace	.20	.04	—
Wheat																
cream of, cooked	1 cup	245	89.5	102.9	3.2	.2	21.3	—	9.8	29.4	352.8	7.4	22.1	.74	.39	—
Flours																
Buckwheat flour																
dark	1 cup	100	12.0	357.0	11.7	2.5	72.0	1.6	33.0	347.0	—	—	—	2.80	2.65	—
light	1 cup	100	12.0	354.0	6.4	1.2	79.5	.5	11.0	88.0	1.0	48.0	320.0	1.00	2.56	.70
Quinoa flour	1 cup	100	12.0	354.0	10.4	4.0	71.1	3.8	94.0	129.0	—	—	—	5.60	—	—
Rye flour																
dark	1 cup	100	11.0	350.0	16.3	1.4	68.1	2.4	54.0	536.0	1.0	115.0	860.0	4.50	7.19	.66
light	1 cup	100	11.0	362.0	9.4	1.4	77.9	.4	22.0	185.0	1.0	73.0	156.0	1.10	—	.42
Wheat flour																
white, enriched	1 cup	110	12.0	400.4	11.6	1.1	83.7	.3	17.6	95.7	2.2	—	104.5	3.19	.77	—
whole	1 cup	133	14.0	480.1	17.7	3.5	94.4	3.1	54.5	494.8	4.0	199.8	492.1	4.39	3.19	—

	Fat-Soluble Vitamins		Water-Soluble Vitamins						
Food Item Name	*Vitamin A (IU)*	*Vitamin E (Alpha Tocopherol) (mg)*	*Vitamin C (mg)*	*Thiamine (mg)*	*Riboflavin (mg)*	*Niacin (mg)*	*Pantothenic Acid (mg)*	*Vitamin B_6 (Pyridoxine) (mg)*	*Folacin (Folic Acid) (mcg)*
Breakfast Cereals									
Oats									
rolled (oatmeal), cooked	0	5.36	0	.20	.05	.24	—	—	—
Rice									
cream of, cooked	0	—	0	.02	Trace	.22	—	—	—
Wheat									
cream of, cooked	0	—	0	.10	.07	.98	—	—	—
Flours									
Buckwheat flour									
dark	0	—	0	.58	.15	2.90	1.45	.58	44.00
light	0	—	0	.08	.04	.40	—	—	44.00
Quinoa flour	0	—	0	.19	.24	.70	—	—	—
Rye flour									
dark	0	—	0	.61	.22	2.70	1.34	.30	78.00
light	0	—	0	.15	.07	.60	.72	.09	78.00
Wheat flour									
white, enriched	0	—	0	.48	.29	3.85	—	—	23.10
whole	0	—	0	.73	.16	5.72	1.46	.45	71.82

SOURCE: Ensminger, A. H.; Ensminger, M. E.; Konland, G. E.; and Robson, J. R. K., *Foods and Nutrition Encyclopedia*. (Clovis, Calif.: Pegus Press, 1983).

Table A.4 Nutritive Value of Selected Legumes

Food Item Name	Approximate Measure	Weight (g)	Moisture (%)	Food Energy Calories (kcal)	Protein (g)	Fats (g)	Carbohydrates (g)	Fiber (g)	Minerals (Macro) Calcium (mg)	Phosphorus (mg)	Sodium (mg)	Magnesium (mg)	Potassium (mg)	Minerals (Micro) Iron (mg)	Zinc (mg)	Copper (mg)
Adzuki Bean																
dried	⅓ cup	100	15.0	324.0	21.1	1.0	59.5	3.9	82.0	313.0	14.0	—	1500.0	6.40	—	—
Common Beans, Dry																
baked	1 cup	300	68.5	360.0	18.9	1.5	69.0	4.2	204.0	363.0	1014.0	111.0	804.0	6.00	—	—
black, brown, & sayo, cooked	1 cup	185	11.2	224.4	14.4	.9	39.6	—	87.0	272.0	—	103.6	—	5.18	—	—
red, cooked	1 cup	250	69.0	295.0	19.5	1.3	53.5	3.8	95.0	350.0	7.5	—	850.0	6.00	2.50	.90
white, unsalted, cooked	1 cup	200	69.0	236.0	15.6	1.2	42.4	3.0	100.0	296.0	14.0	—	832.0	5.40	2.00	—
Garbanzos or Chick-Peas																
dry, cooked or canned	1 cup	140	—	250.6	14.3	3.4	42.4	—	105.0	231.0	—	75.6	—	4.76	—	—
flour	1 oz	28	2.5	103.1	5.6	1.8	16.7	.7	28.0	96.6	2.8	—	281.8	2.0	—	—
Green Beans																
raw	1 cup	100	90.1	32.0	1.9	.2	7.1	1.0	56.0	44.0	7.0	32.0	243.0	.80	.40	—
fresh, boiled in water, drained	1 cup	125	92.4	31.3	2.0	.2	6.8	1.3	62.5	46.3	5.0	—	188.8	.75	.38	—
Lentils																
dry, whole, cooked	1 cup	150	72.0	159.0	11.7	(.6)	29.0	1.8	37.5	178.5	(18.9)	(38.1)	373.5	3.15	1.50	(.27)
Lima Beans																
immature seeds, boiled, drained	1 cup	184	71.1	204.2	14.0	.9	36.4	3.3	86.5	222.6	1.8	—	776.5	4.60	—	—
frozen, boiled, drained	1 cup	160	73.5	158.4	9.6	.2	30.6	2.6	32.0	144.0	161.6	76.8	681.6	2.72	.77	10

Food Item Name	Fat-Soluble Vitamins: Vitamin A (IU)	Fat-Soluble Vitamins: Vitamin E (Alpha Tocopherol) (mg)	Water-Soluble Vitamins: Vitamin C (mg)	Thiamine (mg)	Riboflavin (mg)	Niacin (mg)	Pantothenic Acid (mg)	Vitamin B_6 (Pyridoxine) (mg)	Folacin (Folic Acid) (mcg)
Adzuki Bean									
dried	—	—	0	.45	.15	2.20	—	—	—
Common Beans, Dry									
baked	180.0	—	6.00	.21	.12	1.80	—	—	—
black, brown, & sayo, cooked	18.5	—	0	.35	.13	1.48	—	.32	—
red, cooked	—	—	—	.28	.15	1.75	1.63	—	92.50
white, unsalted, cooked	0	.94	0	.28	.14	1.40	—	—	60.00
Garbanzos or Chick-Peas									
dry, cooked or canned	35.0	—	0	.21	.10	1.40	—	.38	142.80
flour	9.4	—	0	.03	.09	.2	—	—	—
Green Beans									
raw	600.0	—	19.00	.08	.11	.50	.19	.08	27.50
fresh, boiled in water, drained	675.0	—	15.00	.09	.11	.63	—	—	50.00
Lentils									
dry, whole, cooked	30.0	—	0	.11	.09	.90	(.50)	(.24)	—
Lima Beans									
immature seeds, boiled, drained	515.2	—	31.28	.33	.18	2.39	—	—	—
frozen, boiled, drained	368.0	—	27.20	.11	.08	1.60	.29	.16	104.00

Table A.4 *(continued)*

Food Item Name	Approximate Measure	Weight (g)	Moisture (%)	Food Energy Calories (kcal)	Protein (g)	Fats (g)	Carbohydrates (g)	Fiber (g)	Minerals (Macro) Calcium (mg)	Phosphorus (mg)	Sodium (mg)	Magnesium (mg)	Potassium (mg)	Minerals (Micro) Iron (mg)	Zinc (mg)	Copper (mg)
Mung Beans																
sprouted seeds, uncooked	1 cup	210	85.9	111.3	9.0	.4	13.9	1.3	27.3	134.4	10.5	33.6	468.3	4.00	1.89	—
Peas																
mature seeds, dry, whole boiled	1 cup	248	—	256.4	16.9	.7	47.6	11.7	60.0	669.8	33.0	75.4	671.1	6.71	2.73	.45
mature seeds, dry, split, w/o seed coat, cooked	1 cup	200	70.0	230.0	16.0	.6	41.6	.8	22.0	178.0	26.0	—	592.0	3.40	—	—
edible, podded, raw	1 cup	133	83.3	70.5	4.5	.3	16.0	1.0	82.5	119.7	—	8.0	226.1	.93	1.8	—
edible, podded, boiled, drained	1 cup	150	86.6	64.5	4.4	.3	14.3	1.8	84.0	114.0	—	—	178.5	.75	1.9	—
green, immature, raw	1 cup	133	78.0	111.7	8.4	.5	19.2	2.7	34.6	154.3	2.7	46.6	420.3	2.53	1.20	.06
green, immature, sweet, boiled, drained	1 cup	150	81.5	106.5	8.1	.6	18.2	3.0	34.5	148.5	1.5	(31.8)	294.0	2.70	1.05	(.24)
Soybeans																
dry, cooked	1 cup	180	71.0	234.0	19.8	10.3	19.4	2.9	131.4	322.2	3.6	—	972.0	4.86	—	—
flour, full fat	1 cup	72	8.0	303.1	25.8	14.6	21.9	1.7	143.3	401.8	.7	177.8	1195.2	6.05	—	—
flour, defatted	1 cup	138	8.0	449.9	64.9	1.2	52.6	3.2	365.7	903.9	1.4	427.8	2511.6	15.32	6.72	2.39
Tofu																
bean curd	3½ oz	100	84.8	72.0	7.0	4.2	2.4	.1	128.0	126.0	7.0	111.0	42.0	1.90	—	—

	Fat-Soluble Vitamins		*Water-Soluble Vitamins*						
Food Item Name	*Vitamin A (IU)*	*Vitamin E (Alpha Tocopherol) (mg)*	*Vitamin C (mg)*	*Thiamine (mg)*	*Riboflavin (mg)*	*Niacin (mg)*	*Pantothenic Acid (mg)*	*Vitamin B_6 (Pyridoxine) (mg)*	*Folacin (Folic Acid) (mcg)*
Mung Beans									
sprouted seeds, uncooked	42.0	—	42.00	.29	.38	2.31	—	—	—
Peas									
mature seeds, dry, whole boiled	336.0	Trace	Trace	—	—	3.22	—	—	—
mature seeds, dry, split, w/o seed coat, cooked	80.0	—	—	.30	.18	1.80	—	—	14.00
edible, podded, raw	904.4	—	27.93	.37	.16	—	1.09	.20	33.25
edible, podded, boiled, drained	915.0	—	21.00	.33	.17	—	—	—	—
green, immature, raw	851.2	.13	35.91	.47	.19	3.86	1.00	.21	33.25
green, immature, sweet, boiled, drained	810.0	.83	30.00	.42	.17	3.45	(.50)	(.17)	—
Soybeans									
dry, cooked	54.0	—	0	.38	.16	1.08	—	—	—
flour, full fat	79.2	—	0	.61	.22	1.51	1.26	.41	228.96
flour, defatted	55.2	—	0	1.50	.47	3.59	3.06	1.00	438.84
Tofu									
bean curd	0	—	0	.06	.03	.10	—	—	—

SOURCE: Ensminger, A. H.; Ensminger, M. E.; Konland, G. E.; and Robson, J. R. K., *Foods and Nutrition Encyclopedia*. (Clovis, Calif.: Pegus Press, 1983).

Table A.5 Nutritive Value of Selected Nuts and Seeds

Food Item Name	Approximate Measure	Weight (g)	Moisture (%)	Food Energy Calories (kcal)	Protein (g)	Fats (g)	Carbohydrates (g)	Fiber (g)	Minerals (Macro) Calcium (mg)	Phosphorus (mg)	Sodium (mg)	Magnesium (mg)	Potassium (mg)	Minerals (Micro) Iron (mg)	Zinc (mg)	Copper (mg)
Almonds																
unsalted	1 cup	142	—	910.2	27.0	76.5	28.4	4.3	355.0	681.6	4.3	383.4	979.8	5.68	—	—
roasted & salted	1 cup	157	.07	984.4	29.2	90.6	30.6	4.1	369.0	791.3	310.9	—	1213.6	7.38	4.02	—
dried, shelled, whole	1 cup	142	4.7	849.2	26.4	77.0	27.7	3.7	332.3	715.7	5.7	415.6	1097.7	6.67	4.45	2.00
Brazil Nuts																
shelled	1 cup	140	4.6	1001.0	20.0	95.5	15.3	4.3	260.4	970.2	1.4	444.5	1001.0	4.76	5.92	3.34
Cashew Nuts																
unsalted	1 cup	140	5.2	834.4	24.1	63.8	41.0	2.0	53.2	522.1	21.0	373.8	649.6	5.32	6.13	—
Chestnuts																
fresh	1 cup	200	52.5	408.0	5.8	5.4	84.2	2.2	54.0	176.0	12.0	84.0	908.0	3.40	—	.12
dried	1 cup	100	8.4	377.0	6.7	4.1	78.6	2.5	52.0	162.0	12.0	—	875.0	3.30	—	—
Coconuts																
meat, fresh, grated	1 cup	130	50.9	481.9	4.4	46.2	12.2	5.2	16.9	123.5	29.9	59.8	332.8	2.21	.07	.03
meat, dried, unsweetened	1 cup	130	3.5	860.6	9.4	84.4	29.9	5.1	33.8	243.1	68.9	117.0	764.4	4.29	—	(.87)
meat, dried, sweetened, shredded	1 cup	130	3.3	712.4	4.7	50.8	69.2	5.3	20.8	145.6	23.4	100.1	458.9	2.60	—	—
milk	1 cup	244	65.7	614.9	7.8	60.8	12.7	—	39.0	244.0	129.3	—	463.6	3.90	—	—
water	1 cup	244	94.2	53.7	.7	.5	11.5	—	48.8	31.7	61.0	68.3	358.7	0.73	—	—
Filberts (Hazelnuts)																
whole, shelled	1 cup	135	5.8	945.0	17.1	87.3	22.5	4.1	282.2	455.0	2.7	234.8	950.4	4.59	3.29	1.73
Flaxseed																
dried	1 oz	28	6.3	139.4	5.0	9.4	10.4	2.5	75.9	129.4	—	—	—	12.26	—	—
Macadamia Nuts																
shelled	1 cup	140	3.0	1086.4	10.9	106.0	22.3	3.5	67.2	225.4	—	—	369.6	2.80	2.39	—

	Fat-Soluble Vitamins		Water-Soluble Vitamins						
Food Item Name	*Vitamin A (IU)*	*Vitamin E (Alpha Tocopherol) (mg)*	*Vitamin C (mg)*	*Thiamine (mg)*	*Riboflavin (mg)*	*Niacin (mg)*	*Pantothenic Acid (mg)*	*Vitamin B_6 (Pyridoxine) (mg)*	*Folacin (Folic Acid) (mcg)*
Almonds									
unsalted	0	21.30	—	.03	.10	(4.97)	—	.16	136.32
roasted & salted	0	—	0	.08	1.44	5.50	.39	.15	—
dried, shelled, whole	0	39.62	—	.34	1.31	4.97	.67	.14	—
Brazil Nuts									
shelled	0	9.10	14.00	1.34	.17	2.24	.32	.24	5.60
Cashew Nuts									
unsalted	140.0	—	—	.60	.35	2.52	1.82	—	—
Chestnuts									
fresh	160.0	1.00	12.00	.44	.44	1.20	.95	.66	—
dried	—	—	—	.32	.38	1.20	—	—	—
Coconuts									
meat, fresh, grated	0	.91	3.90	.07	.03	.65	.26	.06	31.20
meat, dried, unsweetened	0	—	0	.08	.05	.78	.26	—	—
meat, dried, sweetened, shredded	0	—	0	.05	.04	.52	.26	—	—
milk	0	—	4.88	.07	—	1.95	—	—	—
water	0	—	4.88	—	—	.24	.12	.08	—
Filberts (Hazelnuts)									
whole, shelled	144.5	28.35	4.05	.62	.73	1.21	1.55	.74	97.20
Flaxseed									
dried	0	—	—	.05	.05	.39	—	—	—
Macadamia Nuts									
shelled	0	—	0	.48	.15	1.82	—	—	—

Table A.5 *(continued)*

									Minerals (Macro)					Minerals (Micro)		
Food Item Name	*Approximate Measure*	*Weight (g)*	*Moisture (%)*	*Food Energy Calories (kcal)*	*Protein (g)*	*Fats (g)*	*Carbohydrates (g)*	*Fiber (g)*	*Calcium (mg)*	*Phosphorus (mg)*	*Sodium (mg)*	*Magnesium (mg)*	*Potassium (mg)*	*Iron (mg)*	*Zinc (mg)*	*Copper (mg)*
Peanuts																
raw, w/skins	1 cup	150	5.6	846.0	39.0	71.3	27.9	3.6	103.5	601.5	7.5	237.5	1011.0	3.15	4.86	1.18
raw, w/o skins	1 cup	142	5.4	806.6	37.3	70.6	25.0	2.7	83.8	580.8	7.1	292.5	957.1	2.84	(4.12)	(.38)
roasted, salted	1 cup	144	1.6	842.4	37.4	71.7	27.1	3.4	106.6	577.4	601.9	252.0	970.6	3.02	(4.26)	(.39)
butter, creamy	1 tbls	32	—	190.0	8.1	16.2	5.4	(5.9)	(11.8)	105.7	190.0	(57.6)	200.0	(.67)	.93	(.22)
Pecans																
unsalted	1 cup	108	3.4	797.7	10.2	77.1	15.8	2.5	78.8	312.1	11.9	118.8	651.2	2.59	4.43	1.19
Pinenuts																
pignolias	1 tbls	7	5.6	44.1	2.2	3.6	.8	.1	—	—	—	—	—	—	—	—
Pistachio Nuts																
shelled	1 cup	125	5.3	793.8	23.6	67.0	23.8	2.4	163.8	625.0	—	197.5	1215.0	9.13	—	—
Pumpkin & Squash Seed Kernels																
dry	1 cup	140	—	774.2	40.6	65.4	21.0	2.7	71.4	1601.6	—	—	—	15.68	10.30	—
Sesame Seeds																
dry, whole	1 oz	28	5.4	157.6	5.2	13.7	6.0	1.8	324.8	172.5	16.8	50.7	203.0	2.94	2.80	—
dry, decorticated	1 oz	28	4.8	163.0	7.4	15.3	2.6	.8	36.7	217.3	11.2	97.1	114.0	2.18	2.87	—
Sunflower Seed Kernels																
dry, hulled	1 cup	145	4.8	812.0	33.4	68.6	28.9	5.5	174.0	1213.7	43.5	55.1	1334.0	10.30	6.64	2.57
Walnuts																
black, shelled, chopped	1 cup	125	3.1	847.5	25.6	74.5	18.5	2.1	—	712.5	3.8	237.5	575.0	7.50	4.28	—
Persian or English, shelled, chopped	1 cup	120	3.5	832.8	18.0	76.1	19.0	2.5	118.8	456.0	2.4	172.8	540.0	3.72	3.84	1.68

Food Item Name	Fat-Soluble Vitamins: Vitamin A (IU)	Fat-Soluble Vitamins: Vitamin E (Alpha Tocopherol) (mg)	Water-Soluble Vitamins: Vitamin C (mg)	Thiamine (mg)	Riboflavin (mg)	Niacin (mg)	Pantothenic Acid (mg)	Vitamin B_6 (Pyridoxine) (mg)	Folacin (Folic Acid) (mcg)
Peanuts									
raw, w/skins	24.0	14.55	0	1.71	.20	25.80	4.20	—	—
raw, w/o skins	0	13.77	0	1.41	.19	22.44	3.98	(.75)	(156.21)
roasted, salted	0	13.97	0	.46	.19	24.77	3.02	.58	152.64
butter, creamy	0	(1.49)	Trace	(.05)	(.04)	(4.89)	(.74)	(.16)	(16.90)
Pecans									
unsalted	140.4	1.30	2.16	.93	.14	.97	1.84	.20	25.92
Pinenuts									
pignolias	—	—	—	.04	—	—	—	—	—
Pistachio Nuts									
shelled	287.5	—	0	.84	—	1.75	—	—	72.50
Pumpkin & Squash Seed Kernels									
dry	98.0	—	—	.34	.27	3.36	—	.13	—
Sesame Seeds									
dry, whole	8.4	—	0	.27	.07	1.51	—	—	—
dry, decorticated	18.5	—	0	.20	.02	1.31	.19	.04	—
Sunflower Seed Kernels									
dry, hulled	72.5	18.85	—	2.84	.33	7.83	2.03	1.81	—
Walnuts									
black, shelled, chopped	375.0	—	—	.28	.14	.88	—	—	—
Persian or English, shelled, chopped	36.0	.48	2.40	.40	.16	1.08	1.08	.88	79.20

SOURCE: Ensminger, A. H.; Ensminger, M. E.; Konland, G. E.; and Robson, J. R. K., *Foods and Nutrition Encyclopedia*. (Clovis, Calif.: Pegus Press, 1983).

References

Chapter 1

1. Eaton, S. B., and Konner, M. 1985. "Paleolithic Nutrition: A Consideration of Its Nature and Current Implications." *New England Journal of Medicine* 312: 283–89.
2. Ryde, D. 1985. "What Should Humans Eat?" *Practitioner* 232: 415–18.
3. Ibid.
4. Eaton and Konner, "Paleolithic Nutrition," op. cit.
5. Trowell, H., and Burkitt, D. 1981. *Western Diseases: Their Emergence and Prevention*. Cambridge, Mass.: Harvard University Press. Trowell, H.; Burkitt, D.; and Heaton, K. 1985. *Dietary Fibre, Fibre-depleted Foods and Disease*. New York: Academic Press. Department of Health and Human Services. 1988. *The Surgeon General's Report on Nutrition and Health*. Rocklin, Calif.: Prima. National Research Council. 1989. *Diet and Health: Implications for Reducing Chronic Disease Risk*. Washington, D.C.: National Academy Press.
6. Ibid.
7. Price, W. 1939. *Nutrition and Physical Degeneration*. La Mesa, Calif.: Price-Pottinger Foundation (reprint 1970).
8. National Research Council, *Diet and Health*, op. cit.
9. Ibid.
10. Physicians Committee for Responsible Medicine. 1991. "The New Four Food Groups." P.O. Box 6322, Washington, D.C., 20015.
11. Robbins, J. 1987. *Diet for a New America*. Walpole, N.H.: Stillpoint Publishing.

Chapter 2

1. Newberne, P., and Conner, M. W. 1986. "Food Additives and Contaminants: An Update." *Cancer* 58: 1851–62.
2. Feingold, N. 1975. *Why Your Child Is Hyperactive*. New York: Random House.
3. Conners, C.; Goyette, C.; Southwick, D.; Lees, J.; and Andrulonis, P. 1976. "Food Additives and Hyperkinesis: A Double-blind Experiment." *Pediatrics* 58: 154–66. Goyette, C.; Conners, C.; Petti, T.; and Curtis, L. 1978. "Effects of Artificial Colors on Hyperkinetic Children: A Double-blind Challenge Study." *Psychopharmacology Bulletin* 14: 39–40. Conners, C. 1980. *Food Additives and Hyperactive Children*. New York: Plenum Press. Harley, J.; Ray, R.; Tomasi, L.; et al. 1978. "Hyperkinesis and Food Additives: Testing the Feingold Hypothesis." *Pediatrics* 61: 811–17, 1978. Rowe, K.; Hopkins, I.; and Lynch, B. 1979. "Ar-

tificial Food Colourings and Hyperkinesis." *Australian Paediatrics Journal* 15: 202. Levy, F.; Dumbrell, S.; Hobbes, G.; et al. 1978. "Hyperkinesis and Diet: A Double-blind Crossover Trial with Tartrazine Challenge." *Medical Journal of Australia* 1: 61–64.

4. Rowe, K. 1984. "Food Additives." *Australian Paediatrics Journal* 20: 171–74. Swanson, J., and Kinsbourne, M. 1980. "Food Dyes Impair Performance of Children on a Laboratory Learning Task." *Science* 207: 1485–87. Weiss, B.; Williams, J.; Margen, S.; et al. 1980. "Behavioral Responses to Artificial Food Colours." *Science* 207: 1487–89. Weiss, B. 1982. "Food Additives and Environmental Chemicals as Sources of Childhood Behavior Disorders." *Journal of American Academy of Child Psychiatry* 21: 144–52. Schauss, A. 1984. "Nutrition and Behavior: Complex Interdisciplinary Research." *Nutritional Health* 3: 9–37. Rippere, V. 1983. "Food Additives and Hyperactive Children: A Critique of Conners." *British Journal of Clinical Psychology* 22: 19–32. Rimland, B. 1983. "The Feingold Diet: An Assessment of the Reviews by Mattes, by Kavale and Forness and Others." *Journal of Learning Disabilities* 16: 331–33.
5. Lipton, M., and Mayo, J. 1983. "Diet and Hyperkinesis—An Update." *Journal of American Dietetic Association* 83: 132–34. Anonymous. 1982. "Defined Diets and Childhood Hyperactivity. Consensus Conference: Office for Medical Applications of Research, National Institutes of Health." *Journal of American Medical Association* 248: 290–92.
6. Rowe, Hopkins, and Lynch, "Artificial Food Colourings and Hyperkinesis," op. cit. Levy, Dumbrell, Hobbes, et al., "Hyperkinesis and Diet," op. cit. Rowe, "Food Additives," op. cit. Swanson and Kinsbourne, "Food Dyes Impair Performance," op. cit. Weiss, Williams, Margen, et al., "Behavioral Responses to Artificial Food Colours," op. cit.
7. Conners, Goyette, Southwick, Lees, and Andrulonis, "Food Additives and Hyperkinesis," op. cit. Harley, Ray, Tomasi, et al., "Hyperkinesis and Food Additives," op. cit.
8. Rowe, Hopkins, and Lynch, "Artificial Food Colourings and Hyperkinesis," op. cit. Rowe, "Food Additives," op. cit. Weiss, Williams, Margen, et al., "Behavioral Responses to Artificial Food Colours," op. cit. Cook, P., and Woodhill, J. 1976. "The Feingold Dietary Treatment of the Hyperkinetic Syndrome." *Medical Journal of Australia* 2: 85–90. Salzman, L. 1976. "Allergy Testing, Psychological Assessment and Dietary Treatment of the Hyperactive Child Syndrome." *Medical Journal of Australia* 2: 248–51.
9. Mayron, L.; Ott, J.; Nations, R.; and Mayron, E. 1974. "Light, Radiation and Academic Behavior." *Academic Therapy* 10: 33–47. Mattes, J. 1983. "The Feingold Diet: A Current Reappraisal." *Journal of Learning Disabilities* 16: 319–23.
10. Furia, T., ed. 1980. *CRC Handbook of Food Additives*, vols. 1 and 2. Boca Raton, Fla.: CRC Press.
11. Ibid.
12. Newberne and Conner, "Food Additives and Contaminants," op. cit.
13. Golightly, L. K.; Smolinske, S. S.; Bennett, M. L.; et al. 1988. "Pharmaceutical Excipients: Adverse Effects Associated with Inactive Ingredients in Drug Products." *Medical Toxicology* 3: 128–65.
14. Furia, *CRC Handbook of Food Additives*, op. cit.
15. Collins-Williams, C. 1985. "Clinical Spectrum of Adverse Reactions to Tartrazine." *Journal of Asthma* 22: 139–43. Neuman, I.; Elian, R.; Nahum, H.; et al. 1978. "The Danger of 'Yellow Dyes' (Tartrazine) to Allergic Subjects." *Clinical Allergy* 8: 65–68.
16. Ibid.
17. Natbony, S. F.; Phillips, M. E.; Elias, J. M.; et al. 1983. "Histologic Studies of Chronic Idiopathic Urticaria." *Journal of Allergy and Clinical Immunology* 71: 177–83.
18. Warrington, R. J.; Sauder, P. J.; and McPhillips, S. 1986. "Cell-mediated Immune Responses to Artificial Food Additives in Chronic Urticaria." *Clinical Allergy* 16: 527–33.
19. Michaelsson, G., and Juhlin, L. 1973. "Urticaria Induced by Preservatives and Dye Additives to Food and Drugs." *British Journal of Dermatology* 88: 525–34. Thune, P., and Granhold, A. 1975. "Provocation Tests with Anti-phlogistic and Food Additives in Recurrent Urticaria." *Dermatologica* 151: 360–72. Ros, A. M.; Juhlin, L.; and Michaelsson, G. 1976. "A Follow-up Study of Patients with Recurrent Urticaria and Hypersensitivity to Aspirin, Benzoates and Azo Dyes." *British Journal of Dermatology* 95: 19–24. Warin, R. P., and Smith, R. J. 1976. "Challenge Test Battery in Chronic Urticaria." *British Journal of Dermatology* 94: 401–10. Kaaber, K. 1978. "Colouring and Preservative Agents and Chronic Ur-

ticaria: Value of a Provocative Trial and Elimination Diet." *Ugeskr. Laeger* 140: 1473–76. Meynadier, J.; Guilhou, J.; Meynadier, J.; et al. 1979. "Chronic Urticaria." *Annals of Dermatology and Venereology* 106: 153–58. Lindemayr, H., and Schmidt, J. 1979. "Intolerance to Acetylsalicylic Acid and Food Additives in Patients Suffering from Chronic Urticaria." *Wein. Klin. Wochenschr.* 91: 817–22. Gibson, A., and Clancy, R. 1980. "Management of Chronic Idiopathic Urticaria by the Identification and Exclusion of Dietary Factors." *Clinical Allergy* 10: 699–704. Doeglas, H. M. G. 1975. "Reactions to Aspirin and Food Additives in Patients with Chronic Urticaria, Including the Physicial Urticaria." *British Journal of Dermatology* 93: 135–44. Settipane, G. A.; Chafee, F. H.; Postman, H.; et al. 1976. "Significance of Tartrazine Sensitivity in Chronic Urticaria of Unknown Etiology." *Journal of Allergy and Clinical Immunology* 57: 541–49. Juhlin, L. 1986. "Recurrent Urticaria: Clinical Investigation of 330 Patients." *British Journal of Dermatology* 104: 369–81. Ortolani, C.; Pastorello, E.; Luraghi, M. T.; et al. 1984. "Diagnosis of Intolerance to Food Additives." *Annals of Allergy* 53: 587–91. Juhlin, L. 1987. "Additives and Chronic Urticaria." *Annals of Allergy* 59: 119–23. Supramaniam, G., and Warner, J. O. 1986. "Artificial Food Additive Intolerance in Patients with Angio-oedema and Urticaria." *Lancet* 2: 907–9.

20. Ibid.
21. Stellman, S. D., and Garfinkel, L. 1986. "Artificial Sweetener Use and One-year Weight Change Among Women." *Preventive Medicine* 15: 195–202.
22. Blundell, J. E., and Hill, A. J. 1986. "Paradoxical Effect of an Intense Sweetener (Aspartame) on Appetite." *Lancet* 1: 1092–93. Tordoff, M. G., and Alleva, A. M. 1990. "Oral Stimulation with Aspartame Increases Hunger." *Physiology and Behavior* 47: 555–59.
23. Cohen, S. M. 1986. "Saccharin: Past, Present, and Future." *Journal of American Dietetic Association* 86: 929–31. Council on Scientific Affairs. 1985. "Saccharin: Review of Safety Issues." *Journal of American Medical Association* 24: 2622–24.
24. Arnold, D. L. 1984. "Toxicology of Saccharin." *Fundamentals of Applied Toxicology* 4: 675–85.
25. Council on Scientific Affairs, "Saccharin," op. cit.
26. Blundell and Hill, "Paradoxical Effect of an Intense Sweetener," op. cit.
27. Council on Scientific Affairs. 1985. "Aspartame: Review of Safety Issues." *Journal of American Medical Association* 254: 400–2.
28. Hidehiko, Y.; Roberst, C.; Caballero, B.; and Wurtman, R. 1984. "Effects of Aspartame and Glucose Administration on Brain and Plasma Levels of Large Neutral Amino Acids and Brain 5-hydroxyindoles." *American Journal of Clinical Nutrition* 40: 1–7.
29. Ibid. Coulombe, R. A., and Sharma, R. P. 1986. "Neurobiochemical Alterations Induced by the Artificial Sweetener Aspartame (NutraSweet)." *Toxicology and Applied Pharmacology* 83: 79–85.
30. Monte, W. 1984. "Aspartame: Methanol and Public Health." *Journal of Applied Nutrition* 36: 42–54.
31. Ibid.
32. Bradstock, M. K.; Serdula, M. K.; Marks, J. S.; et al. 1986. "Evaluation of Reactions to Food Additives: The Aspartame Experience." *American Journal of Clinical Nutrition* 43: 464–69.
33. Koehler, S. M., and Glaros, A. 1988. "The Effect of Aspartame on Migraine Headache." *Headache* 28: 10–13.
34. Llaurado, J. G. 1985. "The Saga of BHT and BHA in Life Extension Myths." *Journal of American College of Nutrition* 4: 481–84.
35. Newberne and Conner, "Food Additives and Contaminants," op. cit.
36. Ibid.
37. Michaelsson and Juhlin, "Urticaria Induced by Preservatives," op. cit. Thune and Granhold, "Provocation Tests," op. cit. Ros, Juhlin, and Michaelsson, "A Follow-up Study," op. cit. Warin and Smith, "Challenge Test Battery in Chronic Urticaria," op. cit. Kaaber, "Coloring and Preservative Agents and Chronic Urticaria," op. cit. Meynadier, Guilhou, Meynadier, et al. "Chronic Urticaria," op. cit. Lindemayr and Schmidt, "Intolerance to Acetylsalicylic Acid and Food Additives," op. cit. Gibson and Clancy, "Management of Chronic Idiopathic Urticaria," op. cit. Doeglas, "Reactions to Aspirin and Food Additives," op. cit.

38. Simon, R. A. 1986. "Sulfite Sensitivity." *Annals of Allergy* 56: 281–88.
39. Quillin, P. 1990. *Safe Eating.* New York: Evans. Fan, A. M., and Jackson, R. J. 1989. "Pesticides and Food Safety." *Regulatory Toxicology and Pharmacology* 9: 158–74. Sterling, T., and Arundel, A. V. 1986. "Health Effects of Phenoxy Herbicides." *Scandinavian Journal of Work Environment Health* 12: 161–73.
40. Wigle, D. T.; Semenciw, R. M.; Wilkins, K; et al. "Mortality Study of Canadian Male Farm Operators: Non-Hodgkin's Lymphoma Mortality and Agricultural Practices in Saskatchewan. *Journal of National Cancer Institute* 82: 575–82.
41. Fan and Jackson, "Pesticides and Food Safety," op. cit. Sterling and Arundel, "Health Effects of Phenoxy Herbicides," op. cit.
42. Mott, L., and Broad, M. 1984. *Pesticides in Food.* San Francisco, Calif.: Natural Resources Defense Council.
43. Simon, "Sulfite Sensitivity," op. cit.
44. Fan and Jackson, "Pesticides and Food Safety," op. cit.
45. Mott and Broad, *Pesticides in Food,* op. cit.
46. Quillin, *Safe Eating,* op. cit.
47. Ibid.
48. American Medical Association. 1984. *Drinking Water and Human Health.* Chicago, Ill.: American Medical Association.
49. Quillin, *Safe Eating,* op. cit.

Chapter 3

1. The information presented in this chapter is based in large part on the following sources: Brown, M. B., ed. 1990. *Present Knowledge in Nutrition,* 6th ed. Washington, D.C.: Nutrition Foundation. Linder, M. C., ed. 1991. *Nutritional Biochemistry and Metabolism.* New York: Elsevier. Mahan, L. K., and Arlin, M. 1992. *Krause's Food, Nutrition, and Diet Therapy,* 8th ed. Philadelphia: W. B. Saunders. National Research Council. 1989. *Recommended Dietary Allowances,* 10th ed. Washington, D.C.: National Academy Press. National Research Council. 1989. *Diet and Health: Implications for Reducing Chronic Disease Risk.* Washington, D.C.: National Academy Press. Shils, M. E., and Young, V. R. 1988. *Modern Nutrition in Health and Disease,* 7th ed. Philadelphia, Penn.: Lea & Febiger. Whitney, E. N., and Cataldo, C. B. 1983. *Understanding Normal and Clinical Nutrition.* St. Paul, Minn.: West Publishing.

Chapter 4

1. Taussig, S., and Batkin S. 1988. "Bromelain, the Enzyme Complex of Pineapple (*Ananas comosus*) and Its Clinical Application: An Update." *Journal of Ethnopharmacology* 22: 191–203. Murray, M. T. 1991. *Healing Power of Herbs.* Rocklin, Calif.: Prima Press. Miller, J., and Opher, A. 1964. "The Increased Proteolytic Activity of Human Blood Serum After Oral Administration of Bromelain." *Experimental Medical Surgery* 22: 277–80.
2. Murray, *Healing Power of Herbs,* op. cit. Olson, J. A. 1990. "Vitamin A." In *Present Knowledge in Nutrition,* 6th ed., ed. by M. B. Brown (Washington, D.C.: Nutrition Foundation), pp. 96–107.
3. Titgemeyer, E. C.; Bourquin, L. D.; Fahey, G. C.; and Garleb K. A. 1991. "Fermentability of Various Fiber Sources by Human Fecal Bacteria in Vitro." *American Journal of Clinical Nutrition* 53: 1418–24. Taussig and Batkin, "Bromelain," op. cit. Murray, *Healing Power of Herbs,* op. cit. Miller and Opher, "Increased Proteolytic Activity," op. cit. Alexander, M.; Newmark, H.; and Miller, R. G. 1985. "Oral beta-Carotene Can Increase the Number of OKT4+ Cells in Human Blood." *Immunological Letters* 9: 221–24. Cutler, R. G. 1984. "Ca-

rotenoids and Retinol: Their Possible Importance in Determining Longevity of Primate Species." *Proceedings of National Academy of Science* 81: 7627–31.

4. Titgemeyer et al., "Fermentability of Various Fiber Sources," op. cit. Taussig and Batkin, "Bromelain," op. cit. Murray, *Healing Power of Herbs*, op. cit. Miller and Opher, "Increased Proteolytic Activity," op. cit.
5. Titgemeyer et al., "Fermentability of Various Fiber Sources," op. cit.
6. Taussig and Batkin, "Bromelain," op. cit.
7. Ibid. Murray, *Healing Power of Herbs*, op. cit.
8. Miller and Opher, "Increased Proteolytic Activity," op. cit. Izaka, K.; Yamada, M.; Kawano, T.; and Suyama, T. 1972. "Gastrointestinal Absorption and Anti-inflammatory Effect of Bromelain." *Japanese Journal of Pharmacology* 22: 519–34. Seifert, J.; Ganser, R.; and Brendel, W. 1979. "Absorption of a Proteolytic Enzyme of Plant Origin from the Gastrointestinal Tract into the Blood and Lymph of Adult Rats." *Journal of Gastroenterology* 17: 1–18.
9. Olson, "Vitamin A," op. cit.
10. Ibid. Bendich, A., and Olson, J. A. 1989. "Biological Actions of Carotenoids." *FASEB Journal* 3: 1927–32.
11. Olson, "Vitamin A," op. cit.
12. Ibid. Ziegler, R. G. 1989. "A Review of Epidemiologic Evidence That Carotenoids Reduce the Risk of Cancer." *Journal of Nutrition* 119: 116–22.
13. Olson, "Vitamin A," op. cit. Bendich and Olson, "Biological Actions of Carotenoids," op. cit. Krinsky, N. I. 1989. "Carotenoids and Cancer in Animal Models." *Journal of Nutrition* 119: 123–26. Bendich, A. 1989. "Carotenoids and the Immune Response." *Journal of Nutrition* 119: 112–15.
14. Cutler, "Carotenoids and Retinol," op. cit.
15. Linder, M. C. 1991. *Nutritional Biochemistry and Metabolism*. New York: Elsevier. Micozzi, M. S.; Beecher, G. R.; Taylor, P. R.; and Khachik, F. 1990. "Carotenoid Analysis of Selected Raw and Cooked Foods Associated with a Lower Risk for Cancer." *Journal of National Cancer Institute* 82: 282–85.
16. Bendich, A. 1988. "The Safety of beta-Carotene." *Nutrition and Cancer* 11: 207–14.
17. Cody, V.; Middleton, E.; Harborne, J. B.; and Beretz, A. 1988. *Plant Flavonoids in Biology and Medicine*, vol. 2: *Biochemical, Pharmacological, and Structure-activity Relationships*. New York: Alan R. Liss. Kuhnau, J. 1976. "The Flavonoids: A Class of Semi-essential Food Components: Their Role in Human Nutrition." *World Review of Nutrition and Diet* 24: 117–91. Havsteen, B. 1983. "Flavonoids, a Class of Natural Products of High Pharmacological Potency." *Biochemical Pharmacology* 32: 1141–48.
18. Ibid.
19. Kuhnau, "The Flavonoids," op. cit.
20. Blau, L. W. 1950. "Cherry Diet Control for Gout and Arthritis." *Texas Report on Biology and Medicine* 8: 309–11. Wegrowski, J.; Robert, A. M.; and Moczar, M. 1984. "The Effect of Procyanidolic Oligomers on the Composition of Normal and Hypercholesterolemic Rabbit Aortas. *Biochemical Pharmacology* 33: 3491–97.
21. Amella, M.; Bronner, C.; Briancon, F.; et al. 1985. "Inhibition of Mast Cell Histamine Release by Flavonoids and Biflavonoids." *Planta Medica* 51: 16–20. Busse, W. W.; Kopp, D. E.; and Middleton, E. 1984. "Flavonoid Modulation of Human Neutrophil Function." *Journal of Allergic and Clinical Immunology* 73: 801–9.
22. Rafsky, H. A., and Krieger, C. I. 1945. "The Treatment of Intestinal Diseases with Solutions of Water-soluble Chlorophyll." *Review of Gastroenterology* 15: 549–53. Smith, L., and Livingston, A. 1943. "Chlorophyll: An Experimental Study of Its Water Soluble Derivatives in Wound Healing." *American Journal of Surgery* 62: 358–69.
23. Nahata, M. C.; Sleccsak, C. A.; and Kamp, J. 1983. "Effect of Chlorophyllin on Urinary Odor in Incontinent Geriatric Patients." *Drug Intelligence and Clinical Pharmacology* 17: 732–34. Young, R. W., and Beregi, J. S. 1980. "Use of Chlorophyllin in the Care of Geriatric Patients." *Journal of American Geriatric Society* 28: 46–47.
24. Patek, A. 1936. "Chlorophyll and Regeneration of the Blood." *Archives of Internal Medicine* 57: 73–76. Gubner, R., and Ungerleider, H. E. 1944. "Vitamin K Therapy in Menorrhagia." *Southern Medical Journal* 37: 556–58.

25. Ong, T.; Whong, W. Z.; Stewart, J.; and Brockman, H. E. 1986. "Chlorophyllin: A Potent Antimutagen Against Environmental and Dietary Complex Mixtures." *Mutation Research* 173: 111–15.
26. Ohyama, S.; Kitamori, S.; Kawano, H.; et al. 1987. "Ingestion of Parsley Inhibits the Mutagenicity of Male Human Urine Following Consumption of Fried Salmon." *Mutation Research* 192: 7–10.
27. Pizzorno, J. E., and Murray, M. T. 1988. "Carnitine." In *A Textbook of Natural Medicine.* (Seattle: Bastyr College Publications). Bremer, J. 1983. "Carnitine—Metabolism and Function." *Physiology Review* 63: 1420–80. Borum, P. R. 1983. "Carnitine." *Annual Review of Nutrition* 3: 233–59.
28. Ibid.
29. Pizzorno and Murray, "Carnitine," op. cit.
30. Zeisel, S. H.; Da Costa, R. D.; Franklin, P. D.; et al. 1991. "Choline, an Essential Nutrient for Humans." *FASEB Journal* 5: 2093–98.
31. Gaby, A. 1988. "Coenzyme Q10." In *A Textbook of Natural Medicine.* (Seattle: Bastyr College Publications). Folkers, K., and Yamamura, Y., eds. 1984. *Biomedical and Clinical Aspects of Coenzyme Q,* vols. 1–4. Amsterdam: Elsevier Science Publications.
32. Ibid.
33. Ibid.
34. Ibid.
35. Gegersen, G.; Harb, H.; Helles, A.; and Christensen, J. 1983. "Oral Supplementation of Myoinositol: Effects on Peripheral Nerve Function in Human Diabetics and on the Concentration in Plasma, Erythrocytes, Urine and Muscle Tissue in Human Diabetics and Normals." *Acta Neurologica Scandinavia* 67: 164–71.
36. National Research Council. 1989. *Diet and Health: Implications for Reducing Chronic Disease Risk.* Washington, D.C.: National Academy Press. Steinmetz, K. A., and Potter, J. D. 1991. "Vegetables, Fruit, and Cancer. II. Mechanisms." *Cancer Causes and Control* 2: 427–42.
37. Ibid.
38. Steinmetz and Potter, "Vegetables, Fruit, and Cancer," op. cit.
39. American Cancer Society. 1984. *Nutrition and Cancer: Cause and Prevention.* New York: American Cancer Society.
40. Smart, R. C.; Huang, M. T.; Chang, R. L.; et al. 1986. "Effect of Ellagic Acid and 3-0-decylellagic Acid on the Formation of Benzo[a]pyrene DNA Adducts in Vivo and on the Tumorigenicity of 3-Methylcholanthrene in Mice." *Carcinogenesis.* 7: 1669–75.
41. Majid, S.; Khanduja, K. L.; Gandhi, R. K.; et al. 1991. "Influence of Ellagic Acid on Antioxidant Defense System and Lipid Peroxidation in Mice." *Biochemical Pharmacology* 42: 1441–45.
42. Jones, D. P.; Coates, R. J.; Flagg, E. W.; et al. 1992. "Glutathione in Foods Listed in the National Cancer Institute's Health Habits and History Food Frequency Questionnaire." *Nutrition and Cancer* 17: 57–75.

Chapter 5

1. Cheng, K. K.; Day, N. E.; Duffy, S. W.; et al. 1992. "Pickled Vegetables in the Aetiology of Oesophageal Cancer in Hong Kong Chinese." *Lancet* 339: 1314–18.
2. Yamashita, K.; Kawai, K.; and Itakura, M. 1984. "Effects of Fructo-oligosaccharides on Blood Glucose and Serum Lipids in Diabetic Subjects." *Nutrition Research* 4: 491–96.
3. Maros, T.; Racz, G.; Katonaj, B.; and Kovacs, V. 1966 (1st communication), 1968. "The Effects of *Cynara Scolymus* Extracts on the Regeneration of the Rat Liver." *Arzneim.-Forsch* 16: 127–29; 18: 884–86. Montini, M.; Levoni, P.; Angoro, A.; and Pagani, G. 1975. "Controlled Trial of Cynarin in the Treatment of the Hyperlipemic Syndrome." *Arzneim.-Forsch* 25: 1311–14. Pristautz, H. 1975. "Cynarin in the Modern Treatment of Hyperlipemias." *Wiener Medizinische Wocheschrift* 1223: 705–9.
4. Maros, Racz, Katonaj, and Kovacs, "Effects of *Cynara scolymus* Extracts," op. cit.

5. Montini, Levoni, Angoro, and Pagani, "Controlled Trial of Cynarin," op. cit. Pristautz, "Cynarin in Modern Treatment of Hyperlipemias," op. cit.
6. Manousos, O.; Day, N. E.; Trichopoulus, D.; et al. 1983. "Diet and Colorectal Cancer: A Case-control Study in Greece." *International Journal of Cancer* 32: 1–5.
7. Gallaher, D. D.; Locket, P.; and Gallaher, C. M. 1992. "Bile Acid Metabolism in Rats Fed Two Levels of Corn Oil and Brans of Oat, Rye, and Barley and Sugar Beet Fiber." *Journal of Nutrition* 122: 473–81.
8. Welihinda, J.; Karunanaya, E. H.; Sheriff, M. H. R.; and Jayasinghe, K. S. A. 1986. "Effect of *Momardica charantia* on the Glucose Tolerance in Maturity Onset Diabetes." *Journal of Ethnopharmacology* 17: 277–82. Welihinda, J.; Arvidson, G.; Gylfe, E.; et al. 1982. "The Insulin-releasing Activity of the Tropical Plant *Momardica charantia*." *Acta Biologica Medica Germania* 41: 1229–40.
9. Jifka, C.; Strifler, B.; Fortner, G. W.; et al. 1983. "In Vivo Antitumor Activity of the Bitter Melon (*Momardica charantia*)." *Cancer Research* 43: 5151–55.
10. National Research Council. 1989. *Diet and Health: Implications for Reducing Chronic Disease Risk*. Washington, D.C.: National Academy Press. Rogers, A. E., and Longnecker, M. P. 1988. "Biology of Disease: Dietary and Nutritional Influences on Cancer: A Review of Epidemiologic and Experimental Data." *Laboratory Investigations* 59: 729–59. Steinmetz, K. A., and Potter, J. D. 1991. "Vegetables, Fruit, and Cancer. II. Mechanisms." *Cancer Causes and Control* 2: 427–42.
11. Cheney, G. 1949. "Rapid Healing of Peptic Ulcers in Patients Receiving Fresh Cabbage Juice." *California Medicine* 70: 10–14. Cheney G. 1950. "Anti-peptic Ulcer Dietary Factor." *Journal of American Dietetic Association* 26: 668–72.
12. Wald, N. J.; Thompson, S. G.; Densem, J. W.; et al. 1988. Serum beta-Carotene and Subsequent Risk of Cancer: Results from the BUPA Study." *British Journal of Cancer* 57: 428–33. Harris, R. W. C.; Key, T. J. A.; Silcocks, P. B.; et al. 1991. A Case-control Study of Dietary Carotene in Men with Lung Cancer and in Men with Other Epithelial Cancers." *Nutrition and Cancer* 15: 63–68.
13. Murray, M. T. 1991. *Healing Power of Herbs*. Rocklin, Calif.: Prima Press.
14. Ibid.
15. Ibid.
16. Ibid.
17. Ibid.
18. Sainani, G. S.; Desai, D. B.; Gohre, N. H.; et al. 1979. "Effect of Dietary Garlic and Onion on Serum Lipid Profile in Jain Community." *Indian Journal of Medical Research* 69: 776–80.
19. Rumessen, J. J.; Bode, S.; Hamberg, O.; and Hoyer, E. 1990. "Fructans of Jerusalem Artichokes: Intestinal Transport, Absorption, Fermentation, and Influence on Blood Glucose, Insulin, and C-peptide Responses in Healthy Subjects." *American Journal of Clinical Nutrition* 52: 675–81.
20. Ibid.
21. Ibid.
22. Murray, *Healing Power of Herbs*, op. cit.
23. Ibid.
24. Ibid.
25. Ibid.
26. Keswani, M. H.; Vartak, A. M.; Patil, A.; and Davies, J. W. L. 1990. "Histological and Bacteriological Studies of Burn Wounds Treated with Boiled Potato Peel Dressings." *Burns* 16: 137–43.

Chapter 6

1. Gregersen, S.; Rasmussen, O.; Larsen, S.; and Hermansen, K. 1992. "Glycaemic and Insulinaemic Responses to Orange and Apple Compared with White Bread in Non-insulin-dependent Diabetic Subjects." *European Journal of Clinical Nutrition* 46: 301–3. Crapo,

P. A.; Kolterman, O. G.; and Olefsky, J. M. 1980. "Effect of Oral Fructose in Normal, Diabetic, and Impared Glucose Tolerance Subjects." *Diabetes Care* 3: 575–82.

2. Rodin, J. 1991. "Effects of Pure Sugar vs. Mixed Starch Fructose Loads on Food Intake." *Appetite* 17: 213–19. Rodin, J. 1990. "Comparative Effects of Fructose, Aspartame, Glucose, and Water Preloads on Calorie and Macronutrient Intake." *American Journal of Clinical Nutrition* 51: 428–35. Spitzer, L., and Rodin, J. 1987. "Effects of Fructose and Glucose Preloads on Subsequent Food Intake." *Appetite* 8: 135–45.
3. Anderson, J. W. 1985. "Physiological and Metabolic Effects of Dietary Fiber." *Federation Proceedings* 44: 2902–6. El-Shebini, S. M.; Hanna, L. M.; Topouzada, S. T.; et al. 1988. "The Role of Pectin as a Slimming Agent." *Journal of Clinical Biochemical Nutrition* 4: 255–62.
4. Best, R.; Lewis, D. A.; and Nasser, N. 1984. "The Anti-ulcerogenic Activity of the Unripe Plantain Banana (*Musa* species)." *British Journal of Pharmacology* 82: 107–16.
5. Murray, M. T. 1991. *Healing Power of Herbs.* Rocklin, Calif.: Prima Press.
6. Ibid.
7. Carper, J. 1989. *The Food Pharmacy.* New York: Bantam.
8. Pinski, S. L., and Maloney, J. D. 1990. "Adenosine: A New Drug for Acute Termination of Supraventricular Tachycardia." *Cleveland Clinical Journal of Medicine* 57: 383–88.
9. Sobota, A. E. "Inhibition of Bacterial Adherence by Cranberry Juice: Potential Use for the Treatment of Urinary Tract Infections." *Journal of Urology* 131: 1013–16.
10. Ibid.
11. Ofek, I.; Goldhar, J.; et al. 1991. "Anti-escherichia Activity of Cranberry and Blueberry Juices." *New England Journal of Medicine* 324: 1599.
12. Ibid.
13. Masquelier, J. 1981. "Pycnogenols: Recent Advances in the Therapeutic Activity of Procyanidins." In *Natural Products as Medicinal Agents,* vol. 1 (Stuttgart: Hippokrates-Verlag), pp. 243–56.
14. Cerda, J.; Robbins, F. L.; Burgin, C. W.; et al. 1988. "The Effects of Grapefruit Pectin on Patients at Risk for Coronary Heart Disease Without Altering Diet or Lifestyle." *Clinical Cardiology* 11: 589–94.
15. Robbins, R. C.; Martin, F. G.; and Roe, J. M. 1988. "Ingestion of Grapefruit Lowers Elevated Hematocrits in Human Subjects. *International Journal of Vitamin Nutrition Research* 58: 414–17.
16. Ibid.
17. Kodama, R.; Yano, T.; Furukawa, et al. 1976. "Studies on the Metabolism of d-Limonene." *Xenobiotica* 6: 377–89. Wattenberg, L. W. 1983. "Inhibition of Neoplasia by Minor Dietary Constituents." *Cancer Research* 43 (Supplement): 2448s–53s.
18. Carper, *The Food Pharmacy,* op. cit.
19. Leung, A. 1980. *Encyclopedia of Common Natural Ingredients Used in Food, Drugs, and Cosmetics.* New York: John Wiley & Sons.
20. Taussig, S. J.; Szekerczes, J.; and Batkin, S. 1985. "Inhibition of Tumour Growth in Vitro by Bromelain, an Extract of the Pineapple Plant (*Ananas comosus*)." *Planta Medica* 52: 538–39.

Chapter 7

1. Ensminger, A. H.; Ensminger, M. E.; Konland, G. E.; and Robson, J. R. K. 1983. *Foods and Nutrition Encyclopedia.* Clovis, Calif.: Pegus Press.
2. Ibid.
3. Yoshino, G.; Kazumi, T.; Amano, M.; et al. 1989. "Effects of gamma-Oryzanol on Hyperlipidemic Subjects." *Current Therapeutic Research* 45: 543–52. Gorent, R. C.; 1983. "Pituitary and Thyroid Hormone Responses of Heifers after Ferulic Acid Administration." *Journal of Dairy Science* 66: 624–29.
4. Ensminger, Ensminger, Konland, and Robson, *Foods and Nutrition Encyclopedia,* op. cit.

5. Ibid.
6. Ripsin, C. M.; Keenan, J. M.; Jacobs, D. R.; et al. 1992. "Oat Products and Lipid Lowering, a Meta-analysis." *Journal of American Medical Association* 267: 3317–25.
7. Ensminger, Ensminger, Konland, and Robson, *Foods and Nutrition Encylopedia,* op. cit.
8. Ibid.
9. Ibid.
10. Ibid.

Chapter 8

1. Young, V. R. 1991. "Soy Protein in Relation to Human Protein and Amino Acid Nutrition." *Journal of American Dietetic Association* 91: 828–35.
2. Ibid. Scrimshaw, N. S.; Wayler, A. H.; Murray, E.; et al. 1983. "Nitrogen Balance Response in Young Men Given One of Two Isolated Soy Proteins or Milk Proteins." *Journal of Nutrition* 113: 2492–97.
3. Carrol, K. K. 1991. "Review of Clinical Studies on Cholesterol-lowering Response to Soy Protein. *Journal of American Dietetic Association* 91: 820–27. Van Raaij, J. M. A.; Katan, M. B.; West, C. E.; and Hautvast, J. G. A. 1982. "Influence of Diets Containing Casein, Soy Protein Isolate, and Soy Concentrate on Serum Cholesterol and Lipoproteins in Middle-aged Volunteers." *American Journal of Clinical Nutrition* 35: 925–34. Redgrave, T. G. 1984. "Dietary Proteins and Atherosclerosis." *Atherosclerosis* 52: 349–51. Beynen, A. C.; Van der Meer, R.; and West, C. E. 1986. "Mechanism of Casein-induced Hypercholesterolemia: Primary and Secondary Features." *Atherosclerosis* 60: 291–93.
4. Carrol, "Review of Clinical Studies," op. cit.
5. Beynen, Van der Meer, and West, "Mechanism of Casein-induced Hypercholesterolemia," op. cit.
6. Hanin, I., and Ansell, G. B., eds. 1987. *Lecithin: Technological, Biological, and Therapeutic Aspects.* New York: Plenum Press.
7. Ibid.
8. Tilvis, R. S., and Miettinen, T. A. 1986. "Serum Plant Sterols and Their Relation to Cholesterol Absorption." *American Journal of Clinical Nutrition* 43: 92–97.
9. Messina, M., and Barnes, S. 1991. "The Roles of Soy Products in Reducing Risk of Cancer." *Journal of National Cancer Institute* 83: 541–46. Messina, M., and Messina, V. 1991. "Increasing the Use of Soyfoods and Their Potential Role in Cancer Prevention." *Journal of American Dietetic Association* 91: 836–40.
10. Ibid.
11. Ibid.
12. Titscher, R., and Wrba, H. 1975. "Local Therapy of Malignant Pleural Effusions, Further Observations and Results. *Zeit Onkol.* 1: 19–21.
13. Ransberger, K. 1986. "Enzyme Treatment of Immune Complex Disorders." *Arthritis and Rheumatism* 8: 16–19.
14. Moley, J. E. 1990. "Appetite Regulation by Gut Peptides." *Annual Review of Nutrition* 10: 383–95.
15. Messina and Barnes, "The Roles of Soy Products," op. cit. Messina and Messina, "Increasing the Use of Soyfoods," op. cit.
16. Ibid.
17. Messina and Barnes, "The Roles of Soy Products," op. cit.
18. Ibid.
19. Lin, H. C.; Moller, N. A.; Wolinsky, M. M.; et al. 1992. "Sustained Slowing Effect of Lentils on Gastric Emptying of Solids in Humans and Dogs." *Gastrology* 102: 787–92.

Chapter 9

1. Ensminger, A. H.; Ensminger, M. E.; Konland, G. E.; and Robson, J. R. K. 1983. *Foods and Nutrition Encyclopedia.* Clovis, Calif.: Pegus Press.
2. Ibid.
3. Fraser, G. E.; Sabate, J.; Beeson, W. L.; and Strahan, T. M. 1992. "A Possible Protective Effect of Nut Consumption on Risk of Coronary Heart Disease." *Archives of Internal Medicine* 152: 1416–24.
4. Weller, D. P.; Zaneveld, J. D.; and Farnsworth, N. R. 1985. "Gossypol: Pharmacology and Current Status as a Male Contraceptive." *Economic and Medicinal Plant Research* 1: 87–112.
5. Griffith, R.; DeLong, D.; and Nelson, J. 1981. "Relation of Arginine-Lysine Antagonism to *Herpes simplex* Growth in Tissue Culture." *Chemotherapy* 27: 209–13.
6. Ensminger, Ensminger, Konland, and Robson, *Foods and Nutrition Encyclopedia,* op. cit.
7. Adlercreutz, H.; Fotsis, T.; Bannwart, C.; et al. 1986. "Determination of Urinary Lignans and Phytoestrogen Metabolites, Potential Antiestrogens and Anticarcinogens, in Urine of Women in Various Habitual Diets." *Journal of Steroid Biochemistry* 25: 791–97.
8. Serraino, M., and Thompson, L. U. 1991. "The Effect of Flaxseed Supplementation on Early Risk Markers for Mammary Carcinogenesis." *Cancer Letters* 60: 135–42.
9. Simpoulos, A. P. 1989. "Summary of the NATO Advanced Research Workshop on Dietary ω3 and ω6 Fatty Acids: Biological Effects and Nutritional Essentiality." *Journal of Nutrition* 119: 521–28. Leaf, A., and Weber, P. C. 1988. "Cardiovascular Effects of n-3 Fatty Acids." *New England Journal of Medicine* 318: 549–57. Murray, M. T., and Pizzorno, J. E. 1991. *Encyclopedia of Natural Medicine.* Rocklin, Calif.: Prima Press.
10. Ensminger, Ensminger, Konland, and Robson, *Food and Nutrition Encyclopedia,* op. cit.
11. Ibid.
12. Caster, W. O.; Burton, T. A.; Irvin, T. R.; and Tanner, M. A. 1986. "Dietary Aflatoxins, Intelligence and School Performance in Southern Georgia." *International Journal of Vitamin and Nutrition Research* 56: 291–95.
13. Murray and Pizzorno, *Encyclopedia of Natural Medicine,* op. cit. Fahim, M.; Fahim, Z.; Der, R.; and Harman, J. 1976. "Zinc Treatment for the Reduction of Hyperplasia of the Prostate." *Federation Proceedings* 35: 361.
14. Carper, J. 1989. *The Food Pharmacy.* New York: Bantam.
15. Fukuda, Y.; Osawa, T.; and Namike, M. 1985. "Studies on Antioxidative Substances in Sesame Seed." *Agricultural Biological Chemistry* 49: 301–6.
16. Hirose, N.; Inoue, T.; Nishihara, K.; et al. 1991. "Inhibition of Cholesterol Absorption and Synthesis in Rats by Sesamin." *Journal of Lipid Research* 32: 629–38.

Chapter 10

1. The information in this chapter is largely derived from the following sources: Duke, J. A. 1985. *Handbook of Medicinal Herbs.* Boca Raton, Fla.: CRC Press. Grieve, M. 1971. *A Modern Herbal.* New York: Dover Publications. Kowalchik, C., and Hylton, W. H., eds. 1987. *Rodale's Illustrated Encyclopedia of Herbs.* Emmaus, Penn.: Rodale Press. Leung, A. 1980. *Encyclopedia of Common Natural Ingredients Used in Food, Drugs, and Cosmetics.* New York: John Wiley & Sons. Lust, J. 1974. *The Herb Book.* New York: Bantam Books. Murray, M. T. 1991. *Healing Power of Herbs.* Rocklin, Calif.: Prima Press. Murray, M. T., and Pizzorno, J. E. 1991. *Encyclopedia of Natural Medicine.* Rocklin, Calif.: Prima Press. Willard, T. *Wild Rose Scientific Herbal.* 1991. Calgary, Alta.: Wild Rose College of Natural Healing.

Chapter 11

1. The information in this chapter is largely derived from the following sources: Mahan, L. K., and Arlin, M. 1992. *Krause's Food, Nutrition, and Diet Therapy,* 8th ed. Philadelphia: W. B. Saunders. Shils, M. E., and Young, V. R. 1988. *Modern Nutrition in Health and Disease,* 7th ed. Philadelphia: Lea & Febiger. Whitney, E. N., and Cataldo, C. B. 1983. *Understanding Normal and Clinical Nutrition.* St. Paul, Minn.: West Publishing.

Chapter 12

1. Shils, M. E., and Young, V. R. 1988. *Modern Nutrition in Health and Disease,* 7th ed. Philadelphia: Lea & Febiger. Bray, G. A. 1985. "Obesity: Definition, Diagnosis and Disadvantages." *Medical Journal of Australia* 142: 52–58. Raymond, C. A. 1986. "Biology, Culture, Dietary Changes Conspire to Increase Incidence of Obesity." *Journal of American Medical Association* 256: 2157–58.
2. Shils and Young, *Modern Nutrition,* op. cit. Bray, "Obesity," op. cit.
3. Kolata, G. 1985. "Why Do People Get Fat?" *Science* 227: 1327–28.
4. Bennett, W., and Gurin, J. 1982. *The Dieter's Dilemma.* New York: Basic Books.
5. Ibid.
6. Trowell, H.; Burkitt, D.; and Heaton, K. 1985. *Dietary Fiber, Fiber-depleted Foods and Disease.* New York: Academic Press.
7. Thompson, J. K.; Jarvie, G. J.; Lahey, B. B.; and Cureton, K. J. 1982. "Exercise and Obesity: Etiology, Physiology, and Intervention." *Psychology Bulletin* 91: 55–79.
8. Pollack, M. L.; Wilmore, J. H.; and Fox, S. M. 1984. *Exercise in Health and Disease.* Philadelphia: W. B. Saunders, pp. 131, 141–47, 219–21, 228–34, 378, 382, 384–85, 457–58.
9. American College of Sports Medicine. 1983. "Position Statement on Proper and Improper Weight Loss Programs." *Medical Science Sports and Exercise* 15: ix–xiii.
10. Oscai, L. B., and Holloszy, J. O. 1969. "Effects of Weight Changes Produced by Exercise, Food Restriction or Overeating on Body Composition." *Journal of Clinical Investigation* 48: 2124–28.
11. Lennon, D.; Nagle, F.; Stratman, F.; et al. 1988. "Diet and Exercise Training Effects on Resting Metabolic Rate." *International Journal of Obesity.* 9: 39–47.
12. American College of Sports Medicine. 1986. *Guidelines for Graded Exercise Testing and Prescription,* 3d ed. Philadelphia: Lea & Febiger, pp. 1–4, 22, 36, 48–49, 74–78, 80–83, 456–59.
13. Ibid.
14. Hill, J. O.; Schlundt, D. G.; Sbrocco, T.; et al. 1989. "Evaluation of an Alternating-calorie Diet with and Without Exercise in the Treatment of Obesity." *American Journal of Clinical Nutrition* 50: 238–54.
15. Farmer, M. E.; Locke, B. Z.; Mosciki, E. K.; et al. 1988. "Physical Activity and Depressive Symptomatology: The NHANES 1 Epidemiologic Follow-up Study." *American Journal of Epidemiology* 1328: 1340–51.
16. Gwinup, G.; Chelvam, R.; and Steinberg, T. 1971. "Thickness of Subcutaneous Fat and Activity of Underlying Muscles." *Annals of Internal Medicine,* 74: 408–11. Wilmore, J. H. 1974. "Alterations in Strength, Body Composition and Athropometric Measurements Consequent to a 10-week Weight Training Program." *Medicine Science and Sports* 6: 133–38.
17. Ballor, D. L.; Katch, V. L.; Becque, M. D.; and Marks, C. R. 1988. "Resistance Weight Training During Calorie Restriction Enhances Lean Body Weight Maintenance." *American Journal of Clinical Nutrition* 47: 19–25.
18. Douglass, J. M.; Rasgon, I. M.; Fleiss, P. M.; et al. 1985. "Effects of a Raw Food Diet on Hypertension and Obesity." *Southern Medicinal Journal* 78: 841–44. Anderson, J. W., and Bryant, C. A. 1986. "Dietary Fiber: Diabetes and Obesity." *American Journal of Gastroenterology* 81: 898–906.

19. Bray, "Obesity," op. cit. Raymond, "Biology, Culture, Dietary Changes," op. cit.
20. Shils and Young, *Modern Nutrition*, op. cit. Bray, "Obesity," op. cit.
21. Trowell, Burkitt, and Heaton, *Dietary Fiber*, op. cit.
22. Anderson and Bryant, "Dietary Fiber," op. cit. Rossner, S.; Zweigbergk, D. V.; Ohlin, A.; and Ryttig, K. 1987. "Weight Reduction with Dietary Fibre Supplements: Results of Two Double-blind Studies." *Acta Medica Scandinavia* 222: 83–88. Shearer, R. S. 1976. "Effect of Bulk Producing Tablets on Hunger Intensity and Dieting Pattern." *Current Therapeutic Research* 19: 433–41. Hylander, B., and Rossner, S. 1983. "Effects of Dietary Fiber Intake Before Meals on Weight Loss and Hunger in a Weight-reducing Club." *Acta Medica Scandinavia* 213: 217–20.

Chapter 13

1. Adams, F. 1939. *The Genuine Works of Hippocrates*. Baltimore: Williams & Williams.
2. Wright, J. V. 1984. *Healing with Nutrition*. Emmaus, Penn.: Rodale Press.
3. Dickey, L. D. 1974. *Clinical Ecology*. Springfield, Ill.: C. C. Thomas.
4. Taub, E. L. 1978. *Food Allergy and the Allergic Patient*. Springfield, Ill.: C. C. Thomas.
5. Buckley, R. 1982. "Food Allergy." *Journal of American Medical Association* 248: 2627–29.
6. Hamburger, R. 1982. Proceedings of First International Symposium on Food Allergy. Vancouver, B.C.
7. Bryan, W. T. K., and Bryan, M. P. 1972. "Clinical Examples of Resolution of Some Idiopathic and Other Chronic Disease by Careful Allergic Management." *Laryngoscope* 82: 1231–38.
8. Perelmutter, L. 1984. "Non-IgE Mediated Atopic Disease." *Annals of Allergy* 52: 64–69. Paganelli, R.; Levinsky, R. J.; and Atherton, D. J. 1979. "Detection of Specific Antigen Within Circulating Immune Complexes." *Lancet* i: 1270.
9. Hamburger, Proceedings of First International Symposium, op. cit.
10. McGovern, J. J. 1980. "Correlation of Clinical Food Allergy Symptoms with Serial Pharmacological and Immunological Changes in the Patient's Plasma." *Annals of Allergy* 44: 57–61.
11. Trevino, R. J. 1981. "Immunologic Mechanisms in the Production of Food Sensitivities." *Laryngoscope* 91: 1913–36.
12. Thonnard-Nenmann, E., and Neckers, L. M. 1981. "T-lymphocytes in Migraine." *Annals of Allergy* 47: 325–29. Rivlin, J.; Kuperman, O.; Freier, S.; et al. 1981. "Suppressor T-lymphocyte Activity in Wheezy Children." *Clinical Allergy* 11: 353–56.
13. Minor, J. D.; Tolber, S. G.; and Frick, O. L. 1980. "Leukocyte Inhibition Factor in Delayed-onset Food Sensitivity." *Journal of Allergy and Clinical Immunology* 6: 314–21.
14. Taylor, B.; Norman, A. P.; Orgel, C. R.; et al. 1973. "Transient IgA Deficiency and Pathogenesis of Infantile Atopy." *Lancet* ii: 111–13.
15. Keller, S. E.; Weiss, J. M.; Schleifer, S. J.; et al. 1981. "Suppression of Immunity by Stress: Effect of Graded Series of Stressors on Lymphocyte Stimulation in the Rat." *Science* 213: 1397–400. Ader, R. ed. 1981. *Psychoimmunology*. New York: Academic Press.
16. Hemmings, W. A., and Williams, E. W. 1978. "Transport of Large Breakdown Products of Dietary Protein Through the Gut Wall." *Gut* 19: 715–23.
17. Walker, W. A. 1974. "Uptake and Transport of Macromolecules by the Intestine—Possible Role in Clinical Disorders." *Gastroenterology* 67: 531–50.
18. Grusky, F. L. 1955. "Gastrointestinal Absorption of Unaltered Proteins in Normal Infants." *Pediatrics* 16: 763–68.
19. Dockhorn, R. J., and Smith, T. C. 1981. "Use of a Chemically Defined Hypoallergenic Diet in the Management of Patients with Suspected Food Allergy." *Annals of Allergy* 47: 264–66. Rowe, A. H., and Rowe, A. 1972. *Food Allergy: Its Manifestations and Control and the Elimination Diets*. Springfield, Ill.: C. C. Thomas.
20. Metcalfe, D. 1984. "Food Hypersensitivity." *Journal of Allergy and Clinical Immunology* 73: 749–61.

21. Coca, A. F. 1945. *Familial Nonreagenic Food Allergy.* Springfield, Ill.: C. C. Thomas.
22. Rinkel, H. J.; Randolph, T.; and Zeller, M. 1951. *Food Allergy.* Springfield, Ill.: C. C. Thomas.
23. Rinkel, H. J. 1948. "Food Allergy IV: The Function and Clinical Application of the Rotary Diversified Diet." *Journal of Pediatrics* 32: 266–74.

Chapter 14

1. Murray, M. T., and Pizzorno, J. E. 1991. *Encyclopedia of Natural Medicine.* Rocklin, Calif.: Prima Press.
2. Ibid.
3. Michaelsson, G.; Juhlin, L.; and Ljunghall, K. 1977. "A Double Blind Study of the Effect of Zinc and Oxytetracycline in Acne Vulgaris." *British Journal of Dermatology* 97: 561–65. Weimar, V.; Puhl, S.; Smith, W.; and Broeke, J. 1978. "Zinc Sulphate in Acne Vulgaris." *Archives of Dermatology* 114: 1776–78.
4. Michaelsson, G.; Vahlquist, A.; and Juhlin, L. 1977. "Serum Zinc and Retinol-binding Protein in Acne." *British Journal of Dermatology* 96: 283–86.
5. Michaelsson, G., and Edqvist, L. 1984. "Erythrocyte Glutathione Peroxidase Activity in Acne Vulgaris and the Effect of Selenium and Vitamin E Treatment." *Acta Dermatologica Venerologie* (StockH) 64: 9–14.
6. Murray and Pizzorno, *Encyclopedia of Natural Medicine,* op. cit.
7. Ibid.
8. Ibid.
9. Ibid.
10. Ibid.
11. Bock, S. A. 1983. "Food-related Asthma and Basic Nutrition." *Journal of Asthma* 20: 377–81. Oehling, A. 1981. "Importance of Food Allergy in Childhood Asthma." *Allergology Immunopathology Supplement* 9: 71–73. Ogle, K. A., and Bullocks, J. D. 1980. "Children with Allergic Rhinitis and/or Bronchial Asthma Treated with Elimination Diet: A Five-year Follow-up." *Annals of Allergy* 44: 273–78. Pelikan, Z. 1988. "Nasal Response to Food Ingestion Challenge." *Archives of Otolaryngology and Head Neck Surgery* 114: 525–30.
12. Freedman, B. J. 1977. "A Diet Free from Additives in the Management of Allergic Disease." *Clinical Allergy* 7: 417–21.
13. Ibid.
14. Ibid. Stevenson, D. D., and Simon, R. A. 1981. "Sensitivity to Ingested Metabisulfites in Asthmatic Subjects." *Journal of Allergy and Clinical Immunology* 68: 26–32.
15. Stevenson and Simon, "Sensitivity to Ingested Metabisulfites," op. cit.
16. Lindahl, O.; Lindwall, L.; Spangberg, A.; et al. 1985. "Vegan Diet Regimen with Reduced Medication in the Treatment of Bronchial Asthma." *Journal of Asthma* 22: 45–55.
17. Spannhake, E. W., and Menkes, H. A. 1983. "Vitamin C—New Tricks for an Old Dog." *American Review of Respiratory Disease* 127: 139–41.
18. Olusi, S. O.; Ojutiku, O. O.; Jessop, W. J. E.; and Iboko, M. I. 1979. "Plasma and White Blood Cell Ascorbic Acid Concentrations in Patients with Bronchial Asthma." *Clinica Chemica Acta* 92: 161–66.
19. Anderson, R.; Hay, I.; Van Wyk, H. A.; and Theron, A. 1983. "Ascorbic Acid in Bronchial Asthma." *South African Medical Journal* 63: 649–52. Mohsenin, V.; Dubois, A. B.; and Douglas, J. S. 1983. "Effect of Ascorbic Acid on Response to Methylcholine Challenge in Asthmatic Subjects." *American Review of Respiratory Disease* 127: 143–47.
20. Personal communication with Jonathan Wright, M.D.
21. Simon, S. W. 1951. "Vitamin B_{12} Therapy in Allergy and Chronic Dermatoses." *Journal of Allergy* 2: 183–85.
22. Garrison, R., and Somer, E. 1985. *The Nutrition Desk Reference,* ch. 5, "Vitamin Research: Selected Topics." New Canaan, Conn.: Keats Publications, pp. 93–94.
23. Murray and Pizzorno, *Encyclopedia of Natural Medicine,* op. cit.

24. Kroker, G. F. 1987. "Chronic Candidiasis and Allergy." In *Food Allergy and Intolerance,* J. Brostoff and S. J. Challacombe, eds. Philadelphia: W. B. Saunders, pp. 850–72. Truss, O. 1983. *The Missing Diagnosis.* P.O. Box 26508, Birmingham, Ala. Crook, W. G. 1984. *The Yeast Connection,* 2d ed. Jackson, Tenn.: Professional Books.
25. Ibid.
26. Adetumbi, M. A., and Lau, B. H. 1983. "*Allium sativum* (Garlic)—A Natural Antibiotic." *Medical Hypothesis* 12: 227–37. Amer, M.; Taha, M.; and Tosson, Z. 1980. "The Effect of Aqueous Garlic Extract on the Growth of Dermatophytes." *International Journal of Dermatology* 19: 285–87. Moore, G. S., and Atkins, R. D. 1977. "The Fungicidal and Fungistatic Effects of an Aqueous Garlic Extract on Medically Important Yeastlike Fungi." *Mycologia* 69: 341–48. Sandhu, D. K.; Warraich, M. K.; and Singh, S. 1980. "Sensitivity of Yeasts Isolated from Cases of Vaginitis to Aqueous Extracts of Garlic." *Mykosen* 23: 691–98. Prasad, G., and Sharma, V. D. 1980. "Efficacy of Garlic (*Allium sativum*) Treatment Against Experimental Candidiasis in Chicks." *British Veterinary Journal* 136: 448–51.
27. Ibid.
28. Murray and Pizzorno, *Encyclopedia of Natural Medicine,* op. cit.
29. Ibid.
30. Thomas, H. C.; Ferguson, A.; McLennan, J. G.; and Mason, D. K. 1973. "Food Antibodies in Oral Disease: A Study of Serum Antibodies to Food Proteins in Aphthous Ulceration and Other Oral Diseases. *Journal of Clinical Pathology* 26: 371–74. Wilson, C. W. M. 1980. "Food Sensitivities, Taste Changes, Aphthous Ulcers and Atopic Symptoms in Allergic Disease." *Annals of Allergy* 44: 302–7.
31. Ferguson, R.; Bashu, M. K.; Asquith, P.; and Cooke, W. T. 1975. "Jejunal Mucosal Abnormalities in Patients with Recurrent Aphthous Ulceration." *British Medical Journal* 1: 11–13. Ferguson, M. M.; Wray, D.; Carmichael, H. A.; et al. 1980. "Coeliac Disease Associated with Recurrent Aphthae." *Gut* 21: 223–26. Wray, D. 1981. "Gluten-sensitive Recurrent Aphthous Stomatitis." *Digestive Disease Science* 26: 737–40. Walker, D. M.; Rhodes, J.; Llewelyn, J.; et al. 1979. "Gluten Hypersensitivity in Recurrent Aphthous Ulceration." *Journal of Dental Research* 58 (Special Issue C): 1271. Wray, D. W.; Ferguson, M. M.; Hutcheon, A. W.; and Dagg, J. H. 1978. "Nutritional Deficiencies in Recurrent Aphthae." *Journal of Oral Pathology* 7: 418–23.
32. Ferguson, Bashu, Asquith, and Cooke, "Jejunal Mucosal Abnormalities," op. cit.
33. Ibid. Ferguson, Wray, Carmichael, et al., "Coeliac Disease," op. cit. Wray, "Gluten-sensitive Recurrent Aphthous Stomatitis," op. cit. Walker, Rhodes, Llewelyn, et al., Gluten Hypersensitivity," op. cit.
34. Wray, Ferguson, Hutcheon, and Dagg, "Nutritional Deficiencies in Recurrent Aphthae," op. cit.
35. Wray, D.; Ferguson, M. M.; Mason, D. K.; et al. 1975. "Recurrent Aphthae: Treatment with Vitamin B_{12}, Folic Acid, and Iron." *British Medical Journal* 2: 490–3.
36. Murray and Pizzorno, *Encyclopedia of Natural Medicine,* op. cit.
37. Ellis, J. M.; Folkers, K.; Shizukuishi, S.; et al. 1982. "Response of Vitamin B_6 Deficiency and the Carpal Tunnel Syndrome to Pyridoxine." *Proceedings of National Academy of Science, USA* 79: 7494–98. Ellis, J.; Folkers, K.; Watabe, T.; et al. 1979. "Clinical Results of a Crossover Treatment with Pyridoxine and Placebo of the Carpal Tunnel Syndrome." *American Journal of Clinical Nutrition* 32: 2040–46. Ellis, J. M.; Azuma, J.; Watanabe, T.; et al. 1977. "Survey and New Data on Treatment with Pyridoxine of Patients Having a Clinical Syndrome Including the Carpal Tunnel and Other Defects." *Research Committee on Clinical Pathology and Pharmacology* 17: 165–67.
38. Ibid. Hamfelt, A. 1982. "Carpal Tunnel Syndrome and Vitamin B_6 Deficiency." *Clinical Chemistry* 28: 721.
39. Phalen, G. S. 1981. "The Birth of a Syndrome, or Carpal Tunnel Syndrome Revisited." *Journal of Hand Surgery* 6: 109–10.
40. Gaby, A. 1984. *The Doctor's Guide to Vitamin B_6.* Emmaus, Penn.: Rodale Press.
41. Murray and Pizzorno, *Encyclopedia of Natural Medicine,* op. cit.
42. Taylor, A. 1989. "Associations Between Nutrition and Cataract." *Nutrition Reviews* 47: 225–33. Jacques, P. F., and Chylack, L. T. 1991. "Epidemiologic Evidence of a Role for the

Antioxidant Vitamin and Carotenoids in Cataract Prevention." *American Journal of Clinical Nutrition* 53: 352S–55S.

43. Ibid.
44. Jones, D. P.; Coates, R. J.; Flagg, E. W.; et al. 1992. "Glutathione in Foods Listed in the National Cancer Institute's Health Habits and History Food Frequency Questionnaire." *Nutrition and Cancer* 17: 57–75.
45. Rathbun, W., and Hanson, S. 1979. "Glutathione Metabolic Pathway as a Scavenging System in the Lens." *Ophthalmology Research* 11: 172–76.
46. Ibid.
47. Atkinson, D. 1952. "Malnutrition as an Etiological Factor in Senile Cataract." *Eye, Ear, Nose and Throat Monthly* 31: 79–83. Bouton, S. 1939. "Vitamin C and the Aging Eye." *Archives of Internal Medicine* 63: 930–45.
48. Atkinson, "Malnutrition as an Etiological Factor," op. cit.
49. Ringvold, A.; Johnsen, H.; and Blika, S. 1985. "Senile Cataract and Ascorbic Acid Loading." *Acta Ophthalmologica* 63: 277–80.
50. Auricchio, S. 1983. "Gluten-sensitive Enteropathy and Infant Nutrition." *Journal of Pediatric Gastroenterology and Nutrition* 2 (Supp. 1): S304–9. Auricchio, S.; Follo, D.; deRitis, G.; et al. 1983. "Does Breast Feeding Protect Against the Development of Clinical Symptoms of Celiac Disease in Children?" *Journal of Pediatric Gastroenterology and Nutrition* 2: 428–33. Cole, S. G., and Kagnoff, M. F. 1985. "Celiac Disease." *Annual Review of Nutrition* 5: 241–66.
51. Cole and Kagnoff, "Celiac Disease," op. cit. Fallstrom, S. P.; Winberg, J.; and Anderson, H. J. 1965. "Cow's Milk Malabsorption as a Precursor of Gluten Intolerance." *Acta Paediatrica Scandinavia* 54: 101–15.
52. Cole and Kagnoff, "Celiac Disease," op. cit. McNicholl, B.; Egan-Mitchell, B.; Stevens, F. M.; et al. 1981. "History, Genetics, and Natural History of Celiac Disease—Gluten Enteropathy." In *Food, Nutrition and Evolution,* D. N. Walker and N. Kretchmer, eds. New York: Masson, pp. 169–78.
53. Cole and Kagnoff, "Celiac Disease," op. cit. Simons, F. J. 1981. "Celiac Disease as a Geographic Problem." In *Food, Nutrition and Evolution,* D. N. Walker and N. Kretchmer, eds. New York: Masson, pp. 179–200.
54. Cole and Kagnoff, "Celiac Disease," op. cit. Kasarda, D. D. 1981. "Toxic Proteins and Peptides in Celiac Disease: Relations to Cereal Genetics." In *Food, Nutrition and Evolution,* D. N. Walker and N. Kretchmer, eds. New York: Masson, pp. 201–16.
55. Murray and Pizzorno, *Encyclopedia of Natural Medicine,* op. cit.
56. Messer, M.; Anderson, C. M.; and Hubbard, L. 1964. "Studies on the Mechanism of Destruction of the Toxic Action of Wheat Gluten in Coeliac Disease by Crude Papain." *Gut* 5: 295–303. Krainick, H. G., and Mohn, G. 1959. "Weitere Untersuchungen uber den schadlichen Weizenmehleffekt bei del Coliakie. 2. Die Wirkung der enzymatischen Abbauprodukte des Gliadin." *Helv. Paediatrica Acta* 14: 124–40.
57. Messer, M., and Baume, P. E. 1976. "Oral Papain in Gluten Intolerance." *Lancet* 2: 1022.
58. Calkins, B. M.; Lilieneld, A. M.; Garland, C. F.; et al. 1984. "Trends in Incidence Rates of Ulcerative Colitis and Crohn's Disease." *Digestive Disease Science* 29: 913–20. Mayberry, J. F. 1985. "Some Aspects on the Epidemiology of Ulcerative Colitis." *Gut* 26: 968–74.
59. Murray and Pizzorno, *Encyclopedia of Natural Medicine,* op. cit.
60. Ibid.
61. Levi, A. J. 1985. "Diet in the Management of Crohn's Disease." *Gut* 26: 985–88. Jarnerot, J.; Jarnmark, I.; and Nilsson, K. 1983. "Consumption of Refined Sugar by Patients with Crohn's Disease, Ulcerative Colitis, or Irritable Bowel Syndrome. *Scandinavian Journal of Gastroenterology* 18: 999–1002. Mayberry, J. F.; Rhodes, J.; and Newcombe, R. G. 1980. "Increased Sugar Consumption in Crohn's Disease." *Digestion* 20: 323–26. Grimes, D. S. 1976. "Refined Carbohydrate, Smooth-muscle Spasm and Diseases of the Colon." *Lancet* 1: 395–97. Thornton, J. R.; Emmett, P. M.; and Heaton, K. W. 1979. "Diet and Crohn's Disease: Characteristics of the Pre-illness Diet." *British Medical Journal* 279: 762–64. Heaton, K. W.; Thornton, J. R.; and Emmett, P. M. 1979. "Treatment of Crohn's Disease with an Unrefined-carbohydrate, Fiber-rich Diet." *British Medical Journal* 279: 764–66.
62. Ibid.

63. Thornton, Emmett, and Heaton, "Diet and Crohn's Disease," op. cit.
64. James, A. H. 1977. "Breakfast and Crohn's Disease." *British Medical Journal* 276: 943–45.
65. Morain, C. O.; Segal, A. W.; and Levi, A. J. 1984. "Elemental Diet as Primary Treatment of Acute Crohn's Disease: A Controlled Trial." *British Medical Journal* 288: 1859–62. Harries, A. D.; Danis, V.; Heatley, R. V.; et al. 1983. "Controlled Trial of Supplemented Oral Nutrition in Crohn's Disease." *Lancet* 1: 887–90. Axelsson, C., and Jarnum, S. 1977. "Assessment of the Therapeutic Value of an Elemental Diet in Chronic Inflammatory Bowel Disease." *Scandinavian Journal of Gastroenterology* 12: 89–95. Voitk, A. J.; Echave, V.; Feller, J. H.; et al. 1973. "Experience with Elemental Diet in the Treatment of Inflammatory Bowel Disease." *Archives of Surgery* 107: 329–33. Workman, E. M.; Jonmes, A.; Wilson, A. J.; and Hunter, J. O. 1984. "Diet in the Management of Crohn's Disease." *Human Nutrition: Applied Nutrition* 38A: 469–73. Jones, V. A.; Workman, E.; Freeman, A. H.; et al. 1985. "Crohn's Disease: Maintenance of Remission by Diet." *Lancet* 2: 177–80. Rowe, A., and Uyeyama, K. 1953. "Regional Enteritis—Its Allergic Aspects." *Gastroenterology* 23: 554–71.
66. Rosenberg, I. H.; Bengoa, J. M.; and Sitrin, M. D. 1985. "Nutritional Aspects of Inflammatory Bowel Disease." *Annual Review of Nutrition* 5: 463–84.
67. Ibid.
68. Ibid.
69. Morain, Segal, and Levi, "Elemental Diet as Primary Treatment," op. cit. Harries, Danis, Heatley, et al., "Controlled Trial of Supplemented Oral Nutrition," op. cit. Axelsson and Jarnum, "Assessment of Therapeutic Value of Elemental Diet," op. cit. Voitk, Echave, Feller, et al., "Experience with Elemental Diet," op. cit. Workman, Jonmes, Wilson, and Hunter, "Diet in Management of Crohn's Disease," op. cit. Jones, Workman, Freeman, et al., "Crohn's Disease," op. cit. Rowe and Uyeyama, "Regional Enteritis," op. cit.
70. Workman, Jonmes, Wilson, and Hunter, "Diet in Management of Crohn's Disease," op. cit. Jones, Workman, Freeman, et al., "Crohn's Disease," op. cit. Rowe and Uyeyama, "Regional Enteritis," op. cit.
71. James, "Breakfast and Crohn's Disease," op. cit.
72. Salyers, A. A.; Kurtitza, A. P.; and McCarthy, R. E. 1985. "Influence of Dietary Fiber on the Intestinal Environment." *Proceedings of Society for Experimental Biological Medicine* 180: 415–21.
73. Jones, Workman, Freeman, et al., "Crohn's Disease," op. cit.
74. Hawthorne, A. B.; Daneshmend, T. K.; Hawkey, C. J.; et al. 1992. "Treatment of Ulcerative Colitis with Fish Oil Supplementation: A Prospective 12 Month Randomised Controlled Trial. *Gut.* 33: 922–28.
75. Salloum, T. K. "Therapeutic Fasting." 1988. In *A Textbook of Natural Medicine,* J. E. Pizzorno and M. T. Murray, eds. Seattle: JBC Publications. Duncan, G. G.; Duncan, T. G.; Schless, G. L.; and Cristofori, F. C. 1965. "Contraindications and Therapeutic Results of Fasting in Obese Patients." *Annals of New York Academy of Science* 131: 632–36. Sorbris, R.; Aly, K. O.; Nilsson-Ehle, P.; et al. 1982. "Vegetarian Fasting of Obese Patients: A Clinical and Biochemical Evaluation." *Scandinavian Journal of Gastroenterology* 17: 417–24. Suzuki, J.; Yamauchi, Y.; Horikawa, M.; and Yamagata, S. 1976. "Fasting Therapy for Psychosomatic Disease with Special Reference to Its Indications and Therapeutic Mechanism." *Tohoku Journal of Experimental Medicine* 118 (Supp.): 245–59. Imamura, M., and Tung, T. 1984. "A Trial of Fasting Cure for PCB Poisoned Patients in Taiwan." *American Journal of Industrial Medicine* 5: 147–53. Lithell, H.; Bruce, A.; Gustafsson, I. B.; et al. 1983. "A Fasting and Vegetarian Diet Treatment Trial on Chronic Inflammatory Disorders." *Acta Dermatologia Venereologia* 63: 397–403. Boehme, D. L. 1977. "Preplanned Fasting in the Treatment of Mental Disease: Survey of the Current Soviet Literature." *Schizophrenia Bulletin* 3 (2): 288–96.
76. Imamura and Tung, "A Trial of Fasting Cure," op. cit.
77. Shakman, R. A. 1974. "Nutritional Influences on the Toxicity of Environmental Pollutants: A Review." *Archives of Environmental Health* 28: 105–33.
78. Murray and Pizzorno, *Encyclopedia of Natural Medicine,* op. cit.
79. Canini, F.; Bartolucci, L.; Cristallini, E.; et al. 1985. "Use of Silymarin in the Treatment of Alcoholic Hepatic Steatosis." *Clinica Terapeutica* 114: 307–14. Salmi, H. A., and Sarna,

S. 1982. "Effect of Silymarin on Chemical, Functional, and Morphological Alteration of the Liver: A Double-blind Controlled Study." *Scandinavian Journal of Gastroenterology* 17: 417–21. Boari, C.; Montanari, M.; Galleti, G. P.; et al. 1985. "Occupational Toxic Liver Diseases: Therapeutic Effects of Silymarin." *Minerva Medicine* 72: 2679–88.

80. Murray and Pizzorno, *Encyclopedia of Natural Medicine*, op. cit.
81. Ibid.
82. Burkitt, D., and Trowell, H. 1981. *Western Diseases: Their Emergence and Prevention*. Cambridge, Mass.: Harvard University Press.
83. Ibid.
84. Anderson, J. W., and Ward, K. 1979. "High-carbohydrate, High-fiber Diets for Insulin-treated Men with Diabetes Mellitus." *American Journal of Clinical Nutrition* 32: 2312–21. Anderson, J. 1981. *Diabetes: A Practical Approach to Daily Living*. New York: Arco Press. Kay, R.; Grobin, W.; and Trace, N. 1981. "Diets Rich in Natural Fiber Improve Carbohydrate Tolerance in Maturity Onset, Noninsulin Dependent Diabetics." *Diabetologia* 20: 12–23. Simpson, H. C. R.; Simpson, R. W.; Lousley, S.; et al. 1981. "A High Carbohydrate Leguminous Fiber Diet Improves All Aspects of Diabetic Control." *Lancet* 1: 1–5. Vahouny, G., and Kritchevsky, D. 1982. *Dietary Fiber in Health and Disease*. New York: Plenum Press.
85. Anderson and Ward, "High-carbohydrate, High-fiber Diets," op. cit. Anderson, *Diabetes*, op. cit.
86. Ibid. Vahouny and Kritchevsky, *Dietary Fiber in Health and Disease*, op. cit.
87. Simpson, Simpson, Lousley, et al. "A High Carbohydrate Leguminous Fiber Diet," op. cit.
88. Vahouny and Kritchevsky, *Dietary Fiber in Health and Disease*, op. cit.
89. Hughes, T.; Gwynne, J.; Switzer, B.; et al. 1984. "Effects of Caloric Restriction and Weight Loss on Glycemic Control, Insulin Release and Resistance and Atherosclerotic Risk in Obese Patients with Type II Diabetes Mellitus." *American Journal of Medicine* 77: 7–17.
90. Ibid.
91. Murray and Pizzorno, *Encyclopedia of Natural Medicine*, op. cit.
92. Ibid.
93. Saarinen, U. M. 1982. "Prolonged Breast Feeding as Prophylaxis for Recurrent Otitis Media." *Acta Pediatrica Scandinavia* 71: 567–71.
94. Editor. 1983. "Breast Feeding Prevents Otitis Media." *Nutrition Review* 41: 241–42.
95. McMahan, J. T.; Calenoff, E.; Croft, D. J.; et al. 1981. "Chronic Otitis Media with Effusion and Allergy: Modified RAST Analysis of 119 Cases." *Otology Head Neck Surgery* 89: 427–31. Viscomi, G. J. 1975. "Allergic Secretory Otitis Media: An Approach to Management." *Laryngoscope* 85: 751–58. Van Cauwenberge, P. B. 1982. "The Role of Allergy in Otitis Media with Effusion. *Ther. Umschau.* 39: 1011–16. Bellionin, P.; Cantani, A.; and Salvinelli, F. 1987. "Allergy: A Leading Role in Otitis Media with Effusion." *Allergology Immunology* 15: 205–8.
96. McMahan, Calenoff, Croft, et al., "Chronic Otitis Media," op. cit.
97. Sampson, H. 1983. "Role of Immediate Food Hypersensitivity in the Pathogenesis of Atopic Dermatitis." *Journal of Allergy and Clinical Immunology* 71: 473–80. Sloper, K. S.; Wadsworth, J.; and Brostoff, J. 1991. "Children with Atopic Eczema. I. Clinical Response to Food Elimination and Subsequent Double-blind Food Challenge." *Quarterly Journal of Medicine* 80: 677–93. Atherton, D. J. 1988. "Diet and Atopic Eczema." *Clinical Allergy* 18: 215–18.
98. Jacobs, A. 1976. "Atopic Dermatitis: Clinical Expression and Management." *Pediatric Annals* 5: 763–71.
99. Sloper, Wadsworth, and Brostoff, "Children with Atopic Eczema," op. cit.
100. Manku, M.; Horrobin, D.; Morse, N.; et al. 1982. "Reduced Levels of Prostaglandin Precursors in the Blood of Atopic Patients: Defective delta-6-Desaturase Function as a Biochemical Basis for Atopy." *Prostaglandins Leukotrienes and Medicine* 9: 615–28. Biagi, P. L.; Bordini, A.; Masi, M.; et al. 1988. "A Long-term Study on the Use of Evening Primrose Oil (Efamol) in Atopic Children." *Drugs Experimental Clinical Research* 4: 285–90.
101. Murray and Pizzorno, *Encyclopedia of Natural Medicine*, op. cit.

102. Mann, C., and Staba, E. J. 1986. "The Chemistry, Pharmacology, and Commercial Formulation of Chamomile." *Herbs, Spices, and Medicinal Plants: Recent Advances in Botany, Horticulture, and Pharmacology* 1: 235–80. Evans, F. Q. 1958. "The Rational use of Glycyrrhetinic Acid in Dermatology." *British Journal of Clinical Practice* 12: 269–74.
103. Falck, F.; Ricci, A.; Wolff, M. S.; et al. 1992. "Pesticides and Polychlorinated Biphenyl Residues in Human Breast Lipids and Their Relation to Breast Cancer." *Archives of Environmental Health* 47: 143–46.
104. Petrakis, N. L., and King, E. B. 1981. "Cytological Abnormalities in Nipple Aspirates of Breast Fluid from Women with Severe Constipation." *Lancet* 2: 1203–5.
105. Hentges, D. J. 1980. "Does Diet Influence Human Fecal Microflora Composition?" *Nutrition Review* 38: 329–36.
106. Goldin, B.; Aldercreutz, H.; Dwyer, J.; et al. 1981. "Effect of Diet on Excretion of Estrogens in Pre- and Postmenopausal Women." *Cancer Research* 41: 3771–73.
107. Boyle, C. A.; Berkowitz, G. S.; LiVolsi, V. A.; et al. 1984. "Caffeine Consumption and Fibrocystic Breast Disease: A Case-control Epidemiologic Study." *Journal of National Cancer Institute* 72: 1015–19. Minton, J. P.; Abou-Issa, H.; Reiches, N.; and Roseman, J. M. 1981. "Clinical and Biochemical Studies on Methylxanthine-related Fibrocystic Breast Disease." *Surgery* 90: 299–304. Minton, J. P.; Foecking, M. K.; Webster, D. J. T.; and Matthews, R. H. 1979. "Caffeine, Cyclic Nucleotides, and Breast Disease." *Surgery* 86: 105–9. Ernster, V. L.; Mason, L.; Goodson, W. H.; et al. 1982. "Effects of Caffeine-free Diet on Benign Breast Disease: A Random Trial." *Surgery* 91: 263–67.
108. Minton, Abou-Issa, Reiches, and Roseman, "Clinical and Biochemical Studies," op. cit.
109. London, R. S.; Sundaram, G. S.; Schultz, M.; et al. 1981. "Endocrine Parameters and alpha-Tocopherol Therapy of Patients with Mammary Dysplasia." *Cancer Research* 41: 3811–13. London, R. S.; Sundaram, G.; Manimekalai, S.; et al. 1984. "The Effect of alpha-Tocopherol on Premenstrual Symptomatology: A Double-blind Study. II. Endocrine Correlates." *Journal of American College of Nutrition* 3: 351–56.
110. Trowell, H.; Burkitt, D.; and Heaton, K. 1985. *Dietary Fibre, Fibre-depleted Foods and Disease.* New York: Academic Press.
111. Pixley, F.; Wilson, D.; McPherson, K.; et al. 1985. "Effect of Vegetarianism on Development of Gallstones in Women." *British Medical Journal* 291: 11–12.
112. Breneman, J. C. 1968. "Allergy Elimination Diet as the Most Effective Gallbladder Diet." *Annals of Allergy* 26: 83–87.
113. Ibid.
114. Murray and Pizzorno, *Encyclopedia of Natural Medicine,* op. cit.
115. Ibid.
116. Ibid.
117. Faller, J., and Fox, I. H. 1982. "Ethanol-induced Hyperuricemia." *New England Journal of Medicine* 307: 1598–602.
118. Murray and Pizzorno, *Encyclopedia of Natural Medicine,* op. cit.
119. Ibid.
120. Ibid.
121. Blau, L. W. 1950. "Cherry Diet Control for Gout and Arthritis." *Texas Report on Biology and Medicine* 8: 309–11.
122. Bindoli, A.; Valente, M.; and Cavallini, L. 1985. "Inhibitory Action of Quercetin on Xanthine Oxidase and Xanthine Dehydrogenase Activity." *Pharmacology Research Committee* 17: 831–39. Busse, W. W.; Kopp, D. E.; and Middleton, E. 1984. "Flavonoid Modulation of Human Neutrophil Function." *Journal of Allergy and Clinical Immunology* 73: 801–9.
123. Appelboom, T., and Bennett, J. C. 1986. "Gout of the Rich and Famous." *Journal of Rheumatology* 13: 618–22.
124. Murray and Pizzorno, *Encyclopedia of Natural Medicine,* op. cit.
125. Mansfield, L. E.; Vaughan, T. R.; Waller, S. T.; et al. 1985. "Food Allergy and Adult Migraine: Double-blind and Mediator Confirmation of an Allergic Etiology." *Annals of Allergy* 55: 126–29. Carter, C. M.; Egger, J.; and Soothill, J. F. 1985. "A Dietary Management of Severe Childhood Migraine." *Human Nutrition: Applied Nutrition* 39A: 294–303. Hughes, E. C.; Gott, P. S.; Weinstein, R. C.; and Binggeli, R. 1985. "Migraine: A Diag-

nostic Test for Etiology of Food Sensitivity by a Nutritionally Supported Fast and Confirmed by Long-term Report." *Annals of Allergy* 55: 28–32. Egger, J.; Carter, C. M.; Wilson, J.; et al. 1983. "Is Migraine Food Allergy?" *Lancet* 2: 865–69. Monro, J.; Brostoff, J.; Carini, C.; and Zilkha, K. 1980. "Food Allergy in Migraine." *Lancet* 2: 1–4. Grant, E. C. G. 1979. "Food Allergies and Migraine." *Lancet* 1: 966–69.

126. Littlewood, J.; Glover, V.; Petty, R.; et al. 1982. "Platelet Phenolsulphotransferase Deficiency in Dietary Migraine." *Lancet* 1: 983–86.
127. Littlewood, J. T.; Glover, V.; and Sandler, M. 1985. "Red Wine Contains a Potent Inhibitor of Phenolsulphotransferase." *British Journal of Clinical Pharmacology* 19: 275–78.
128. Johnson, E. S.; Kadam, N. P.; Hylands, D. M.; and Hylands, P. J. 1985. "Efficacy of Feverfew as Prophylactic Treatment of Migraine." *British Medical Journal* 291: 569–73.
129. Murray and Pizzorno, *Encyclopedia of Natural Medicine,* op. cit.
130. Ibid.
131. National Research Council. 1989. *Diet and Health: Implications for Reducing Chronic Disease Risk.* Washington, D.C.: National Academy Press.
132. Arntzenius, A.C. 1991. "Regression of Atherosclerosis." *Acta Cardiologica* 46: 431–38. Ornish, D.; Brown, S.E.; Scherwitz, L. W.; et al. 1990. "Can Lifestyle Changes Reverse Coronary Heart Disease?" *Lancet* 336: 129–33.
133. Ornish, Brown, Scherwitz, et al., "Can Lifestyle Changes Reverse Coronary Heart Disease?" op. cit.
134. Rosenthal, M. B.; Barnard, R. J.; Rose, D. P.; et al. 1985. "Effects of a High-complex-carbohydrate, Low-fat, Low-cholesterol Diet on Levels of Serum Lipids and Estradiol." *American Journal of Medicine* 78: 23–27. Fisher, M.; Levine, P. H.; Weiner, B.; et al. 1986. "The Effect of Vegetarian Diets on Plasma Lipid and Platelet Levels." *Archives of International Medicine* 146: 1193–97.
135. Robertson, J.; Brydon, W. G.; Tadesse, K.; et al. 1979. "The Effect of Raw Carrot on Serum Lipids and Colon Function." *American Journal of Clinical Nutrition* 32: 1889–92.
136. Stanto, J. L., and Keast, D. R. 1989. "Serum Cholesterol, Fat Intake, and Breakfast Consumption in the United States Adult Population." *Journal of American College of Nutrition* 8: 567–72.
137. National Research Council, *Diet and Health,* op. cit. Yudin, J. 1978. "Dietary Factors in Atherosclerosis: Sucrose." *Lipids* 13: 370–72.
138. Wood, D. A.; Butler, S.; Riemersma, R. A.; et al. 1984. "Adipose Tissue and Platelet Fatty Acids and Coronary Heart Disease in Scottish Men." *Lancet* 2: 117–21.
139. Murray and Pizzorno, *Encyclopedia of Natural Medicine,* op. cit. National Research Council, *Diet and Health,* op. cit. Simpoulos, A. P. 1989. "Summary of the NATO Advanced Research Workshop on Dietary w3 and w6 Fatty Acids: Biological Effects and Nutritional Essentiality." *Journal of Nutrition* 119: 521–28.
140. Murray and Pizzorno, *Encyclopedia of Natural Medicine,* op. cit. National Research Council, *Diet and Health,* op. cit. Riemersma, R. A.; Oliver, M.; Elton, R. A.; et al. 1989. "Plasma Antioxidants and Coronary Heart Disease: Vitamins C and E, and Selenium." *European Journal of Clinical Nutrition* 44: 143–50. Gerster, H. 1991. "Potential Role of beta-Carotene in the Prevention of Cardiovascular Disease." *International Journal of Vitamin and Nutrition Research* 61: 277–91.
141. Murray and Pizzorno, *Encyclopedia of Natural Medicine,* op. cit.
142. Ibid.
143. Ibid.
144. Ibid. Burkitt and Trowell, *Western Diseases,* op. cit.
145. Murray and Pizzorno, *Encyclopedia of Natural Medicine,* op. cit. Moesgaard, F.; Nielsen, M. L.; Hansen, J. B.; and Knudsen, J. T. 1982. "High-fiber Diet Reduces Bleeding and Pain in Patients with Hemorrhoids." *Diseases of Colon and Rectum* 25: 454–56.
146. Webster, D. J.; Gough, D. C.; and Craven, J. L. 1978. "The Use of Bulk Evacuation in Patients with Hemorrhoids." *British Journal of Surgery* 65: 291–92.
147. Rubenstein, E., and Federman, D. D., eds., "Scientific American Medicine," *Scientific American* 7(26): 1–9.
148. Griffith, R.; DeLong, D.; and Nelson, J. 1981. "Relation of Arginine–Lysine Antagonism to Herpes Simplex Growth in Tissue Culture." *Chemotherapy* 27: 209–13. DiGiovanna, J.,

and Blank, H. 1984. "Failure of Lysine in Frequently Recurrent Herpes Simplex Infection." *Archives of Dermatology* 120: 48–51.

149. DiGiovanna and Blank, "Failure of Lysine," op. cit. Griffith, R. S.; Walsh, D. E.; Myrmel, K. H.; et al. 1987. "Success of L-lysine Therapy in Frequently Recurrent Herpes Simplex Infection." *Dermatologica* 175: 183–90.
150. Pompei, R.; Pani, A.; Flore, O.; et al. 1980. "Antiviral Activity of Glycyrrhizic Acid." *Experientia* 36: 304.
151. Murray and Pizzorno, *Encyclopedia of Natural Medicine,* op. cit.
152. Kaplan, N. M. 1989. "Nonpharmacological Control of High Blood Pressure." *American Journal of Hypertension* 2: 55S–59S.
153. Miettinen, T. A. 1985. "Multifactorial Primary Prevention of Cardiovascular Diseases in Middle-aged Men: Risk Factor Changes, Incidence, and Mortality." *Journal of American Medical Association* 254: 2097–2102. Multiple Risk Factor Intervention Trial Research Group. 1985. "Baseline Rest Electrocardiographic Abnormalities, Antihypertensive Treatment, and Mortality in the Multiple Risk Factor Intervention Trial." *American Journal of Cardiology* 55: 1–15.
154. Murray and Pizzorno, *Encyclopedia of Natural Medicine,* op. cit. Burkitt and Trowell, *Western Diseases,* op. cit. Trowell, Burkitt, and Heaton, *Dietary Fibre, Fibre-depleted Foods and Disease,* op. cit.
155. Burkitt and Trowell, *Western Diseases,* op. cit. Trowell, Burkitt, and Heaton, *Dietary Fibre, Fibre-depleted Foods and Disease,* op. cit.
156. National Research Council, *Diet and Health,* op. cit.
157. Murray and Pizzorno, *Encyclopedia of Natural Medicine,* op. cit. Rouse, I. L.; Beilin, L. J.; Mahoney, D. P.; et al. 1983. "Vegetarian Diet and Blood Pressure." *Lancet* 2: 742–43.
158. Miettinen, "Multifactorial Primary Prevention of Cardiovascular Diseases," op. cit. Havlik, R.; Hubert, H.; Fabsitz, R.; and Feinleib, M. 1983. "Weight and Hypertension." *Annals of Internal Medicine* 98: 855–59.
159. Miettinen, "Multifactorial Primary Prevention of Cardiovascular Diseases," op. cit. Iimura, O.; Kijima, T.; Kikuchi, K.; et al. 1981. "Studies on the Hypotensive Effect of High Potassium Intake in Patients with Essential Hypertension." *Clinical Science* 61 (Supp. 7): 77s–80s. Khaw, K. T., and Barrett-Connor, E. 1984. "Dietary Potassium and Blood Pressure in a Population." *American Journal of Clinical Nutrition* 39: 963–68. Skrabal, F.; Aubock, J.; and Hortnagl, H. 1981. "Low Sodium/High Potassium Diet for Prevention of Hypertension: Probable Mechanisms of Action." *Lancet* 2: 895–900.
160. Hodges, R., and Rebello, T. 1983. "Carbohydrates and Blood Pressure." *Annals of Internal Medicine* 98: 838–41.
161. Miettinen, "Multifactorial Primary Prevention of Cardiovascular Diseases," op. cit. McCarron, D. A., and Morris, C. D. 1986. "Epidemiological Evidence Associating Dietary Calcium and Calcium Metabolism with Blood Pressure." *American Journal of Nephrology* 6 (Supp. 1): 3–9. Whelton, P. K., and Klag, M. J. 1989. "Magnesium and Blood Pressure: Review of the Epidemiologic and Clinical Trial Experience." *American Journal of Cardiology* 63: 26G–30G.
162. Ibid.
163. Yoshioka, M.; Matsushita, T.; and Chuman, Y. 1984. "Inverse Association of Serum Ascorbic Acid Level and Blood Pressure or Rate of Hypertension in Male Adults Aged 30–39 Years." *International Journal of Vitamin Nutrition Research* 54: 343–47.
164. Pierkle, J. L.; Schwartz, J.; Landis, J. R.; and Harlan, W. R. 1985. "The Relationship Between Blood Lead Levels and Blood Pressure and Its Cardiovascular Risk Implications." *American Journal of Epidemiology* 121: 246–58.
165. Glauser, S.; Bello, C.; and Glauser, E. 1976. "Blood-cadmium Levels in Normotensive and Untreated Hypertensive Humans." *Lancet* 1: 717–18.
166. Murray and Pizzorno, *Encyclopedia of Natural Medicine,* op. cit. Czarnetzki, B. M. 1986. *Urticaria.* New York: Springer-Verlag.
167. Ibid.
168. Murray and Pizzorno, *Encyclopedia of Natural Medicine,* op. cit. Pachor, M. L.; Andri, L.; Nicolis, F.; et al. 1986. "Elimination Diet and Challenge Test in Diagnosis of Food Intolerance." *Italian Journal of Medicine* 2: 1–6.

169. Warrington, R. J.; Sauder, P. J.; and McPhillips, S. 1986. "Cell-mediated Immune Responses to Artificial Food Additives in Chronic Urticaria," 16: 527–33.
170. Natbony, S. F.; Phillips, M. E.; Elias, J. M.; et al. 1983. "Histologic Studies of Chronic Idiopathic Urticaria." *Journal of Allergy and Clinical Immunology* 71: 177–83.
171. Murray and Pizzorno, *Encyclopedia of Natural Medicine,* op. cit. Czarnetzki, *Urticaria,* op. cit. Winkelmann, R. K. 1987. "Food Sensitivity and Urticaria or Vasculitis." In *Food Allergy and Intolerance,* J. Brostoff and S. J. Challacombe, eds. Philadelphia: W. B. Saunders, pp. 602–17.
172. Czarnetzki, *Urticaria,* op. cit.
173. Ormerod, A. D.; Reid, T. M. S.; and Main, R. A. 1987. "Penicillin in Milk—Its Importance in Urticaria." *Clinical Allergy* 17: 229–34. Wicher, K., and Reisman, R. E. 1980. "Anaphylactic Reaction to Penicillin in a Soft Drink." *Journal of Allergy and Clinical Immunology* 66: 155–57. Schwartz, H. J., and Sher, T. H. 1984. "Anaphylaxis to Penicillin in a Frozen Dinner." *Annals of Allergy* 52: 342–43.
174. Boonk, W. J., and Van Ketel, W. G. 1982. "The Role of Penicillin in the Pathogenesis of Chronic Urticaria." *British Journal of Dermatology* 106: 183–90.
175. Ormerod, A. D.; Reid, T. M. S.; and Main, R. A. 1987. "Penicillin in Milk—Its Importance in Urticaria." *Clinical Allergy* 17: 229–34.
176. Lindemayr, H.; Knobler, R.; Kraft, D.; and Baumgartner, G. 1981. "Challenge of Penicillin Allergic Volunteers with Penicillin Contaminated Meat." *Allergy* 36: 471–78.
177. Ormerod, Reid, and Main, "Penicillin in Milk," op. cit.
178. Green, G.; Koelsche, G.; and Kierland, R. 1965. "Etiology and Pathogenesis of Chronic Urticaria." *Annals of Allergy* 23: 30–36.
179. Schertzer, C. L., and Lookingbill, D. P. 1987. "Effects of Relaxation Therapy and Hypnotizability in Chronic Urticaria." *Archives of Dermatology* 123: 913–16.
180. Murray and Pizzorno, *Encyclopedia of Natural Medicine,* op. cit.
181. Palmblad, J.; Hallberg, D.; and Rossner, S. 1977. "Obesity, Plasma Lipids and Polymorphonuclear (PMN) Granulocyte Functions." *Scandinavian Journal Haematology* 19: 293–303.
182. Ibid.
183. Sanchez, A.; Reeser, J.; Lau, H.; et al. 1973. "Role of Sugars in Human Neutrophilic Phagocytosis." *American Journal of Clinical Nutrition* 26: 1180–84. Ringsdorf, W.; Cheraskin, E.; and Ramsay, R. 1976. "Sucrose, Neutrophil Phagocytosis and Resistance to Disease." *Dentistry Survey* 52: 46–48.
184. Bernstein, J.; Alpert, S.; Nauss, K.; and Suskind, R. 1977. "Depression of Lymphocyte Transformation Following Oral Glucose Ingestion." *American Journal of Clinical Nutrition* 30: 613–19.
185. Mann, G., and Newton, P. 1975. "The Membrane Transport of Ascorbic Acid," *Annals of New York Academy of Science* 258: 243–51.
186. Stich, H.; Stich, W.; Rosin, M.; and Vallejera, M. 1984. "Use of the Micronucleus Test to Monitor the Effect of Vitamin A, beta-Carotene and Canthaxanthin on the Buccal Mucosa of Betel Nut/Tobacco Chewers." *International Journal of Cancer* 34: 745–50. Garewal, H. S. 1991. "Potential Role of beta-Carotene in Prevention of Oral Cancer." *American Journal of Clinical Nutrition* 53: 294S–97S. Garewal, H. S.; Meyskens, F. L.; Killen, D.; et al. 1990. "Response of Oral Leukoplakia to beta-Carotene." *Journal of Clinical Oncology* 8: 1715–20.
187. Stich, Stich, Rosin, and Vallejera, "Use of the Micronucleus Test," op. cit.
188. Baird, I.; Hughes, R.; Wilson, H.; et al. 1979. "The Effects of Ascorbic Acid and Flavonoids on the Occurrence of Symptoms Normally Associated with the Common Cold." *American Journal of Clinical Nutrition* 32: 1686–90. Anderson, T.; Reid, D.; and Beaton, G. 1972. "Vitamin C and the Common Cold: A Double Blind Trial." *Canadian Medical Association Journal* 107: 503–8. Cheraskin, E.; Ringsdorf, W. M.; and Sisley, E. L. 1983. *The Vitamin C Connection.* New York: Bantam Books. Anderson, T. W. 1975. "Large Scale Trials of Vitamin C." *Annals of New York Academy of Science* 258: 494–505.
189. Murray and Pizzorno, *Encyclopedia of Natural Medicine,* op. cit. Scott, J. 1982. "On the Biochemical Similarities of Ascorbic Acid and Interferon." *Journal of Theoretical Biology* 98: 235–38.

190. Sundstrom, H.; Korpela, H.; Sajanti, E.; and Kauppila, A. 1989. "Supplementation with Selenium, Vitamin E and Their Combination in Gynaecological Cancer During Cytotoxic Chemotherapy." *Carcinogenesis* 10: 273–78. Hoffman, F. A. 1985. "Micronutrient Requirements of Cancer Patients." *Cancer* 55: 295–300.
191. Fuchs, J.; Ochsendorf, F.; Schofer, H.; et al. 1991. "Oxidative Imbalance in HIV Infected Patients." *Medical Hypothesis* 36: 60–64.
192. Sundstrom, Korpela, Sajanti, and Kauppila, "Supplementation with Selenium," op. cit. Hoffman, "Micronutrient Requirements of Cancer Patients," op. cit. Judy, W. V.; Hall, J. H.; Dugan, W.; et al. 1984. "Coenzyme Q10 Reduction of Adriamycin Cardiotoxicity." In *Biomedical and Clinical Aspects of Coenzyme Q*, vol. 4, K. Folkers and Y. Yamamura, eds. Amsterdam: Elsevier Science Publications, pp. 231–41.
193. Wu, J.; Levy, E. M.; and Black, P. H. 1989. "2-Mercaptoethanol and n-Acetylcysteine Enhance T Cell Colony Formation in AIDS and ARC." *Clinical Experimental Immunology* 77: 7–10.
194. Dausch, J. G., and Nixon, D. W. 1990. "Garlic: A Review of Its Relationship to Malignant Disease." *Preventive Medicine* 19: 346–61.
195. Ibid.
196. Murray and Pizzorno, *Encyclopedia of Natural Medicine*, op. cit.
197. Ibid.
198. Ibid.
199. Jones, V.; McLaughlin, P.; Shorthouse, M.; et al. 1982. "Food Intolerance: A Major Factor in the Pathogenesis of Irritable Bowel Syndrome." *Lancet* 2: 1115–18. Petitpierre, M.; Gumowski, P.; and Girard, J. 1985. "Irritable Bowel Syndrome and Hypersensitivity to Food." *Annals of Allergy* 54: 538–40.
200. Murray and Pizzorno, *Encyclopedia of Natural Medicine*, op. cit.
201. Ibid. Trowell, Burkitt, and Heaton, *Dietary Fibre, Fibre-depleted Foods and Disease*, op. cit.
202. Ibid. Burkitt and Trowell, *Western Diseases*, op. cit.
203. Robertson, W.; Peacock, M.; and Marshall, D. 1982. "Prevalence of Urinary Stone Disease in Vegetarians." *European Urology* 8: 334–39. Rose, G., and Westbury, E. 1975. "The Influence of Calcium Content of Water, Intake of Vegetables and Fruit and of Other Food Factors upon the Incidence of Renal Calculi." *Urological Research* 3: 61–66.
204. Shaw, P.; Williams, G.; and Green, N. 1980. "Idiopathic Hypercalciuria: Its Control with Unprocessed Bran." *British Journal of Urology* 52: 426–29.
205. Murray and Pizzorno, *Encyclopedia of Natural Medicine*, op. cit.
206. Ulmann, A.; Aubert, J.; Bourdeau, A.; et al. 1982. "Effects of Weight and Glucose Ingestion on Urinary Calcium and Phosphate Excretion: Implications for Calcium Urolithiasis." *Journal of Clinical Endocrinology and Metabolism* 54: 1063–67. Rao, N.; Gordon, C.; Davis, D.; and Blacklock, N. 1982. "Are Stone Formers Maladaptive to Refined Carbohydrates?" *British Journal of Urology* 54: 575–77.
207. Johansson, G.; Backman, U.; Danielson, B.; et al. 1980. "Biochemical and Clinical Effects of the Prophylactic Treatment of Renal Calcium Stones with Magnesium Hydroxide." *Journal of Urology* 124: 770–74. Wunderlich, W. 1981. "Aspects of the Influence of Magnesium Ions on the Formation of Calcium Oxalate." *Urological Research* 9: 157–60. Hallson, P.; Rose, G.; and Sulaiman, S. 1982. "Magnesium Reduces Calcium Oxalate Crystal Formation in Human Whole Urine. *Clinical Science* 62: 17–19.
208. Prien, E., and Gershoff, S. 1974. "Magnesium Oxide-Pyridoxine Therapy for Recurrent Calcium Oxalate Calculi." *Journal of Urology* 112: 509–12. Gershoff, S., and Prien, E. 1967. "Effect of Daily MgO and Vitamin B_6 Administration to Patients with Recurring Calcium Oxalate Stones." *American Journal of Clinical Nutrition* 20: 393–99.
209. Seeling, M. S. 1983. "Vitamin D—Risk vs. Benefit." *Journal of American College of Nutrition* 4: 109–10.
210. Dharmsathaphorn, K.; Freeman, D.; Binder, H.; and Dobbins, J. 1982. "Increased Risk of Nephrolithiasis in Patients with Steatorrhea." *Digestive Disease Science* 27: 401–5.
211. Pak, C. Y. C., and Fuller, C. 1986. "Idiopathic Hypocitraturic Calcium-Oxalate Nephrolithiasis Successfully Treated with Potassium Citrate." *Annals of Internal Medicine* 104: 33–37.

212. Murray and Pizzorno, *Encyclopedia of Natural Medicine,* op. cit. Scott, R.; Cunningham, C.; McLelland, A.; et al. 1982. "The Importance of Cadmium as a Factor in Calcified Upper Urinary Tract Stone Disease—A Prospective 7-year Study." *British Journal of Urology* 54: 584–89.
213. Murray and Pizzorno, *Encyclopedia of Natural Medicine,* op. cit.
214. Swank, R. L. 1991. "Multiple Sclerosis: Fat-Oil Relationship." *Nutrition* 7: 368–76. Swank, R. L., and Pullen, M. H. 1977. *The Multiple Sclerosis Diet Book.* Garden City, N.Y.: Doubleday.
215. Ibid.
216. Millar, Z. H. D.; Zilkha, K. J.; Langman, M. J. S.; et al. 1973. "Double-blind Trial of Linolate Supplementation of the Diet in Multiple Sclerosis." *British Medical Journal* 1: 765–68. Bates, D.; Fawcett, P. R. W.; Shaw, D. A.; and Weightman, D. 1978. "Polyunsaturated Fatty Acids in Treatment of Acute Remitting Multiple Sclerosis." *British Medical Journal* 2: 1390–91. Paty, D. W.; Cousin, H. K.; Read, S.; and Adlakkha, K. 1978. "Linoleic Acid in Multiple Sclerosis: Failure to Show Any Therapeutic Benefit." *Acta Neurologica Scandinavia* 58: 53–58.
217. Taussig, S. 1980. "The Mechanism of the Physiological Action of Bromelain." *Medical Hypothesis* 6: 99–104. Ransberger, K. 1986. "Enzyme Treatment of Immune Complex Diseases." *Arthritis and Rheumatism* 8: 16–19.
218. Ransberger, K., and van Schaik, W. 1986. "Enzyme Therapy in Multiple Sclerosis." *Der Kassenarzt* 41: 42–45.
219. Murray and Pizzorno, *Encyclopedia of Natural Medicine,* op. cit.
220. Ibid.
221. Ibid.
222. Sullivan, M. X., and Hess, W. C. 1935. "Cystine Content of Finger Nails in Arthritis." *Journal of Bone and Joint Surgery* 16: 185–88.
223. Senturia, B. D. 1934. "Results of Treatment of Chronic Arthritis and Rheumatoid Conditions with Colloidal Sulphur." *Journal of Bone and Joint Surgery* 16: 119–25.
224. Childers, N. F., and Russo, G. M. 1973. *The Nightshades and Health.* Somerville, N.J.: Horticulture Publications.
225. Murray and Pizzorno, *Encyclopedia of Natural Medicine,* op. cit.
226. Nicar, M. J., and Pak, C. Y. C. 1985. "Calcium Bioavailability from Calcium Carbonate and Calcium Citrate. *Journal of Clinical Endocrinology and Metabolism* 61: 391–93.
227. Murray and Pizzorno, *Encyclopedia of Natural Medicine,* op. cit.
228. Ellis, F.; Holesh, S.; and Ellis, J. 1972. "Incidence of Osteoporosis in Vegetarians and Omnivores." *American Journal of Clinical Nutrition* 25: 55–58. Marsh, A.; Sanchez, T.; Chaffe, F.; et al. 1983. "Bone Mineral Mass in Adult Lacto-ovo-vegetarian and Omnivorous Adults." *American Journal of Clinical Nutrition* 37: 453–56.
229. Licata, A.; Bou, E.; Bartter, F.; and West, F. 1981. "Acute Effects of Dietary Protein on Calcium Metabolism in Patients with Osteoporosis." *Journal of Gerontology* 36: 14–19.
230. Thom, J.; Morris, J.; Bishop, A.; and Blacklock, N. J. 1978. "The Influence of Refined Carbohydrate on Urinary Calcium Excretion." *British Journal of Urology* 50: 459–64.
231. Bitensky, L.; Hart, J. P.; Catterall, A.; et al. 1988. "Circulating Vitamin K Levels in Patients with Fractures." *Journal of Bone and Joint Surgery* 70-B: 663–64.
232. Neilsen, F. H.; Hunt, C. D; Mullen, L. M.; and Hunt, J. R. 1987. "Effect of Dietary Boron on Mineral, Estrogen, and Testosterone Metabolism in Postmenopausal Women." *FASEB Journal* 1: 394–97.
233. Murray and Pizzorno, *Encyclopedia of Natural Medicine,* op. cit.
234. Abraham, G. E. 1983. "Nutritional Factors in the Etiology of the Premenstrual Tension Syndromes." *Journal of Reproductive Medicine* 28: 446–64.
235. Horrobin, D. F.; Manku, M. S.; Brush, M.; et al. 1991. "Abnormalities in Plasma Essential Fatty Acid Levels in Women with Premenstrual Syndrome and with Non-malignant Breast Disease." *Journal of Nutritional Medicine* 2: 259–64.
236. Bennett, F. C., and Ingram, D. M. 1990. "Diet and Female Sex Hormone Concentrations: An Intervention Study for the Type of Fat Consumed." *American Journal of Clinical Nutrition* 52: 808–12.

237. Facchinetti, F.; Borella, P.; Sances, G.; et al. 1991. "Oral Magnesium Successfully Relieves Premenstrual Mood Changes." *Obstetrics and Gynecology* 78: 177–81.
238. Murray and Pizzorno, *Encyclopedia of Natural Medicine,* op. cit.
239. Horrobin, Manku, Brush, et al. "Abnormalities in Plasma Essential Fatty Acid Levels," op. cit.
240. Murray and Pizzorno, *Encyclopedia of Natural Medicine,* op. cit.
241. Ibid. Brush, M. G.; Bennett, T.; and Hansen, K. 1988. "Pyridoxine in the Treatment of Premenstrual Syndrome: A Retrospective Survey in 630 Patients." *British Journal of Clinical Practice* 42: 448–52.
242. Murray and Pizzorno, *Encyclopedia of Natural Medicine,* op. cit. Fahim, M.; Fahim, Z.; Der, R.; and Harman, J. 1976. "Zinc Treatment for the Reduction of Hyperplasia of the Prostate." *Federation Proceedings* 35: 361.
243. Wallace, A. M., and Grant, J. K. 1975. "Effect of Zinc on Androgen Metabolism in the Human Hyperplastic Prostate." *Biochemistry Society Transcripts* 3: 540–42.
244. Hart, J. P., and Cooper, W. L. 1941. "Vitamin F in the Treatment of Prostatic Hyperplasia." Report Number 1, Lee Foundation for Nutritional Research, Milwaukee, Wis.
245. Scott, W. W. 1945. "The Lipids of the Prostatic Fluid, Seminal Plasma and Enlarged Prostate Gland of Man." *Journal of Urology* 53: 712–18. Boyd, E. M., and Berry, N. E. 1939. "Prostatic Hypertrophy as Part of a Generalized Metabolic Disease: Evidence of the Presence of a Lipopenia." *Journal of Urology* 41: 406–11.
246. Murray and Pizzorno, *Encyclopedia of Natural Medicine,* op. cit.
247. Ibid.
248. Ibid.
249. Champlault, G.; Patel, J. C.; and Bonnard, A. M. 1984. "A Double-blind Trial of an Extract of the Plant *Serenoa repens* in Benign Prostatic Hyperplasia." *British Journal of Clinical Pharmacology* 18: 461–62. Tasca, A.; Barulli, M.; Cavazzana, A.; et al. 1985. "Treatment of Obstructive Symptomatology Caused by Prostatic Adenoma with an Extract of *Serenoa repens:* Double-blind Clinical Study vs. Placebo." *Minerva Urology and Nefrology* 37: 87–91. Boccafoschi, C., and Annoscia, S. 1983. "Comparison of *Serenoa repens* Extract with Placebo by Controlled Clinical Trial in Patients with Prostatic Adenomatosis." *Urologia* 50: 1257–59.
250. Murray and Pizzorno, *Encyclopedia of Natural Medicine,* op. cit.
251. Ibid.
252. Proctor, M.; Wilkenson, D.; Orenberg, E.; et al. 1979. "Lowered Cutaneous and Urinary Levels of Polyamines with Clinical Improvement in Treated Psoriasis." *Archives of Dermatology* 115: 945–49.
253. Ibid.
254. Rosenberg, E., and Belew, P. 1982. "Microbial Factors in Psoriasis." *Archives of Dermatology* 118: 1434–44.
255. Monk, B. E., and Neill, S. M. 1986. "Alcohol Consumption and Psoriasis." *Dermatologica* 173: 57–60.
256. Bittiner, S. B.; Tucker, W. F. G.; Cartwright, I.; and Bleehen, S. S. 1988. "A Double-blind, Randomized, Placebo-controlled Trial of Fish Oil in Psoriasis." *Lancet* 1: 378–80. Ziboh, V. A.; Cohen, K. A.; Ellis, C. N.; et al. 1986. "Effects of Dietary Supplementation of Fish Oil on Neutrophil and Epidermal Fatty Acids." *Archives of Dermatology* 122: 1277–82. Maurice, P. D. L.; Allen, B. R.; Barkley, A. S. J.; et al. 1987. "The Effects of Dietary Supplementation with Fish Oil in Patients with Psoriasis." *British Journal of Dermatology* 1117: 599–606.
257. Lithell, H.; Bruce, A.; Gustafsson, B.; et al. 1983. "A Fasting and Vegetarian Diet Treatment Trial on Chronic Inflammatory Disorders." *Acta Dermatologica Venerologica* (StockH) 63: 397–403.
258. Weber, G., and Galle, K. 1983. "The Liver, a Therapeutic Target in Dermatoses." *Med Welt* 34: 108–11.
259. Murray and Pizzorno, *Encyclopedia of Natural Medicine,* op. cit.
260. Ibid.
261. Ibid.

262. Darlington, L. G.; Ramsey, N. W.; and Mansfield, J. R. 1986. "Placebo-controlled, Blind Study of Dietary Manipulation Therapy in Rheumatoid Arthritis." *Lancet* 1: 236–38. Hicklin, J. A.; McEwen, L. M.; and Morgan, J. E. 1980. "The Effect of Diet in Rheumatoid Arthritis." *Clinical Allergy* 10: 463–67. Panush, R. S. 1986. "Delayed Reactions to Foods: Food Allergy and Rheumatic Disease." *Annals of Allergy* 56: 500–503.
263. Skoldstam, L.; Larsson, L.; and Lindstrom, F. D. 1979. "Effects of Fasting and Lacto-vegetarian Diet on Rheumatoid Arthritis." *Scandinavian Journal of Rheumatology* 8: 249–55. Kroker, G. P.; Stroud, R. M.; Marshall, R. T.; et al. 1984. "Fasting and Rheumatoid Arthritis: A Multicenter Study." *Clinical Ecology* 2: 137–44. Kjeldsen-Kragh, J.; Haugen, M.; Borchgrevink, C. F.; et al. 1991. "Controlled Trial of Fasting and One-year Vegetarian Diet in Rheumatoid Arthritis." *Lancet* 338: 899–902.
264. Ibid.
265. Kremer, J.; Michaelek, A. V.; Lininger, L.; et al. 1985. "Effects of Manipulation of Dietary Fatty Acids on Clinical Manifestation of Rheumatoid Arthritis." *Lancet* 1: 184–87. Lucas, P., and Power, L. 1981. "Dietary Fat Aggravates Active Rheumatoid Arthritis." *Clinical Research* 29: 754A. Ziff, M. 1983. "Diet in the Treatment of Rheumatoid Arthritis." *Arthritis and Rheumatism* 26: 457–61. Magaro, M.; Altomonte, L.; Zoli, A.; et al. 1988. "Influence of Diet with Different Lipid Composition on Neutrophil Chemiluminescence and Disease Activity in Patients with Rheumatoid Arthritis." *Annals of Rheumatic Disease* 47: 793–96.
266. Darlington, L. G. 1988. "Do Diets Rich in Polyunsaturated Fatty Acids Affect Disease Activity in Rheumatoid Arthritis?" *Annals of Rheumatic Disease* 47: 169–72. Jantti, J.; Nikkari, T.; Solakivi, T.; et al. 1989. "Evening Primrose Oil in Rheumatoid Arthritis: Changes in Serum Lipids and Fatty Acids." *Annals of Rheumatic Disease* 48: 124–27.
267. Murray and Pizzorno, *Encyclopedia of Natural Medicine,* op. cit.
268. Srivastava, K. C., and Mustafa, T. 1989. "Ginger (*Zingiber officinale*) and Rheumatic Disorders." *Medical Hypothesis* 29: 25–28.
269. Ibid.
270. Siegel, J. 1974. "Gastrointestinal Ulcer—Arthus Reaction!" *Annals of Allergy* 32: 127–30. Andre, C.; Moulinier, B.; Andre, F.; and Daniere, S. 1983. "Evidence for Anaphylactic Reactions in Peptic Ulcer and Varioliform Gastritis." *Annals of Allergy* 51: 325–28. Siegel, J. 1977. "Immunologic Approach to the Treatment and Prevention of Gastrointestinal Ulcers." *Annals of Allergy* 38: 27–29. Rebhun, J. 1975. "Duodenal Ulceration in Allergic Children." *Annals of Allergy* 34: 145–49.
271. Siegel, "Gastrointestinal Ulcer," op. cit. Rebhun, "Duodenal Ulceration in Allergic Children," op. cit.
272. Rydning, A.; Berstad, A.; Aadland, E.; and Odegaard, B. 1982. "Prophylactic Effects of Dietary Fiber in Duodenal Ulcer Disease." *Lancet* 2: 736–39.
273. Glick, L. 1982. "Deglycrrhizinated Liquorice in Peptic Ulcer." *Lancet* 2: 817. Tewari, S. N., and Wilson, A. K. 1972. "Deglycyrrhizinated Liquorice in Duodenal Ulcer." *Practitioner* 210: 820–25.
274. Morgan, A. G.; McAdam, W. A. F.; Pacsoo, C.; and Darnborough, A. 1982. "Comparison Between Cimetidine and Caved-S in the Treatment of Gastric Ulceration, and Subsequent Maintenance Therapy." *Gut* 23: 545–51. Kassir, Z. A. 1985. "Endoscopic Controlled Trial of Four Drug Regimens in the Treatment of Chronic Duodenal Ulceration." *Irish Medical Journal* 78: 153–56.
275. Murray and Pizzorno, *Encyclopedia of Natural Medicine,* op. cit.
276. Burkitt and Trowell, *Western Diseases,* op. cit. Trowell, Burkitt, and Heaton, *Dietary Fibre, Fibre-depleted Foods and Disease.*
277. Latto, C.; Wilkinson, R. W.; and Gilmore, O. J. A. 1973. "Diverticular Disease and Varicose Veins." *Lancet* 1: 1089–90.
278. Pourrat, H. 1977. "Anthocyanidin Drugs in Vascular Disease." *Plant Medicine Phytotherapy* 11: 143–51.
279. Kreysel, H. W.; Nissen, H. P.; and Enghoffer, E. 1983. "A Possible Role of Lysosomal Enzymes in the Pathogenesis of Varicosis and the Reduction in Their Serum Activity by Venostasin." *VASA* 12: 377–82.

280. Visudhiphan, S.; Poolsuppasit, S.; Piboonnakarintr, O.; and Tumliang, S. 1982. "The Relationship Between High Fibrinolytic Activity and Daily Capsicum Ingestion in Thais." *American Journal of Clinical Nutrition* 35: 1452–58. Bordia, A. K.; Josh, H. K.; and Sanadhya, Y. K. 1977. "Effect of Garlic Oil on Fibrinolytic Activity in Patient with CHD." *Atherosclerosis* 28: 155–59. Baghurst, K. I.; Raj, M. J.; and Truswell, A. S. 1977. "Onions and Platelet Aggregation." *Lancet* 1: 101. Srivastava, K. 1984. "Effects of Aqueous Extracts of Onion, Garlic and Ginger on the Platelet Aggregation and Metabolism of Arachidonic Acid in the Blood Vascular System: In Vitro Study." *Prostatic Leukotriene Medicine* 13: 227–35.
281. Ako, H.; Cheung, A.; and Matsura, P. 1981. "Isolation of a Fibrinolysis Enzyme Activator from Commercial Bromelain." *Archives of Internal Pharmacodynamics* 254: 157–67.

Glossary

Achlorhydria. Absence of gastric acid.
Acute. Having a rapid onset, severe symptoms, and a short course; not chronic.
Adrenaline. A hormone, secreted by the adrenal gland, that produces the "fight or flight" response. Also called *epinephrine.*
Aldosterone. A hormone, secreted by the adrenal gland, that causes the retention of sodium and water.
Alkaloids. A group of nitrogen-containing substances found in plants.
Allopathy. The conventional method of medicine, which combats disease by using substances and techniques specifically against the disease and its symptoms.
Amebiasis. An intestinal infection characterized by severe diarrhea, caused by the parasite *Entamoeba histolytica.*
Amino acids. A group of nitrogen-containing chemical compounds that form the basic structural units of proteins.
Analgesic. A substance that reduces the sensation of pain.
Androgens. Hormones that stimulate male characteristics.
Anemia. A condition in which the oxygen-carrying pigment hemoglobin in the blood is below normal limits.
Anorexia. The medical term for loss of appetite.
Anthocyanidin. A particular class of flavonoids that gives plants, fruits, and flowers colors ranging from red to blue.
Antibody. Proteins manufactured by the body that bind to antigens to neutralize, inhibit, or destroy them.
Antigen. Any substance that, when introduced into the body, causes the formation of antibodies against it.
Antihypertensive. Having a blood-pressure-lowering effect.
Antioxidant. A compound that prevents free-radical or oxidative damage.

Artery. A blood vessel that carries oxygen-rich blood away from the heart.

Atherosclerosis. A process in which fatty substances (cholesterol and triglycerides) are deposited in the walls of medium to large arteries, eventually leading to blockage of the artery.

Atopy. A predisposition to various allergic conditions, including eczema and asthma.

Auto-immune. Causing antibodies to develop against the body's own tissues.

Basal metabolic rate. The rate of metabolism when the body is at rest.

Basophil. A type of white blood cell that is involved in allergic reactions.

Benign. Not serious; a mild disorder that is usually not fatal.

beta-Carotene. Pro-vitamin A—a plant carotene that can be converted to two vitamin A molecules.

beta-Cell. The cells in the pancreas that manufacture insulin.

Bilirubin. The breakdown product of the hemoglobin molecule of red blood cells.

Biofeedback. A technique for developing conscious control over various involuntary functions, including heart rate, intestinal motility, and body temperature.

Bleeding time. The time required for the cessation of bleeding from a small skin puncture as a result of platelet disintegration and blood vessel constriction; ranges from 1 to 4 minutes.

Blood–brain barrier. A special barrier that prevents the passage of materials from the blood to the brain.

Blood pressure. The force exerted by blood as it presses against and attempts to stretch blood vessels.

Bromelain. The protein-digesting enzyme found in pineapple.

Bursa. A sac or pouch that contains a special fluid for lubricating joints.

Calorie. A unit of heat; 1 nutritional Calorie is the amount of heat necessary to raise 1 kg of water 1°C.

Candida albicans. A yeast common to the intestinal tract.

Candidiasis. A complex medical syndrome produced by a chronic overgrowth of the yeast *Candida albicans*.

Carbohydrate. Sugars and starches.

Carcinogen. Any agent or substance capable of causing cancer.

Carcinogenesis. The development of cancer through the actions of certain chemicals, viruses, and unknown factors on primarily normal cells.

Cardiac output. The volume of blood pumped from the heart in 1 minute.

Cardiopulmonary. Pertaining to the heart and lungs.

Cardiotonic. A compound that tones and strengthens the heart.

Carotenes. Fat-soluble plant pigments, some of which can be converted into vitamin A by the body.

Cartilage. A type of connective tissue that acts as a shock absorber at joint interfaces.
Cathartic. A substance that stimulates the movement of the bowels; more powerful than a laxative.
Cholagogue. A compound that stimulates the contraction of the gallbladder.
Choleretic. A compound that promotes the flow of bile.
Cholinergic. Pertaining to the parasympathetic portion of the autonomic nervous system and to the release of acetylcholine as a transmitter substance.
Chronic. Long-term or frequently recurring.
Cirrhosis. A severe disease of the liver characterized by the replacement of liver cells with scar tissue.
Coenzyme. A necessary nonprotein component of an enzyme; usually a vitamin or a mineral.
Cold sore. A small skin blister anywhere around the mouth caused by the *Herpes simplex* virus.
Colic. Severe, spasmodic pain that occurs in waves of increasing intensity, reaches a peak, then abates for a short time before returning.
Colitis. Inflammation of the colon; usually associated with diarrhea that contains blood and mucus.
Collagen. The protein that serves as the main component of connective tissue.
Congestive heart failure. A chronic disease that results when the heart is incapable of supplying the oxygen needs of the body.
Connective tissue. The type of tissue that provides support, structure, and cellular cement to the body.
Coronary artery disease. A condition in which the heart receives inadequate supplies of blood and oxygen, due to atherosclerosis.
Corticosteroid drugs. A group of drugs, similar to the natural corticosteroid hormones, that are used primarily to treat inflammation and to suppress the immune system.
Corticosteroid hormones. A group of hormones, produced by the adrenal glands, that control the body's use of nutrients and its excretion of salt and water in the urine.
Cushing's syndrome. A condition caused by a hypersecretion of cortisone; characterized by spindly legs, "moon face," "buffalo hump," abdominal obesity, flushed facial skin, and poor wound healing.
Dehydration. Excessive loss of water from the body.
Dementia. Senility. Loss of mental function.
Demineralization. Loss of minerals from the bone.
Dermatitis. Inflammation of the skin, sometimes due to allergy.

Diastolic. The second number in a blood-pressure reading, measuring the pressure in the arteries during the relaxation phase of the heart beat.
Disaccharide. A sugar composed of two monosaccharide units.
Diuretic. A compound that causes increased urination.
Diverticuli. Saclike outpouchings of the wall of the colon.
Double-blind study. A way of controlling against experimental bias by ensuring that neither the researcher nor the subject knows whether an active agent or a placebo is being used.
Down's syndrome. A genetic disorder marked by moderate to severe retardation, a short flattened skull, slanting eyes, and an extra twenty-first chromosome.
Dysfunction. Abnormal function.
Edema. Accumulation of fluid in tissues (swelling).
Eicosapentaenoic acid (EPA). An omega-3 fatty acid found primarily in cold-water fish.
Electroencephalogram. A machine that measures and records brain waves.
Elimination diet. A diet that eliminates allergenic foods.
Emulsify. To disperse large fat globules into smaller uniformally distributed particles.
Encephalitis. Inflammation of the brain, usually due to viral infection.
Endometrium. The mucous membrane lining of the uterus.
Enteric-coated. A special way of coating a tablet or capsule to ensure that it does not dissolve in the stomach, so that it can reach the intestinal tract.
Enzyme. An organic catalyst that speeds chemical reactions.
Epidemiology. The study of the occurrence and distribution of diseases in human populations.
Epinephrine. See **Adrenaline**.
Epithelium. The cells that cover the body's entire surface and line most of the internal organs.
Essential fatty acids. Fatty acids that the body cannot manufacture—linoleic and linolenic acids.
Estrogens. Hormones that stimulate female characteristics.
Excretion. The process of eliminating waste products from a cell, a tissue, or the entire body.
Extracellular. Involving the space outside the cell composed of fluid.
Fibrin. A white insoluble protein, formed by the clotting of blood, that serves as the starting point for wound repair and scar formation.
Fibrinolysis. The dissolution of fibrin or of a blood clot by the action of enzymes that convert insoluble fibrin into soluble particles.
Flavonoids. Plant pigments that exert various physiological effects in the human body.

Free radicals. Highly reactive molecules, characterized by an unpaired electron, that can bind to and destroy cellular compounds.
Gerontology. The study of aging.
Glucose. A monosaccharide found in the blood that serves as one of the body's primary energy sources.
Gluten. A protein in wheat and certain other grains that gives dough its tough, elastic character.
Goblet cell. A goblet-shaped cell that secretes mucus.
Ground substance. The thick, gellike material in which cells, fibers, and blood capillaries of cartilage, bone, and connective tissue are embedded.
Helper T-cells. Lymphocytes that help in the immune response.
Hematocrit. An expression of the percentage of blood occupied by blood cells.
Holistic medicine. A form of therapy aimed at treating the whole person, and not just the part or parts in which symptoms occur.
Hormone. A secretion of an endocrine gland that controls and regulates body functions.
Huntington's chorea. A hereditary nerve disease of adults marked by progressive mental deterioration and dementia.
Hyperglycemia. High blood sugar.
Hypersecretion. Excessive secretion.
Hypertension. High blood pressure.
Hypochlorhydria. Insufficient gastric acid output.
Hypoglycemia. Low blood sugar.
Hypolipidemic. A substance that lowers the levels of cholesterol and/or triglycerides in the blood.
Hypotension. Low blood pressure.
Immunoglobulins. Antibodies.
Incidence. The number of new cases of a disease that occur during a given period (usually years) in a defined population.
Incontinence. The inability to control urination or defecation.
Infarction. Death to a localized area of tissue due to lack of oxygen supply.
Insulin. A hormone, secreted by the pancreas, that lowers blood-sugar levels.
Interferon. A potent immune-enhancing substance that is produced by the body's cells to fight off viral infection and cancer.
Jaundice. A condition caused by an elevated level of bilirubin in the body and characterized by yellowing of the skin.
Keratin. An insoluble protein found in hair, skin, and nails.
Korsakoff's syndrome. A form of mental deterioration seen in chronic alcoholics, caused by thiamine deficiency.

Lactase. A enzyme that breaks down lactose into the monosaccharides glucose and galactose.
Lactose. One of the sugars present in milk. It is a disaccharide.
Lesion. Any localized, abnormal change in tissue formation.
Lethargy. A feeling of tiredness, drowsiness, or lack of energy.
Leukocyte. White blood cell.
Leukoplakia. A precancerous lesion usually seen in the mouth and characterized by a white-colored patch.
Leukotrienes. Inflammatory compounds produced when oxygen interacts with polyunsaturated fatty acids.
Lipids. Fats, phospholipids, steroids, and prostaglandins.
Lipotropic. Promoting the flow of lipids to and from the liver.
Lymph. Fluid contained in lymphatic vessels that flows through the lymphatic system to be returned to the blood.
Lymphocyte. A type of white blood cell found primarily in lymph nodes.
Malabsorption. Impaired absorption of nutrients, most often due to diarrhea.
Malaise. A vague feeling of sickness or of physical discomfort.
Malignant. Of a condition, tending to worsen and eventually causing death.
Mast cell. A cell, found in many tissues of the body, that contributes greatly to allergic and inflammatory processes by secreting histamine and other inflammatory particles.
Metabolism. All of the chemical processes that take place in the body.
Metabolite. A product of a chemical reaction.
Metalloenzyme. An enzyme that contains a metal at its active site.
Microbe. A popular term for *microorganism.*
Molecule. The smallest complete unit of a substance that can exist independently and still retain the characteristic properties of the substance.
Monosaccharide. A simple, one-unit sugar such as fructose or glucose.
Mortality rate. The number of deaths per 100,000 members of the population per year.
Mucosa. Another term for mucous membrane.
Mucous membrane. The soft, pink, tissue that lines most of the cavities and tubes in the body, including the respiratory tract, gastrointestinal tract, genitourinary tract, and eyelids; the mucous membranes secrete mucus.
Mucus. A slick, slimy fluid, secreted by the mucous membranes, that acts as a lubricant and as a mechanical protector of the mucous membranes.
Mycotoxins. Toxins from yeast and fungi.
Myelin sheath. A white fatty substance that surrounds nerve cells and aids in nerve impulse transmission.

Neoplasia. A medical term for tumor formation, characterized by progressive, abnormal replication of cells.
Neurofibrillary tangles. Clusters of degenerated nerves.
Neurotransmitters. Substances that modify or transmit nerve impulses.
Night blindness. The inability to see well in dim light or at night.
Nocturia. The disturbance of a person's sleep at night by the need to pass urine.
Oligoantigenic diet. See **Elimination diet**.
Otitis media. Acute infection of the middle ear.
Pancreatin. A product, obtained from the pancreas of pigs, that contains a potent concentration of digestive enzymes.
Papain. The protein-digesting enzyme of papaya.
Parkinson's disease. A slowly progressive, degenerative disease of the nervous system, characterized by resting tremor, pill rolling of the fingers, a masklike facial expression, shuffling gait, and muscle rigidity and weakness.
Pathogen. Any agent, particularly a microorganism, that causes disease.
Pathogenesis. The process by which a disease originates and develops—particularly the cellular and physiological processes.
Peristalsis. Successive muscular contractions on the intestines that move food through the intestinal tract.
Physiology. The study of the functioning of the body, including the physical and chemical processes of its cells, tissues, organs, and systems.
Physostigmine. A drug that blocks the breakdown of acetylcholine.
Phytoestrogens. Plant compounds that exert estrogen-like effects.
Pick's disease. A form of presenile dementia that occurs in middle age, characterized by slow disintegration of the intellect, personality, and emotions.
Piles. A common name for hemorrhoids.
Placebo. An inert or inactive substance used to test the efficacy of another substance.
Polysaccharide. A molecule composed of many simple sugar molecules linked together.
Prostaglandins. Hormonelike compounds manufactured from essential fatty acids.
Psychosomatic. Pertaining to the relationship between the mind and the body; commonly used to refer to physiological disorders that are thought to be caused entirely or partly by psychological factors.
Putrefaction. The process of breaking down protein compounds by rotting.
Recommended Dietary Allowance (RDA). The recommended daily intake of a particular essential nutrient.
Saccharide. A sugar molecule.
Satiety. A feeling of fullness or gratification.

Saturated fat. A fat whose carbon atoms are bonded to the maximum number of hydrogen atoms; found in animal products such as meat, milk, milk products, and eggs.
Sclerosis. The process of hardening or scarring.
Senile dementia. Mental deterioration associated with aging.
Submucosa. The tissue just below the mucous membrane.
Suppressor T-cells. Lymphocytes, controlled by the thymus gland, that suppress the immune response.
Syndrome. A group of signs and symptoms that occur together in a pattern characteristic of a particular disease or abnormal condition.
T-cell. A lymphocyte that is under the control of the thymus gland.
Tonic. A substance that exerts a gentle strengthening effect on the body.
Trans-fatty acid. The type of fat found in margarine.
Uremia. The retention of urine by the body, and the presence of high levels of urine components in the blood.
Urinalysis. The analysis of urine.
Urticaria. Hives.
Vasoconstriction. The constriction of blood vessels.
Vitamin. An essential compound that acts as a catalyst in normal processes of the body.
Western diet. A diet characteristic of the type eaten in Western societies—high in fat, refined carbohydrate, and processed foods, and low in dietary fiber.
Wheal. The characteristic lesion in hives; a small welt.

Index